Transforming Healthcare in Africa

Transforming Healthcare in Africa

A Comparative Analysis

Edited by
Robert Dibie

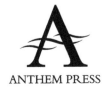

ANTHEM PRESS

Anthem Press
An imprint of Wimbledon Publishing Company
www.anthempress.com

This edition first published in UK and USA 2025
by ANTHEM PRESS
75–76 Blackfriars Road, London SE1 8HA, UK
or PO Box 9779, London SW19 7ZG, UK
and
244 Madison Ave #116, New York, NY 10016, USA

British Library Cataloguing-in-Publication Data
A catalogue record for this book is available from the British Library.

Library of Congress Cataloging-in-Publication Data
A catalog record for this book has been requested.

ISBN-13: 978-1-83999-120-2 (Hbk)
ISBN-10: 1-83999-120-8 (Hbk)

Cover Credit: Robert Dibie

This title is also available as an e-book.

This book is dedicated to my late parents Mr. David Jones Dibie, Mrs. Sarah Eloh Dibie, my lovely wife Dr. Josephine Dibie, and my children Ajiri and Kome.

CONTENTS

LIST OF FIGURES

LIST OF TABLES

ABOUT THE EDITOR

Robert Dibie, Ph.D. is a Distinguished Professor of Public Policy and Public Administration. He also serves as Vice Provost for Academic Affairs at Fort Valley State University. He previously served as Dean, of the School of Public Affairs and Environmental Affairs at Indiana University Kokomo. He also served as the director of graduate programs in public administration at Western Kentucky University. He was honored with the 2023 Peace Education award from the Board of the Center for African Peace and Conflict Resolution at California State University Sacramento in recognition of his exemplary leadership and outstanding contribution to impactful research and publication on peace, security, and social governance in Africa. He is twice the recipient of the prestigious Carnegie African Diaspora Fellowship award by the Institute of International Education, Washington DC. He has published eleven books and more than 120 peer-reviewed journal articles in environmental policy, civil society, public management, sustainable development, public policy, nongovernmental organizations (NGOs), women empowerment, and ethics. latest books includes *Comparative Perspectives on Environmental Policy and Issues* by Routledge Press; *Public Administration: Analysis, Theories and Application* by Babcock University Press; *Comparative Perspectives on Civil Society* by Lexington Press; *Public Management and Sustainable Development in Nigeria* by Ashgate; *Nongovernmental Organizations and Sustainable Development in Sub-Saharan Africa by Lexington Press,* His recent research articles have appeared in the *International Journal of Public Administration; Journal of African Policy Studies, Journal of Developing Societies, Journal of Sociology and Social Welfare; Journal of Social Justice, Journal of African and Asian Studies; Politics Administration and Change Journal, Journal of International Politics and Development, Journal of African Business,* and so on. He has presented more than 140 academic papers at national and international conferences, focusing on issues of sustainable development, public management, public policy, women empowerment, environmental policies, development administration, and NGOs. As a nationally recognized leader in higher education, he has presented many seminars, workshops, and lectures in the areas of Higher Education Leadership, Public Policy, Environmental Policy, Gender Empowerment, and Sustainable Development in a number of universities around the world. He has also developed continuing education materials and taught professional development courses (Executive Leadership, Program Evaluation, and Ethics) for various professional organizations, including Banks, City and County Governments, Nonprofit institutions, NGOs, and some National Governments' Departments in the United States and abroad. He has also consulted for several NGOs and universities in the United States, Europe, Africa, and the Caribbean Islands.

Dibie is committed to the pursuit of knowledge, wisdom, discovery, and creativity. He is a proven student-centered educator and has fostered personal and intellectual growth to prepare students for productive careers, meaningful lives, and responsible citizenship in a global society. Professor Dibie has also supervised more than 62 doctoral and masters' degree dissertations on Public Management, Public Policy, Environmental Policy, NGOs, Economic Development Policy, Sustainable Development, Women Empowerment, Business Administration, Environmental Health and Safety, and Political Science.

Dibie holds a bachelor's degree in business administration (BS), a concentration in marketing management, and international business, and a master's degree in business administration (MBA) with a concentration in strategic management. In addition, he also earned a master's degree in public administration and international relations (MA) from the University of Detroit Mercy, Michigan. He received his Ph.D. in public policy analysis and public administration from Western Michigan University. He also completed several advanced professional diplomas from both the Association of Business Executives in England, and Charted Institute of Marketing, United Kingdom. He also earned a Certificate in Quality Matters in Online Course Development and Teaching.

PREFACE

According to the World Health Organization (2022), the health priorities that nations around the world should explore are children and women's health, environmental pollution, material, nutrition, and venerable diseases. Strides were made in increasing life expectancy and reducing some of the common killers associated with child and maternal mortality. Although, many African countries have made more efforts over the past three decades to fully eradicate a wide range of diseases and address many different persistent and emerging health issues. There have been incremental challenges all over the African continent in appropriating sufficient funding to their health systems, improved sanitation, and hygiene, as well as increasing access to physicians and well-equipped healthcare institutions to save the lives of millions. Despite the fact it has been argued that no government, either local, state, or national, can afford to ignore the health needs of their citizens. How should the government in African countries regulate their health system, or what should they choose to let the private sector or market coordinate the system? *Transforming Healthcare in Africa: A Comparative Analysis* brings together many of Sub-Saharan African leading scholars to address these questions. The book examines the key players in the health system game in many African countries. It explores the regulatory regimes that impact the health systems, such as the Ministry of Health. It also provides a few case studies of the relationship between government, the environment, and their citizens. Apart from filling the gap in the healthcare policy in Africa literature, the authors also seek to examine the impacts of weak health policies and the inability to effectively formulate solid initiatives for capacity building that could lead to enhanced healthcare for all their citizens.

The findings presented in this book will be especially useful to policymakers, public administrators, public policy analysts, readers, researchers, graduate and undergraduate studies in health administration, nurses, doctors, nonprofit, NGOs, development, and public policy disciplines. It examines nature of the healthcare system, expansion of health regulation, the privatization of health corporations, the government, and the citizens' perception of the quality of health services, and access to health institutions, reforming government regulation, and change in citizens lifestyle behaviors and use of examples and embedded content to help students and readers better appreciate the dynamics changes in the healthcare delivery system in the world.

With the wide variety of cases, this book can provide conceptual insights to better understand how healthcare institutions and governments in African countries have not been able to effectively integrate sustainable policies to effectively address poverty and the crisis of preventing the spread of diseases and recovery, and the accomplishment of sustainable development. It reviews the extensive literature on healthcare policies, capacity-building strategies, and regulation policies, as well as examines the implication of sustainable development of countries in the African continent. The chapters present a wide range of new dimensions and variables that are not considered by other health policy books.

Robert A. Dibie, Ph.D.

FOREWORD

Dr. Willie Clark-Okah

The health of the people of Africa is essential in all ramifications to their physical and mental well-being as well as the economies of the 55 countries on the continent. Professor Robert Dibie's new *Transforming Healthcare in Africa: A Comparative Analysis* book will contribute another especially important framework in the human right to healthcare in the African continent. It is directed at examining how globalization, and nations interdependence affects healthcare decisions and processes across many boundaries and borders. It is especially important that students, scholars, and citizens of the world understand how these systems work or do not work. The book is also especially important because healthcare is about life and human right in Africa as well as in the world in general. While some African countries have the capacity to do so much more by understanding the variability of our worldwide health policies and practices others are not capable to do so due to ineffective political institutions, political will, lack of visionary leaders, and lack of funding. The challenge in most African countries is how to think in new ways and produce innovations that will enable them to develop organizations, processes, policies, and best practices that can be in place for a long time as well as sustain a healthy life for all citizens. The major goal of this book is to help students think more deeply about how healthcare is organized and delivered in various countries. Each country in the African continent has invented its healthcare system to respond to a particular set of forces. By examining each of the systems presented in the book, students will come away with new perspectives and ideas of what an ideal health policy should be. In addition, these innovative ideas could then be used as a series of lenses to first get new insights about each person's home country system, and what best practices to adopt. The African countries covered in this book have been successful in their respective ways. However, celebrating and valuing each of these are especially important mechanisms for advancing a better healthcare system for not only African countries but the entire world. Further, examining various approaches could enable readers to understand the connections between and among the variety of health systems. Every country in the world needs a nourishing and good health system and structures that could foster or enhance international sustainable healthcare and wellness for its citizens. It is my hope that readers could see unexpected results, similarities, and differences, as well as be able to produce coherent, new interpretations, and innovative ideas for future health policies, systems, and structures that serve all humanity.

ACKNOWLEDGMENTS

I would like to express my appreciation to many individuals who directly or indirectly graciously played a role in the development of this book. First, I thank many people at Routledge, in particular, my editor David Varley who has strongly supported this project and provided exemplary leadership throughout the revision process. Collectively, they are an extraordinary team that demonstrated extremely lofty standards of excellence in their work.

I am also grateful to the reviewers who took time to review the early draft of my work and provided helpful suggestions for improving the book. Their comments undoubtedly made the book better. My heartfelt thanks to all the scholars that contributed chapters or co-authored chapters with me: Dr. Josephine Dibie, Fort Valley State University, USA; Dr. Leonard Gadzekpo, Southern Illinois University Carbondale, USA; Professor Kealeboga J. Maphunye, University of South Africa; Professor Ayandiji D. Aina, Babcock University Nigeria; Dr. Chinyeaka Igbokwe-Ibeto Nnamdi Azikiwe University, Nigeria; Dr. Yusuf Nur Indiana University Kokomo, USA; Dr. Willie Clark-Okah Canada International Development Agency. Dr. Peter Nwafu, Albany State University, USA; Dr. Mariam Konete, Western Michigan University; Professor Idrissa Quedraogo, University of Ouagadougou, Burkina Faso; Dr. Muawya Hussien, Dufar University, Oman; Dr. Halima Khunoethe; and Dr. Lusanda Juta Northwest University in the Republic of South Africa; Professor Jacob Oboreh, Delta State University of Science and Technology, Ozoro, Nigeria, and Professor Edwin Ijeoma Fort Hare University, Eastern Cape, South Africa.

I wish to thank my colleagues and graduate students at Indiana University Kokomo, USA, Babcock University, Nigeria, The University of the West Indies, Jamaica, Fort Hare University South Africa, Central Michigan University, USA, Caleb University Lagos, Nigeria, and Fort Valley State University for their continued encouragement and interest in comparative health system and sustainable development issues.

A special acknowledgment goes to Professor Basil Ikede in Ottawa, Canada; Professor Felix Edoho, Lincoln University Jefferson City, and Dr. Nelson Dibie, Fresno Pacific University, USA, for their insights, and contributions have added to the quality of this book. Additionally, I thank the King of Ozoro Kingdom, Delta State Nigeria, His Royal Highness Barrister Anthony Uvietobore Ogbogbo for his support as I worked my way through this multifaceted international research. I also want to acknowledge the comparative health system scholars whose research and analysis provided the foundation of this book. Their continuing efforts make me optimistic about continued progress in the study of how good health delivery systems and policies could be enacted and effectively regulated to accomplish sustainable development goals in several African countries.

The promulgation of the Universal Health Insurance policies should come as part of the African nations' governments' future attempts to restructure and reform the healthcare sector by introducing improved and effective health policies, purchasing modern medical equipment, refining subsidy reallocation, and launching various healthcare initiatives, that could discourage medical tourism and brain drain of doctors and nurses seek better working conditions in foreign countries. African leaders must be mindful that healthcare is a human right.

Finally, I am especially thankful for the efforts of my lovely wife and best friend Dr. (Mrs.) Josephine Dibie for her time, energy, commitment, and contribution to the quality and success of this book. Dr. Josephine Dibie and I have worked together in one capacity or another for over 30 years, always around health policies, economic development policies, business and government relations, and fiscal and monetary policy issues. This volume represents the most recent culmination of that collaboration.

LIST OF CONTRIBUTORS

Ayandiji Daniel Aina, Ph.D., is a Professor of Political Science and Provost of the Post-graduate School at Babcock University Nigeria. He previously served as Vice Chancellor and President at Caleb University in Lagos, Nigeria. He has also served as Vice Chancellor/President of Adeleke University Ede, Osun State, Nigeria, for three years, and Provost, College of Management and Social Sciences at Babcock University, Ilishan-Remo, Ogun State, Nigeria. He has consulted widely on matters of governance, public policy, and administration for universities, intergovernmental bodies, and NGOs in Nigeria. He is an insightful scholar and writer, who has published several book chapters and peer-reviewed journal articles in the areas of public policy, civil society, public administration, sustainable development, NGOs, international relations, political elections, and good governance. Before going to graduate school, he was a journalist with the *Nigerian Daily Times* Newspaper in Lagos. He received his B.A., Master of Political Science/Public Administration, and Ph.D. degrees in Political Science from the University of Ibadan, as well as a Diploma in Journalism, from the School of Journalism in Lagos, Nigeria. He has presented his research papers in more than 50 international conferences, in the United States, Canada, England, South Africa, Ghana, Kenya, Nigeria, and Cameroon. He is the current Managing Editor of the *Journal of International Politics and Development (JIPAD)*.

Muriel Harris, Ph.D., is an Associate Professor in the Department of Health Promotion and Behavioral Sciences at the University of Louisville, Kentucky in the United States. Her area of special interest is public health programs, policy planning, implementation, evaluation, and community-based participatory research. She teaches and engages in community-based projects with a view to improving the public's health. Over her more than 30-year career in Public Health, she has worked in Sierra Leone, Liberia, the United States, and Ghana. She is the author of a textbook with the title "Evaluating Public and Community Health Programs." Her book is now in its second edition, published by Jossey-Bass. She is also the author of many presentations and publications. Her primary interest and the focus of my research have been the social determinants of health and the factors that influence the health of individuals and communities. This includes an interest in infectious diseases and prevention. She has also worked diligently and engaged in various research projects in respective of the recent Ebola Epidemic in West Africa. She also spent over three months in Sierra Leone and got to see how a small thing like the Ebola virus can transform a nation, a society, a people! She was a Fulbright Scholar at the Kwame Nkrumah University of

Science and Technology Kumasi (KNUST) Ghana, School of Public Health for a year (2015–2016). While she was a Fulbright Scholar at KNUST, she taught two courses per semester in the Department of Health Promotion and Education. She returned to her home University at the School of Public Health and Information Sciences at the University of Louisville (UofL), as an Associate Professor. She is currently the Director of the Master's in Public Health Program as well as Chair of the Commission on Racial Diversity and Equality. In addition to her academic and administrative responsibilities at the University, she mentors students at KNUST and the University of Louisville at the PhD and MPH levels as they work on their dissertations and theses, respectively. She is a Rotarian with the Rotary Club of Prospect/Goshen. Although she is the first female Rotarian of the Rotary Club of Freetown, she is the Chair of the Health Care Committee and former Chair of the Board for the Family Health Centers in Louisville, Kentucky. She is also a proud mother of two phenomenally successful adult sons.

Josephine Dibie, DBA., is an Assistant Professor in Management, Economics, and Accounting at Fort Valley State University Georgia in the United States. She was also an Assistant Professor in Business at Indiana University Kokomo. She has conducted several fields of research in Africa, Jamaica, England, and the United States, respectively. She, previously served as an Executive Analyst for the City of Fresno Government in California, as Assistant Manager at the Universal Investment Corporation, Benin City as well as a Grant Account Specialist with Indiana State University Terre Haute Indiana, United States. She is the author and co-author of more than two dozen articles and book chapters. She has published extensively in the area of NGOs and women empowerment in Africa. Her publications have appeared in the *Journal of Business and Social Sciences, International Journal of Politics and Development, Journal of Asian and African Studies, and the Journal of African Policy Studies.* Her research work has also been published in the following books *Women's Empowerment for Sustainable Development in Africa* edited by Robert Dibie Cambridge Scholars Press, England; *Business and Government Relations in Africa,* edited by Robert Dibie, Routledge Press, New York; and *Comparative Perspective of Environmental Policies and Issues,* edited by Professor Robert Dibie, Taylor and Francis Press, New York. Her research interests are in the areas of corporate executive compensation, the political economy of leadership in Africa, NGOs, women's capacity building and empowerment, sustainable development, economic growth in Africa, and corporate social responsibility in Africa. She holds a Doctorate in Business Administration degree. She also earned a Master of Public Administration degree from Indiana State University; an M.B.A. from the University of Benin; a Master of Arts degree in Economics from the University of Ibadan; and a Bachelor of Science in Statistics from the University of Nigeria, Nnsuka.

Mariam Konaté, Ph.D., is an Associate Professor in the Department of Gender and Women's Studies at Western Michigan University. Her work examines the lives of women of African descent in the West as well in Africa. Her newest research project explores the relevance of father absence to African American women's heterosexual dating experiences. The changing roles of African women who, through the interplay of gender, economics, and power, are redefining themselves in America and postcolonial

African societies are central to her research and teaching. Her book, *Heroism, and the Supernatural in the African Epic* (Routledge, 2010) underscores the crucial role women play in the hero's life and rise to power as well as in her initiation to supernatural powers. Women's empowerment and contribution to economic growth through self-determination is ubiquitous in the writings of many contemporary African and African American women writers whose works Konaté teaches in her courses. Her research work has also been published in the following books *Women's Empowerment for Sustainable Development in Africa* edited by Robert Dibie Cambridge Scholars Press, England, and *Business and Government Relations in Africa*, edited by Robert Dibie, Routledge Press, New York. She holds a Ph.D. degree from Temple University, Philadelphia in the United States.

Hassimi Traore, Ph.D., is a Professor of Chemistry at the University of Wisconsin-Whitewater, where he lectures on Chemistry with expertise in Physical Chemistry. He has a doctorate in Chemistry, a master's degree in applied Math from the University of Iowa, and a master's degree from the University of Ouagadougou in Burkina Faso (West Africa). He is currently enrolled in the master's program for Sustainable Peacebuilding (MSP) at the University of Wisconsin-Milwaukee where he is expecting to receive his master's degree in Summer 2022. He has published results of his Cannabinoid research in Elsevier, in *Australian Journal of Chemistry* and the *Journal de la Société Ouest-Africaine de Chimie*. He is a co-author of the book *Marketing Management in Africa* published in 2018 by Rutledge. He is the recipient of several grants, including a National Science Foundation grant, with which he established a molecular modeling laboratory at the University of Wisconsin-Whitewater. He has also served as a grant reviewer for the National Science Foundation and is professionally active as a consultant for the Higher Learning Commission. In addition, Dr. Traore does non-profit work and is president of Empowering Care for Widows and Children in Burkina Faso (ECWC) to benefit his country of birth, Burkina Faso, and is currently collaborating on a development project in collaboration with faculty from Purdue University.

Leonard Gadzekpo, Ph.D., is an Associate Professor and Chair of the Department of Africana Studies at Southern Illinois University Carbondale. He was born in Cote d'Ivoire and grew up in Ghana. He got his first degree from the University of Science and Technology, Kumasi, Ghana, and taught in Ghana and Nigeria. He spent four years in Germany as an artist working on religious art pieces for the St. Stepanus Katholische Gemeinde in Oldenburg and studied at Universitaet Oldenburg and Salzburg Universitaet, Austria. From 1990 to 1997 he did graduate studies at Bowling Green State University, Bowling Green, Ohio, and earned an M.A. in German, an M.F.A. in Painting, and an Ph.D. in African American Cultural Studies. His writing and research interests are in the areas of Government and the Africana society, empowerment for sustainable development in Africa, and comparative study of Africana history and culture. He has also presented his research papers at many national and international conferences. He is also presently working on a series of paintings dealing with the Africana experience in the world.

Mesay Barekew Liche is a Senior Lecturer at Adama Science and Technology University (ASTU), School of Humanities and Social Science. Currently, he is a graduate program student in the European consortium universities of Danube University of Austria and Tampere University of Finland with a prestigious Erasmus Mundus scholarship. His work focuses on Innovation and policy in Africa. His project work on mitigating graduate student unemployment through entrepreneurship earned him an opportunity to participate in the Mandela-Washington Fellowship (MWF), at Lincoln University, USA, in 2016. The fellowship was an initiative by President Barack Obama to nurture youth leadership in Africa under the umbrella of the Young African Leadership Initiative (YALI). Upon returning to his home country, Ethiopia, he won the MWF Alumni Fund project competition intending to advance transparency, accountability, and ethics in public institutions in East Africa. His current project is on COVID-19. He is a multidisciplinary innovation team member who won a COVID-19 challenge fund competition from the Ministry of Innovation and Technology (MInT) of Ethiopia with UNDP's financial support in 2020. Furthermore, He expanded his service and area of expertise by holding various administrative positions at his university, ASTU, including university-level Associate Dean for Administration from 2015 to 2017. In addition to multiple projects. He has been engaged in research projects. His most recent work includes a book chapter publication titled *Socio-Economic Dimension of Sustainable Livelihood in Subaltern Perspective in Reference to Arsi Zone*, Ethiopia. He presented the paper at an international research conference organized by the International Foundation for Sustainable Development in Africa and Asia (IFSDAA) at HAWK University of Applied Sciences and Arts, Germany, in September 2019. Subsequently, the paper was published on *Trends on Technology for Agriculture, Food and Environment and Health* book.

Chinyeaka Justine Igbokwe-Ibeto, Ph.D., is a Senior Lecturer in the Department of Public Administration, Nnamdi Azikiwe University, Awka, Nigeria. He is also a Research Fellow at the University of Johannesburg, South Africa. He earned a B.Sc. in Public Administration from the Ambrose Alli University, Ekpoma, Edo State in Nigeria. He received a Master of Public Administration degree (MPA), with a specialization in Human Resources Management (HRM) from the Lagos State University, Ojo in Nigeria. His Ph.D. in Public Administration is from the Nnamdi Azikiwe University, Awka, Anambra State in Nigeria. He has published over 80 peer-reviewed journal articles as well as 15 book chapters. He is the author of a book chapter with the title *Government and Business Relations in Tanzania*. In Dibie R. (eds) (2018) *Business and Government Relations in Africa*. New York: Routledge Press. His other research work has appeared in the *International Journal of Business and Management Studies, Routledge Critical Studies in Public Management, CABI International, African Administrative Studies, Journal of Sustainable Development in Africa, Africa's Public Service Delivery and Performance Review, and Review of Public Administration and Management*. He is a consultant to NGOs and external examiner to a number of universities in Nigeria and South Africa. He was a member, 20 Man Think Tank discussion on Reforming Nigeria's Public Service. Member, Development Discourse on Fighting Insecurity in Nigeria, Member, 20 Man Think Tank discussion on Managing the Cost of Governance in Nigeria. He is a Member of the International

Society for Development and Sustainability, Japan, Fellow of the Chartered Institute of Public Management (CIPM), Nigeria. Member Advisory Board of Zainab Arabian Research Society for Multidisciplinary Issues, United Arab Emirates. Editor, *Journal of Local Government Research and Innovation*, Editorial Board Member, *Journal of Human Resource Management*, Editorial Board Member, *Africa's Public Service Delivery and Performance Review*. His research interest is in the areas of Human Resource Management, Public Management, and Economic Development. His research also focuses on sub-Saharan Africa's democratic governance, organizational Behavior, Sustainable Development, and Public Policy Making and Analysis.

Lusanda B. Juta, Ph.D., is an Associate Professor of Public Administration and Public Policy at Northwest University in the Republic of South Africa. She has published in a variety of peer-reviewed journals in the areas of municipal finance, public budgeting in South Africa, socio-economic policy in South Africa, training, and development of employees in local governments, curriculum implementation in schools, affordable human settlements in South Africa, challenges of democratic government, and the challenges public policy implementation in South Africa. She has been a Member of the South African Association of Public Administration and Management (SAAPAM), an Advisory Board Member of THNIC Foundation, a Provincial Committee Member of the African Peer Review Mechanism Country Review Mission, a Committee member of Ngaka Modiri District Municipality Local Economic Development, Member of the Department of Public Service and Administration Northwest Provincial Government, Member Independent Student Electoral Commission and so on. She obtained her Doctoral Degree (Ph.D.) in Public Administration from Northwest University, South Africa, Master of Technology in Public Management from Tshwane University of Technology, South Africa, and Bachelor of Technology in Public Management (Honors) from Cape Peninsula University South Africa, and Diploma in Public Management from Cape Peninsula University South Africa. Her research interest is in the areas of public policy, public management, municipal finance, government relations, local development management, capacity building in new democratic governments in Africa, and civil society organizations in South Africa. Her research also focuses on social justice, capacity building, welfare policy, sustainable development, and economic development and analysis.

Jacob Snapps Oboreh, Ph.D., is a Professor of Operations Research and Management, Delta State University Abraka, Nigeria. He is currently serving as the Vice Chancellor/President of Delta State University of Science and Technology at Ozoro, Delta State in Nigeria. He was the Rector of Delta State Polytechnic at Ozoro for five years. He holds a Higher National Diploma HND (1989) in Business Administration from Federal Polytechnic Ilaro, Nigeria. He also earned a Graduate Associate of Science (GAS)/MBA (1996) from Southland University California in the United States. He holds a Ph.D. in Management with a specialization in Operations Research (2007) from Delta State University Abraka, Nigeria. He is a Member of the Academy of Management Nigeria (MAMN), Member Northeast Business & Economic

Association (NBEA), USA and a Fellow of the Chartered Institute of Administrative Managers Nigeria (F. Inst.AM). Within a period of over 22 years of his teaching experience, he has held high profile roles in higher education institutions such as Head of Department, Business Administration, Rector/CEO, Delta State Polytechnic Ozoro. Currently, he is the Managing Director, Delta State University Investment Limited (DIL). These positions have made him continue to work closely with industries and professional bodies in developing undergraduate and postgraduate programs as well as developing business algorithms for the industries. He has also actively supervised Ph.D. students, and most of his former Ph.D. students now hold academic positions in several universities both in Nigeria and overseas He is well-traveled, having attended several business conferences within Nigeria and abroad. Since 2012, he has served as a referee, guest editor and editorial board member of several academic journals both in Nigeria and overseas. He is also an external examiner/assessor to several universities in his area. His research interests are interrelated with optimizations techniques to resolve business problems and improvement of the student's experience. His current projects include understanding how students make work placement decisions using operations research techniques and investigating the learning experiences of business students working in global virtual teams.

Yusuf Ahmed Nur, Ph.D., is an Associate Professor of strategic management in the School of Business at Indiana University Kokomo. He currently teaches strategic management, international business, and international marketing at the graduate and graduate levels. In his courses, he explores innovative ways to engage students so that they take full responsibility for their learning. His research interests include strategic leadership, culture and leadership, entrepreneurship, and economic development. His research has been published in *Business Horizons*, *Global Business Issues Journal*, and *The Business Renaissance Quarterly*. He holds a Ph.D. in Strategic Management from Indiana University; an M.B.A. from California State University, Fresno; and a Bachelor of Science in Electrical Engineering from Military Technical College in Cairo.

Imisha Gurung, Ph.D., in Health Promotion & Behavioral Sciences from the University of Louisville School of Public Health and Information Sciences in 2023. She also earned a Master of Public Health (MPH) degree. She recently received a prestigious award from Nepal's Prime Minister for becoming the first female to obtain a Ph.D. from her village. She was named a faculty favorite nominee while assisting as a graduate assistant for the program evaluation class. She is certified in Teaching & Learning in Health Professions Education, was an Dr. M. Celeste Nichols award winner, multicultural association of graduate student scholar, and the Department of Health Promotion & Behavioral Sciences Scholar. Her Ph.D. dissertation was on Menstruation stigma: A qualitative exploratory study on lived experiences among Nepali women. She has worked on women's health, maternal and child health, racial equity, immigrant health, health policies, mental health, health equity, and more. She is originally from Nepal and continues to work and advocate for Nepali Women's health equity.

Okonmah I. Emmanuel, Ph.D., is an Associate Professor in the Department of Public Administration at the University of Benin, Nigeria. He holds a Ph.D. degree in Public Administration and Comparative Politics; Master of Science (M.Sc.) in Public Administration; and Bachelor of Science (B.Sc.) in Political Science and Public Administration. He has been in the teaching services of the University of Benin since 2010. His areas of teaching and specialties include Development Administration, Research Methods, Public Finance Management, Public Policy Analysis and Evaluations, and Quality Assurance in Public Policy Implementations and Strategies. His areas of research interest include public policy, sustainable development, bureaucratic performance, ethics and administration, development administration economic development, human rights, and social justice in developing countries. He has quite a number of articles published in local, national, and international journals.

Kealeboga J. Maphunye, Ph.D., is a Political Science Professor and former Chair of the Department of Political Sciences (2018–2020), College of Human Sciences, at the University of South Africa (UNISA) (2018–2020). He holds a doctoral degree in Government from the University of Essex (UK), a Master of Public Administration (MPA) from the University of Botswana, and a B.Sc. Sociology (Hons.) from the University of Zimbabwe. Between 2012 and 2018, he was the inaugural Research Professor of the WIPHOLD-Brigalia Bam Chair in Electoral Democracy (UNISA). A political science and public administration scholar, his areas of research interest include African politics, particularly elections and post-independence bureaucratic performance in developing countries. A member of the South African Association of Political Science (SAAPS), and the South African Association of Public Administration and Management (SAAPAM), he has written policy papers, publications, and presented papers at local and international conferences and conducted research on elections, governance, gender, and democracy in South Africa. He has also conducted public sector training and lectured at the University of the Western Cape, worked for the Human Sciences Research Council (HSRC), and South Africa's Electoral Commission (IEC). Further, he has observed elections and regularly collaborates with peers, election, and policy experts from many countries across Africa, the United States, and Europe. At Unisa, he serves in the Departmental Higher Degrees Committee, participates in numerous academic citizenship activities; and advises the University on national and SRC elections. In Africa, he is consulted regularly by SADC, AU, and ECF (SADC-Electoral Commissions Forum) for advice on election management issues. He also contributes regularly to national and international debates on democracy, elections, and governance through the local and international media (radio, television, print and social media). He also mentors' colleagues, conducts research, provides academic leadership, and supervises master's and doctoral students at Unisa. Since 2013, he has functioned as an external examiner of master's and doctoral degrees and as an academic assessor for the promotion of academic staff to doctoral and professorial levels for local (South Africa) and regional (Zimbabwe and Lesotho) universities.

Rayton Sianjina, Ph.D., is currently serving as the Executive Director of the Office of Internationalization and Global Studies at Fort Valley State University (FVSU). Prior to his current position, since joining FVSU, he has served in various positions which include but are not limited to serving as Director of Assessment in the College of Education and Professional Studies, Interim Provost, and Vice President for Academic Affairs. Transitioning from Delaware State University where he served in various progressive leadership positions, during his 16-year tenure, there. He joined FVSU in August 2014 as Dean of the College of Graduate Studies and Extended Education. As Director of the Office of Global Studies and Engagement, he is responsible for negotiating global partnerships among institutions of higher education. It is through those partnerships that FVSU students encounter experiential and service learning by shadowing leaders in a plethora of industries as well as educational settings. He is also responsible for welcoming students and faculty who come for experiential study abroad programs to the FVSU and surrounding local communities. During his 16-year tenure at Delaware State University, he served in various progressive leadership positions, namely, Assistant Vice President for Online Learning, Associate Dean, Department chairperson and director of Delaware Instructional Technology Association. He is a former found board member for Early College High School located on the Delaware State University campus. He earned his Doctor of Philosophy in Educational Administration Leadership & Supervision. Harding university awarded him his bachelor's and master's degrees in 1984 and 1985, respectively. He is an ardent writer and publisher of educational-related areas. His research interest is in the areas of leadership, intercultural competency, information technology, data analysis, education policy, and human capacity building.

Charles B.A. Ubah, Ph.D., is a Professor of Criminology, Criminal Justice, Law, Sociology, and Public Policy at Georgia College & State University Milledgeville, USA. He has published in a variety of peer-reviewed journals in the areas of criminology, criminal justice, law, sociology, and public policy. He has been active in the American Society of Criminology, Academy of Criminal Justice Sciences, Southern Criminal Justice Association, Criminal Justice Association of Georgia, University System of Georgia Africa Council, and the African Criminology and Justice Association. He obtained his Doctoral Degree (Ph.D.) in Criminology/Sociology from Southern Illinois University, Carbondale, Illinois, Master of Arts in Criminal Justice/Sociology from Lincoln University, Jefferson City, Missouri, and Bachelor of Science (Honors) from Lincoln University, Jefferson City, Missouri. His research interest is in the areas of criminal justice, law, and human resources. His research also focuses on social justice, capacity building, comparative criminology, welfare policy, homeland security and emergency management, sustainable development, and economic development and analysis.

Peter Ngwafu, Ph.D., is a Professor of Public Administration at Albany State University USA. He is also the Dean of the College of Arts and Sciences at Albany State University in Georgia, United States. He previously served as the Director of the Department of Public Administration at Albany State University Georgia. He has consulted for several local government and nonprofit organizations in the United States and many countries in Africa. He has also conducted several fields, of research in Africa. His research interests are in the areas of public administration, human resources management, economic development, and public policy. His research papers have been presented in more than 50 national and international conferences. He is well-published in the areas of business–government relations in Africa.

Halima Khunoethe, Ph.D., is a senior government official in the Government of South Africa who has worked for more than 25 years. She has also served as executive director at the federal, provincial, and district levels of the Republic of South African Government, respectively. She has published three books, two on state capacity and one on gender equality. His Excellency the President of the Government of South Africa Mr. Cyril Ramaphosa has signed all three books, a first for any citizen in the world to have three books signed by a sitting president of their country. She is currently the Head of Capacity Building, and she is a subnational governance specialist. She is also currently a member of the National Governments Capacity Building Forum, which provides advise on capacity building strategies that are implemented by the leaders of the country. In addition, her administrative responsibility includes advising cabinet members of the Government of South Africa including the President of the country on aspects related to the capacity of the nation. She is the Chairperson of the Provincial Capacity Building Forum responsible for the implementation of the National and Provincial capacity building strategy. She obtained her Doctoral Degree (Ph.D.) and Master of Public Administration degree from the University of KwaZulu in South Africa. She also received a National Diploma in Public Administration and an Advance Diploma in Adult Education from the University of KwaZulu. She currently serves on various editorial or advisory committees of publishing houses and journals in South Africa, Malawi, Qatar, Swaziland including Zimbabwe. She is the author/co-author of several publications focusing on inter alia capacity of the state and traditional leadership. Her research interest is in the areas of public management, regional economic development, leadership, public policy, non-profit organization, NGOs, capacity building in new democratic governments in Africa, and civil society organizations in South Africa. Her research also focuses on, capacity building, welfare policy, social justice, sustainable development, and economic development analysis.

Leonda Richardson, Ph.D., candidate at the University of Louisville, Department of Health Promotion & Behavioral Sciences, School of Public Health & Information Sciences. Richardson will complete her Ph.D. in July 2024. She earned a master's of dental hygiene. She is also a registered dental hygienist. While completing her bachelor's in dental hygiene, she developed a passion for educating others, public health and issues involving racial and ethnic diversity within and beyond the field of dental hygiene. Her research interests include health inequities impacting Black and Indigenous People of Color. She is also interested in transforming curricular content of health professions education programs, to that which focuses on social justice, critical/liberation theories, and critical pedagogy.

Muawya Hussien, Ph.D., is a Senior Lecturer and Acting Chairperson of the Department of Accounting and Finance in the College of Commerce and Business Administration at Dhofar University, Salalah, Sultanate of Oman in the Middle East. He earned his doctoral, master's and bachelor's degrees in the business management discipline. He has presented his research paper at several national and international conferences in Ethiopia, Sudan, the United Arab Emirates, and South Africa. He has also published many journal articles relating to economic development, business administration, fiscal management, and development administration in Africa. His research is in accounting, business and government relations in Africa, foreign investment in Africa, finance, international environmental policy, sustainable development, public sector partnership with NGOs, multinational corporations' operations in Africa, and comparative trade policies.

Charles Onochie Ochie, Ph.D., is a Professor of Criminal Justice, at Albany State University Georgia, USA. He is also the Dean of the College of Graduate Studies at the same institution. He was the Department Chairperson for Criminal Justice and Forensic Science for 18 years at Albany State University before he assumed the position of Executive Director of Graduate Studies. He was also instrumental in the development of the Forensic Science program at ASU and directed the Forensic Science program at ASU, including developing the graduate curriculum concentration. He graduated from Albany State University in 1987 with a Bachelor of Science degree in Criminal Justice and a Master of Science degree in Sociology from Valdosta State University in 1989. He earned his Ph.D. in Sociology-Criminology from Oklahoma State University in 1993, and he has taught at the following institutions, that is, Troy University, West State University, before coming to his Alma Mater, Albany State University, in 1997. In his capacity as a Chair for 18 years, he participated in a lot of curriculum development, revisions, academic policy development, etc., and facilitated and supervised the development of the first fully online Master of Science degree in Criminal Justice within the USG. He was also the former President of the African Criminology and Justice Association. He is highly published and has presented papers at several national and internal conferences. His research interest is in the areas of criminal justice, economic development, social justice, public policy, capacity building, and sustainable development. He is also highly active in his community and has been appointed by City and County Commissioners to serve in important community boards and commissions. He and his colleagues champion and advocate for ex-offenders released into the community through their Albany Second Chance Program.

Raphael Dibie, Ph.D., candidate in Accounting at the University of Benin, Nigeria. He is currently a Lecturer in Accounting at the Faculty of Management, Delta State University of Science and Technology, Ozoro, Nigeria. He earned his Master of Science in Accounting degree from Benson Idahosa University in Benin City, Nigeria, and Bachelor of Science in Accounting and Taxation (Honors) from the University of Benin, Nigeria, and a Diploma in Accounting (Certified Accountant) from the Institute of Chartered Accountants of Nigeria (ICAN). He previously worked as a Tax Accountant with the Delta State Polytechnic Ozoro. He also has many years' experience working as a Manager in Accounting with Ascama Tax Advocacy and Consulting Company in Warri, as well as a Transaction Officer with the First Bank of Nigeria. He has presented his research paper at several national professional conferences in Nigeria. He has also published some of his research papers relating to tax compliance, fiscal management, and economic development in journals. His research interest is in accounting, taxation, investment, and economic development in Africa.

Fredah Mainah, Ph.D., is currently a Training Officer with US Citizenship and Immigration Services. Previously she was an Adjunct Instructor at the Institute for Intercultural and Anthropological Studies, Lewis Walker Institute for the Study of Race and Ethnic Relations, and Lee Honors College, at Western Michigan University. While at the Institute she was also a Faculty Development Fellow for part-time instructors. She is the author of a book chapter with the title *Government and Business Relations in Kenya*. In Dibie R. (eds) (2018), *Business and Government Relations in Africa*. New York: Routledge Press. She has published a chapter on Women's Empowerment in Kenya. In Dibie R (eds) (2019) *Women's Empowerment for Sustainability in Africa*. Her research interests include leader and leadership development, Women's Capacity Building in Africa, Economic development Policies in Africa, African philosophy, pedagogical research, and instructional technology.

Robert Dibie, Ph.D., is a Distinguished Professor of Public Policy and Public Administration. He also serves as Vice Provost for Academic Affairs at Fort Valley State University. Dibie was also Dean of the School of Public and Environmental Affairs (SPEA) for many years at Indiana University Kokomo. Previously, he served as the director of graduate programs in public administration at Western Kentucky University. He was honored the 2023 Peace Education award from the Board of the Center for African Peace and Conflict Resolution at California State University Sacramento in recognition of his exemplary leadership and outstanding contribution to impactful research and publication on peace, security, and social governance in Africa. He is twice the recipient of the prestigious Carnegie African Diaspora Fellowship award by the Institute of International Education, Washington DC. He has published 11 books and more than 120 peer-reviewed journal articles in environmental policy, civil society, public management, sustainable development, public policy, NGOs, women empowerment, and ethics. Latest books includes *Comparative Perspectives on Environmental Policy and Issues* by Routledge Press; *Public Administration: Analysis, Theories and Application* by Babcock University Press; *Comparative Perspectives on Civil Society by Lexington Press; Public Management and Sustainable Development in Nigeria* by Ashgate; *Nongovernmental Organizations and Sustainable Development in Sub-Saharan Africa* by Lexington Press. His recent research articles have appeared in the *International Journal of Public Administration; Journal of African Policy Studies, Journal of Developing Societies, Journal of Sociology and Social Welfare; Journal of Social Justice, Journal of African and Asian Studies; Politics Administration and Change Journal, Journal of International Politics and Development, Journal of African Business*, and so on. He has presented more than 140 academic papers in national and international conferences, focusing on issues of sustainable development, public management, public policy, women empowerment, environmental policies, development administration, and NGOs. As a nationally recognized leader in higher education, he has presented many seminars, workshops, and lectures in the areas of Higher Education Leadership, Public Policy, Environmental Policy, Gender Empowerment, and Sustainable Development in a number of universities around the world. He is a member of several professional academic organizations and currently serves on the Editorial Advisory Board of many scholarly journals. He has also consulted for several NGOs, Banks, Book Publishers, and Universities in the United States, Europe, Africa, and the Caribbean Islands. He previously served as the Editor of the *International Journal of Politics and Development*. He is a member of the Rotary Club International.

LIST OF ACRONYMS

AA	Absolute Advantage
ADF	African Development Fund
ADB	Asian Development Bank
AGM	Acquired Group Memberships
AKST	Agricultural knowledge, science, and technology
APEC	Asian Pacific Economic Cooperation
AQL	Acceptable Quality Level
BAU	Business-as-usual
BBC	British Broadcasting Corporation
BCI	Better Cotton Initiative
BSI	Better Sugar Initiative
BONGO	Business Organization Non-Governmental Organization
BWA	Bretton Wood Agreement
CAADP	Comprehensive Africa Agriculture Development Program
CADEC	Catholic Development Commission
CBO	Community-based Organizations
CEDAW	Communique for the Eradication of all Discrimination
AW	Against Women
CIDA	Canadian International Development Agency
CG	Corporate Governance
CGIAR	Consultative Group on International Agricultural Research
CIG	Common Initiative Group
CLS	Customary Law System
COWAN	Country Women's Association of Nigeria
CPE	Centrally Planned Economy
CPI	Consumer Price Index
CSIRO	The Commonwealth Scientific and Industrial Research Organization
CSR	Corporate Social Responsibility
ECB	European Central Bank
EEC	European Economic Community

EMS	European Monetary System
EMC	Export Management Company
ERP	Enterprise Resource Planning
ETC	Export Trading Company
DEFRA	Department for Environment, Food and Rural Affairs (UK)
DRC	Democratic Republic of Congo
EU	European Union
FAO	Food and Agriculture Organization of the United Nations
FAOSTAT	Food and Agriculture Organization Statistical Databases
FASB	Financial Accounting Standard Board
FIBL	German Research Institute of Organic Agriculture
FONGO	Funder Organization Non-Governmental Organization
FTA	Free Trade Area
FTZ	Foreign Trade Zone
FWCW	Fourth World Conference on Women
G8	Group of Eight
GAP	Good Agricultural Practices
GDP	Gross Domestic Product
GEF	Global Environmental Facility
GHG	Greenhouse gas
GMO	Genetically modified organism
GNI	Gross National Income
GNP	Gross National Product
GONGO	Government Organized Non-Governmental Organization
GRID	Global Resource Information Database
GRO	Grassroots Organizations
GSO	Grassroots Support Organizations
HICs	High-Income Countries
HRWWR	Human Rights Watch World Report
IAASTD	International Assessment of Agricultural Knowledge, Science and Technology for Development
ICARDA	International Centre for Agricultural Research in the Dry Areas
IDH	Dutch Sustainable Trade Initiative
IEA	International Energy Agency
IFAD	International Fund for Agricultural Development
IFOAM	International Federation of Organic Agriculture Movements
IFPRI	International Food Policy Research Institute
ILO	International Labor Organization

IMF	International Monetary Fund
IP	Intellectual Property
IPCC	Intergovernmental Panel on Climate Change
IPM	Integrated Pest Management
ITC	International Trade Centre
IITA	International Institute of Tropical Agriculture
INGO	International Non-Government Organization
KANGO	Kenya HIV/AID NGOs Consortium
LICs	Low-Income Countries
LMICs	Lower Middle-Income Countries
MDG	Millennium Development Goal
MSCI	Morgan Stanley Capital International
MSO	Membership Support Organizations
NANGO	National Association of Nongovernmental Organizations
NCAR	National Centre for Atmospheric Research
NFGO	Non for Gain Organization
NGO	Nongovernmental Organizations
NORAD	Norwegian For Development
OAU	Organization of African Unity
ODA	Oversees Development Assistance
ODA	Official Development Assistance
OECD	Organization for Economic Cooperation and Development
OPEC	Organization of Petroleum Exporting Countries
PAHM	Plant and animal health management
PES	Payment for Ecosystem Services
PICS	Purdue Improved Cowpea Storage
PLC	Product Life Cycle
PPP	Public–Private Partnerships
PPP	Purchasing Power Parity
PONGO	Political Non-Governmental Organization
PTE	Private Technology Exchange
QUANGO	Quasi Autonomous Non-Governmental Organizations
RCS	Reverse Culture Shock
R&D	Research and Development
RD	Representative Democracy
ROI	Return on Investment
RSPO	Roundtable on Sustainable Palm Oil
RTRS	Round Table on Responsible Soy

SAM	Sustainable Asset Management AG
SAP	Structural Adjustment Program
SIDA	Swedish International Development Agency
SOM	Soil organic matter
SMO	Social Marketing Orientation
SMO	Strategic Marketing Orientation
SRI	System Rice Intensive
SWFs	Sovereign wealth funds
TANGO	Tanzania Association of Non-Government Organization
TC	Transnational Company
TM	Traditional Medicine
TQM	Total Quality Management
UMICs	Upper Middle-Income Countries
UNCTAD	United Nations Conference on Trade and Development
UN	DESA United Nations Department of Economic and Social Affairs
UN	United Nations
UNCTAD	United Nations Conference on Trade and Development
UNDP	United Nations Development Program
UNEP	United Nations Environment Program
UNESC	ECA United Nations Economic and Social Council, Economic Commission for Africa
VAT	Value Added Tax
WDR	World Development Report
WIPO	World Intellectual Property Organization
WTO	World Trade Organization

BOOK DESCRIPTION

The *Transforming Healthcare in Africa* book explores the impact of historical institutions, multilateral organizations, and informal norms, such as, respectively, colonialism, the World Health Organization, and the Western-inspired biomedical approach to disease on health policy choices, implementation, and results in Africa. In addition, it examines the role of international philanthropy, such as the Bill and Melinda Gates Foundation, Partners in Health, Doctors Without Borders, and the multitude of NGOs that pullulate the African healthcare landscape. The emphasis on these factors, not to mention Cuban medical aid, clearly underscores the "globalization" of healthcare policy in Africa. The case studies of Botswana, Ghana, and Rwanda—three differently endowed countries economically that are also at varying stages of democratic rule—help to shed light on the influence of domestic political institutions and elite agencies on healthcare policy processes across the continent.

Understanding—and improving—governance of African health is more than a matter of prescribing mechanisms intended to increase accountability and transparency. It requires taking stock of how global policies and local politics interact, the transnational channels through which political pressure is exercised, as well as how a broad spectrum of therapeutic alternatives is made available to, or shunned by, health-seekers. Health systems in Africa surpass what is accessible through the public system to encompass a patchwork of providers, whether these are biomedical entrepreneurs, churches, NGOs, or "traditional" healers. Health systems also encompass shifting systems of social solidarity that insure against risk: there may be private health insurance for a few and some free health services here and there, but it is extended social networks (which may be more or less based on varying notions of kinship) that insure against health risk. Thus, it is more apt to speak of a proliferating therapeutic economy where therapeutic transactions may be valued in other than monetary terms, and where affliction is not necessarily understood in a strictly biomedical idiom.

The therapeutic economy is a strikingly hybridized one, where the irrational use of biomedicines coincides with the industrially produced traditional remedies, and where affliction is simultaneously understood and treated in biomedical and spiritual terms. It will be necessary to come to grips with this creolized therapeutic world, as attempts to govern health through a purely biomedical model and the illusion of its rational management are destined to run aground in the messy therapeutic politics of the real world. Conclusion There is recognition that accountability, transparency, and vigorous citizen participation are essential to achieving a viable society, sustainable economic growth, and equitable distribution of benefits and risk of growth. Yet African countries are characterized by persistent and in many cases worsening social, economic, gender, and health inequalities. This theme runs across the articles in this volume 'Governing the African Health System.' Some of the key issues discussed in this volume include corruption in hospitals, transparency in Primary Health Care (PHC) delivery, citizen participation in decision-making regarding health care, and the empowerment of traditional birth attendants, among others. Health sector reforms have also been widely addressed; with decentralization, financing of health care delivery, and traditional medical practice being the key issues. Sama & Nguyen: Governing the Health System in Africa. This volume on Transforming Health Systems in Africa focus on—what will make the health system in African countries transform from Good to Better and then Great in the future. It is our goal to clarify the uses of social science research, to provide evidence on how the health social sciences have influenced our thinking about health care issues, and to underscore some promising and relevant areas of research for the future.

Chapter One

OVERVIEW OF HEALTH SYSTEMS IN AFRICA

Robert Dibie

Introduction

The continent of Africa is considered to be the second largest and second most populous on earth with an estimated population in 2020 of 1,340,598,147 (1.3 billion) people (Human Development Report 2020; World Bank 2023). It is estimated that the African continent's population constitutes over 14% of the world's human population (World Alas, 2020). The continent is also home to 55 recognized independent countries or states. According to the United Nations Human Development Report (2022), Africa also has nine territories and two de facto independent states with very little recognition. Western Sahara is supposed to be the 55th nation in the African continent but its statehood has still been disputed by Morocco. It should be noted however that despite the predicament of its statehood status Western Sahara is a member state of the African Union. In addition, South Sudan is Africa's newest independent state. It gains its independence on July 9, 2011 (Infoplease 2020). Although the African Union was established in July 2002, with the purpose of helping Africa's nations to secure a pragmatic and better-functioning democracy, create an effective common market; sustainable economy, and human rights, as well as end the multiple conflicts in the continent, the organization has not been able to accomplish most of its goals (African Development Bank 2023; Ake 1996; USAID Africa Report 2020).

The African continent is endowed with many mountains, hills, the Sahara, and Sahel deserts. It also contains many famous rivers such as the Nile River, which is the world's longest, the river Niger, and the Congo River (African Development Bank 2023; Human Development Index Report 2020). After the colonial period and the independence of many African countries from various European countries, most of the newly created nations were plagued with ineffective governments, leaders that were dictators, civil wars, coup d'états, ethnic conflicts, and religious insurgencies (Ayana et al. 2023; Dibie 2022, 2017; Hopkins et al. 2009). In addition to the above predicaments, the continent experiences various unfavorable environmental and humanitarian conditions such as famine, drought, flood, and poverty. According to Infoplease (2020), these political, humanitarian, and environmental conditions often lead to displaced refugees, vulnerable forced labor and sexual exploitation of girl children and women, sex trade, inter-ethnic abduction,

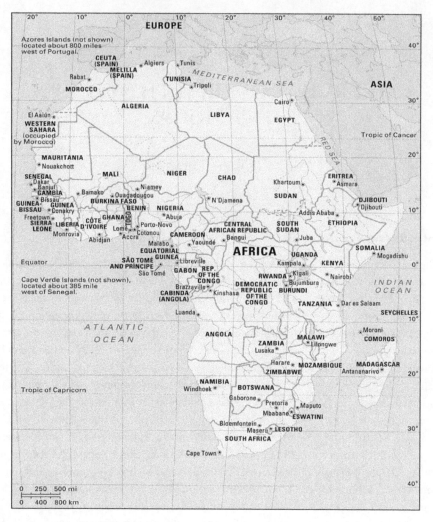

Figure 1: Map of Africa Showing Countries in the Continent.
Source: Map of Africa (2024).

and religious insurgencies. It is mind-boggling to see children begging on the streets when their parents cannot afford to provide a home for them or send the children to school. Furthermore, these humanitarian crises in some countries in the African continent were followed by famine, genocide, malaria, Ebola, HIV/AIDS, COVID-19, tuberculosis, and other diseases (African Development Bank 2023; Human Development Index 2020). Economic development, as used in this book, refers to a process that reinvigorates the social, economic, healthcare services, infrastructure facilities, and technical progress of people in any country (Dibie 2018). Figure 1 shows the Map of Africa. Note that, there are 55 independent countries in the African continent.

According to Coccia (2019) and Nafziger (2005), the major components of development in any nation or society include the improvement of the health of all citizens, the creation of new knowledge and technology, the growth of wealth and the provision of public goods and services that could benefit everyone in the country. Economic and sustainable development could be enhanced in Sub-Saharan African (SSA) countries if their efforts to boost the efficiencies of the economic system are enhanced. Most developed countries such as Japan, South Korea, Singapore, Canada, the United States, and the United Kingdom have done a lot to build state-of-the-art universal healthcare systems (World Bank 2023). Some scholars argued that for industrialization to take place, a nation's capital must be built first and not left to be based on a subsistence practice (Slavin 2020; Nafziger 2005). Therefore, the production capacity of a nation can only be raised by building some plants, equipment, a vibrant health system, and revitalizing production (Mankiw 2024). In addition, governments of African countries must provide an environment that will help them to maintain a vibrant competitive system in order to enhance the law of supply and demand (Hubbard & O'Brien 2021). Further, an environment that could help to boost economic development also requires a good functioning government that could provide an effective legal system where nobody (including the president of the nation) is above the law (Dibie & Dibie 2017). This is because a good legal system could further enhance a functional free-enterprise economy. An effective rule of law system could also enforce business contracts as well as be able to reduce the challenges of bribery by defining the rights and nonrecognition of rights to private ownership (Chenery & Syrquin 1975; Slavin 2020). Unfortunately, most African countries are not considered as developed because of the challenges alluded to above. In the past few decades, there have been opportunities for African political leaders to promote economic development strategies that could help to build plants and industries however greed, corruption, and the lack of foresight have caused such plants or projects not to take place (Ayittey 2005; Daley 2017; Dibie 2022). Thus, it could be argued that some African leaders are their own worst enemies because they often fail to engage in strategic planning and fail to get the right team with professional skills, and ethical experts involved in planning. Furthermore, some African leaders do not have good skills in collaborative governance, steward leadership, and good management (Coccia 2019; Edoho & Dibie 2017).

Health policy as used in this book includes actions that governments in African countries adopt to influence the provision and implementation of healthcare services delivery to all its citizens. Healthcare policy also involves the various government activities that affect or attempt to affect public health and the well-being of all the citizens and residents of a nation (Kraft & Furlong 2021). Furthermore, health policies are the major mechanism through which the government shapes the delivery of healthcare in many nations around the world (Jacob & Skocpol 2016; Shi 2019). Healthcare, as used in this book, refers to the maintenance or improvement of health through the diagnosis, prevention, and treatment of sickness or illness, injury, communicable and noncommunicable diseases, and other physical or mental impairments (Kraft & Furlong 2021). In addition, healthcare includes nursing, medicine, dentistry, psychology, physical therapy, occupational therapy, and traditional medicine (Abdullahi 2011; Dibie 2022).

According to Ayana et al. (2023) and Longest and Darr (2014) policies are adopted in both the public and private sectors. On one hand, members of the national and regional legislative, executive, and judiciary branches of government could enact policies. On the other hand, Chief Executive officers, directors, and managers of private sector companies could also make policies for their staff. It is important to note that policies made in the public sector affect everyone in the nation, while policies established in the private sector are only applicable to staff within the corporation. This book focuses on public sector healthcare policies. There are however going to be some sections where private sector policies might be discussed because health companies also own hospitals and health centers that provide medical services to citizens of many societies. There are African countries that have collaborated with nongovernment organizations (NGOs) and other private donors to fund health services.

In addition, health is a human right and a cornerstone for reinvigorating economies in African countries (Dibie 2022; World Health Organization 2020a). It should be noted that a major principle of democratic government is to facilitate ensure, and promote healthcare delivery as well as the well-being of individuals, and everyone in the societies (Ayana et al. 2023; Longest 2016; Shi 2019). The state of citizens' health and physical and mental well-being is what constitutes a pleasant, meaningful, and productive life. Thus, health is a very important mechanism for the sustainable economic development of any nation. Anna (2020) and Kraft and Furlong (2021) argued that the priority, ethical values, and political will that political leaders, and public administrators, bestowed on their health system will determine the magnitude of the budget that is appropriate to funding healthcare for everyone.

According to the World Bank (2020) and the United States Agency for International Development African (USAID) Report (2020), it is estimated that 1.6 million Africans died of malaria, tuberculosis, and HIV-related illnesses in 2015. Furthermore, the African continent is reported to bear one-quarter of the global disease burden, however, the continent has only 2% of the world's doctors (World Health Organization 2020b). There is no doubt that these diseases can be prevented or treated if many African countries have effective healthcare systems, which could facilitate timely access to appropriate and affordable medicines, vaccines, and other health services (African Development Bank 2020; Yamey et al. 2019). The World Bank (2020) also reported that African countries account for nearly a quarter of all disability and deaths caused by various diseases worldwide, despite these health challenges only 1% of global health expenditures are budgeted. The report also indicated that only 3% of the world's health workers live in the 55 countries in the continent (World Bank 2020).

The major challenge, however, is that less than 2% of drugs consumed in Africa are produced in the continent, meaning that many sick patients do not have access to locally produced drugs and may not afford to buy the imported ones (Atake 2018; USAID 2020; World Health Organization 2020a). Thus, it has been reported that many African countries are challenged with serious social and economic situations that can be classified as dangerous to humanity. The African predicaments include persistent poor health, lower life expectancy, higher mortality rates, and forms of communicable and noncommunicable diseases as well as few specialist doctors and modern health facilities (Adjei 2018; Clausen 2015; Yamey et al. 2019; USAID 2020).

According to the African Development Bank (2020) and United Nations Human Developing Index (2020), Many Africa's countries continue to be classified as one the poorest nations of the world. Despite these negative stigmas, there are quite a few countries that have galvanized their agricultural and manufacturing sectors. It is what noting that African nations such as Egypt, Morocco, Nigeria, and South Africa have made significant economic and social gains over the past 20 years (Dibie 2018; Edoho & Dibie 2017). While many African countries are now shipping manufacturing products all over the world, countries such as Angola, Libya, and Nigeria are also exporting crude oil and generating a lot of revenue to alleviate the standard of living for their citizens, respectively.

According to the African Development Bank (2023) and World Bank (2023), the continent of Africa has six of the world's 10 fastest-growing economies. In addition, the Northern region of the African continent has vast oil and natural gas deposits, while the Sub-Saharan region holds the most strategic nuclear ore, and resources such as coltan, gold, and copper, among many others, are abundant on the continent. According to the United States Agency for International Development Report (2020) and the Human Development Index Report (2020), many democratic nations in Africa such as Algeria, Angola, Cameroon, Chad, Republic of Congo, Egypt, Eritrea, Gabon, Ghana, Kenya, Libya, Nigeria, South Sudan, Sudan, Tunisia, and Mozambique are all rich in crude oil and natural gas (African Development Bank 2023; Dibie 2022). It has also been reported that share of world production from African soil was bauxite 9%; aluminum 5%; chromite 44%; cobalt 57%; copper 5%; gold 21%; iron ore 4%; steel 2%; lead (Pb) 3%; manganese 39%; zinc 2%; cement 4%; natural diamond 46%; graphite 2%; phosphate rock 31%; coal 5%; mineral fuels (including coal) petroleum 13%; and uranium 16% (Dibie 2018, Yamey et al. 2019; World Bank 2020). Thus, the African continent could be regarded as the world's fastest-growing region for foreign direct investment and sustainable development. The deplorable economic situation in the African continent is due to what has been described as an unfair twenty-first-century exploitation (African Development Bank 2023; Ayana et al. 2023; Ayittey 2005; Dibie 2022).

The African continent is endowed with many natural resources and the world's largest agricultural area and a 1.2-billion-person market new (African Development Bank 2023; World Bank 2023). In addition, the continent has the potential to forge a new (World Bank 2023). Despite these great mechanisms of economic development, the extent of government quality and government effectiveness is lower compared with other parts of the world (African Development Bank 2023; Ayana et al. 2023). In addition, the greater corruption index and the lower voice and accountability are issues in Sub-Saharan African countries relative to other parts of the world (Lidetu et al. 2024; Nkalu & Agu 2023). Some scholars contend that the questions of economic policy credibility and policy implementation strategies are also more stimulating problems in SSA countries (Ayana et al. 2023; Dibie 2022; Nkaju & Agu 2023). According to the African Development Bank (2023), the continent's GDP growth rate dropped from 4.8% in 2021 to 3.8%–2.8% in 2022. Despite the slowdown in the economy, the African continent remains resilient with average growth projected to improve to about 4.1% in 2023. Furthermore, as the African continent's economies recover at a faster rate in the near future, appropriate economic development policies should be enacted toward sharing the growth benefits more equally across the population by enhancing capacity building, healthcare, fostering job-friendly economic growth, as well as economic diversification.

Healthcare Policy and Poverty

Environmental conditions such as global climate change, air and water pollution, levels of particles or ozone, sanitation problems, lack of clean water as well as radical human behavior or choice have all directly or indirectly affected the public health in all countries of the world (Kwame & Petrucka 2024). In the past 20–50 years, healthcare for all citizens of the world has increasingly been recognized as an important aspect of human and economic development in many African countries. Millennium Development Goals (MDGs) have also galvanized the momentum to increase investment in actions and reform to improve health outcomes and accelerate initiatives to accomplish the objectives of the healthcare system in many African countries (Friis 2016).

Many scholars have argued that healthy populations could galvanize economic dividends (Dibie 2022; Henderson 2019; Shi 2019; Wilensky & Teitelbaum 2023). This is because healthy people are more productive, and healthy infants and children can develop better and become productive adults (Kwame & Petrucka 2024). In addition, a healthy population can also contribute to a country's economic growth (Kraft & Furlong 2021; Kwame & Petrucka 2024; World Health Organization 2020; WHO 2014). Healthcare policy includes all the actions that governments take to influence the provision of healthcare services and the various government activities that affect or attempt to affect the public health and well-being of all citizens (Dibie 2022; Kraft & Furlong 2021; Lidetu et al. 2023). A vivid assessment of history, social, and economic conditions in many African countries reveals that there is a causal relationship between poor health and poverty in the continent (Lidetu et al. 2023; Wilensky & Teitelbaum 2020).

Further, while many African countries normally have a Ministry or Department of Health, they often fail to establish a public health division within the ministry. Furthermore, some countries do not have a Food and Drug Administration agency to monitor food safety. In some poor countries, it is the Customs and Excise Agency that monitors the importation of drugs and their safety. This overlap in public health has often created more complicated issues in many African countries. It is unfortunate to observe that despite the many natural economic development potentials in Africa, healthcare services have not been adequately funded. In many countries, the health budget has drastically been reduced due to unethical reasons by political leaders (Human Development Index 2020). Evidence of how infectious diseases such as HIV/AIDS, COVID-19, Ebola, malaria, pneumonia, schistosomiasis, tuberculosis, missus, and other communicable and noncommunicable diseases have been properly handled without the help of foreign assistants (Dibie 2022; USAID Report 2020). In addition, diseases that result from environmental pollution, climate change, drought, flood, new lifestyles as a result of urbanization, industrialization, exploration of minerals, and slum growth have often been ignored by the governments of many African countries (Ansah et al. 2024; Atake 2018).

Structural violence includes economic and political structures that constrain human beings. In addition, Anasah et al. (2024) contends that structural conflict occurs when patterned social relationships fail to satisfy basic needs such as healthcare or secure the vital interests of one or both parties. In many African countries, poor citizens suffer severe health issues and die at a younger age. This is because they probably have a higher child–maternal mortality, more serious disease infection, and limited access to hospitals and healthcare services (Kwame & Petrucka 2024; OECD 2023; Wilensky & Teitelbaum 2020). The World Health Organization Report (2020) and Patel and Rushefsky contend that increased investment in health would translate into hundreds of billions of dollars per year of additional income for citizens of any country. In the case of African countries, such an amount of money could be used to improve the living conditions and social infrastructure of all citizens. Some scholars have also argued that for every 10% increase in life expectations. At birth, there is a corresponding rise in economic growth of 0.4% per year (Jacobs & Skocpol 2016; Wilensky & Teitelbaum 2020; Holsinger 2018). One other challenge in many countries in Africa is that economic growth does not benefit the majority of the people on the continent.

According to the World Health Organization Report (2020), poverty is not just the lack of money, it also prevents people not to having basic living needs as well as unpredictable plans for the future. As a result of poverty, my people cannot afford to pay for their medical. In addition, people who live far from hospitals as well as those who believe that their minor ailment does not require going to seek medical consultation often resort to self-medication in Africa (World Economic Forum 2023). Other reasons for resorting to self-medication in many African countries include knowledge about the disease or treatment of the illness, previous experience, cheap availability of medications, mild diseases affordability, and to save time (Dibie 2022; World Economic Forum 2023). The reasons for self-medication vary from one region to another in Africa. Although the practice of self-medication seems to be all over the world, most rich and poor Africans often engage in self-medication. In addition, this practice of improper self-medication has led to dangerous and handful interactions, risk of dependence and abuse, as well as overdose of medication and death (Di Muzio et al. 2017; Esan et al. 2018). Further, it is also a common practice for people in Africa to resort to traditional medicine whenever they are confronted with the difficulties of lack of access to modern medicines (Handley & Nembhard 2020; Mansouri 2024).

Health financing systems in many African countries are regarded as very pluralistic because most of the funds tend to come from several sources such as foreign donors, government, households, employers, private business owners, philanthropies, and nongovernmental organizations (World Health Organization 2013). In addition, many African countries have been reported to engage in low health financing in their annual budget in Africa is normally below 15% of their GDP that they agreed to in the Abuja Declaration in 2001 (African Development Bank 2020; Ateke 2018; ASAID African Report 2020). For example, of some African nations' health budget in the past few years, Nigeria 3.8% (2021), Ghana 3.9% (2020), Ethiopia 3.48% (2020), Zimbabwe 3.4% (2021), Kenya 4.2% (2021), South Africa 8.1% (2020), Botswana 6.1% (2021), Rwanda 6.41% (2019), Uganda 3.8% (2020), Sudan 3.02% (2020), Zambia 5.6% (2021), Burkina Faso 6.72% (2019), Mali 4.3% (2022), and Somalia 1.2% (1999) (World Bank Indicators 2022).

The World Health Organization Report (2022) recommended that each country in the African continent should invest at least US$44 per capita per year for its health system. The data above show that while some African countries have persistently spent over US$ 44 per capita each year, there are some countries that have not been able to meet this goal. Consequently, government financing of the healthcare system including the public health sector is very low. The outcomes are that many citizens do not have access to healthcare, especially, if they are poor and unemployed. In many SSA countries, some governments have enacted and implemented National Health Insurance to cover civil servants and their dependents, members of the army forces, and civil servants' retirees. Unfortunately, employees in the private sector and nongovernmental organizations (NGOs) do not have access to the National Health Insurance, despite the fact they constitute more than 92% of the national workforce (Atake 2018).

Technology and Healthcare Delivery

The United States International Development Agency (USAID) Report (2016) confirms that there has been tremendous growth in access to information and communication technology (ICT), particularly, mobile phones and network connectivity in Africa. The capacity building in information technology has galvanized more opportunities for better healthcare delivery in many African countries. In addition, technology is beginning to transform how healthcare is delivered in many African countries, giving more people in remote areas there and around the world access to better care (Sama & Nguyen 2020). According to Jimenez et al. (2015) and Haddiya et al. (2020) information systems have increasingly become very important for measuring and improving the quality and coverage of health services all over the world in the past three decades. Likewise, easier access to data helps both doctors and policymakers make better-informed decisions about how to continue to improve the system (Jimenez et al. 2015). In some African countries however, it is often ironic that while pharmaceutical shopping malls are equipped with air-conditioning, doctors, and their patients are sweltering in hospitals and medical clinics without a cool and refreshing environment, and the much-needed medical equipment such as MRI machines due to lack of adequate funding (Clausen 2015).

In the twenty-first century, electricity and modern technology allow hospitals, health clinics outpatient facilities, and other parties in the healthcare system of any country to access and analyze patient data from registration to diagnoses to post-discharge helping reshape the way healthcare can be delivered. During the past two decades, several SSA nations have attained a high level of information technology with the use of mobile devices. According to Dibie and Quadri (2019), internet penetration and mobile device usage have become incrementally used as a mechanism for e-healthcare delivery. Information technology is beginning to resolve the major challenges in communication distance between rural and urban regions in many African countries. For example, it has been reported that public health officers in some East and West African countries now use technology systems called mTrac, and telemedicine to report medicine stocks across hospitals and clinics all over their respective nations (Bastos de Morais 2017). Thus, new information technology has increased access and faster response rates in the healthcare system in African countries unlike what it used to be 20 or 30 years (Dibie & Quadri 2019). Despite the advent of information technology in Africa, many doctors and nurses do not have proper training on how to better adapt the new IT into medical practices.

Rwanda is a pioneer in digital health in Africa. The nation's technology successes include the use of artificial intelligence-based algorithms in mobile phones to get a diagnosis, doctors using telemedicine to consult, blood delivery by medical drones, and a central electronic health records system ensuring data is collected accurately (Moyce & Schenker 2018). The insights that other African country's government and private sectors can learn from projects like this are critical to achieving universal healthcare coverage and better access to affordable health promises. It is also reported that in Kenya, Novartis is working on an mHealth pilot in Nairobi and Mombasa to better understand the supply chain cycle and build capabilities to ensure how medicines could be better administered to affected patients in need in the country (Jimenez et al. 2015; USAID 2016). The Rwanda and Kenya technology innovation has spurred the creation of KEA Medicals Pharmaceutics and Technologies, a Republic of Benin-based start-up that uses innovative technology to store and transfer basic medical information that can be accessed in times of emergency (Moyce & Schenker 2018). Furthermore, Vula Mobile in South Africa offers a mobile phone application that aids rural health professionals in providing effective eye care by communicating directly with specialists over a messaging system. The purpose of this modern technology is to reduce the impact of treatable and reversible illnesses (Dibie & Quadri 2019; Moyce & Schenker 2018).

There is doubt that modern technology in the future healthcare system has a lot of potential. Doctors can access their patient's EHR, reviewing medical histories, writing follow-up emails, and sending prescriptions to pharmacies in far and near destinations within a few seconds. iPad and smartphone technologies could also help nurses and doctors to complete various tasks from urban or rural regions in Africa to their health quarters and specialist and medical laboratories around the world (Matchaba 2019). In addition, improved communication could not only save lives but also aid the role of medical billers, allowing them to send text message alerts about payment, as well as schedule outstanding bills and making electronic payments with credit cards or Zelle money transfers (Dibie & Quadri 2019). Some scholars have argued that modern health systems need a technology cloud computing platform system that has a high-performance capacity and can handle big data (Matchaba 2019; Ratchinsky 2016). This is because keeping patients' data secured and confidential is very crucial to the administration of an effective healthcare system.

Health System Governance and Leadership

It has been argued that the value or importance that a nation's leaders and citizens place on the health of their citizens is categorically reflected in the amount of funding, policies, infrastructure, and resources devoted to the pursuit of a vibrant healthcare system in the country (Kraft & Furlong 2021; Longest 2016; Marks et al. 2018). In addition, the objective of any healthcare system is to improve the health of all citizens in a country. A good leader or president of any health system is expected to promote strong ethical and social justice values (Dibie 2022). The moral and social justice values that must be promoted as well as practiced by leaders should involve the integration of the principles of freedom, social and ethnic equality, and the worth and dignity of all the people in the continent of Africa, respectively. The practice of servant and stewardship leadership could ensure a good life for everyone (Dibie 2017; Ferrell et al. 2019). Unfortunately, the health systems in many African countries are in deplorable conditions, rather than their presidents and political elites to solve the dilapidated state of their healthcare system, they frequently travel outside their respective countries to seek better treatment in foreign countries (Daley 2017; Harrison 2016). According to the Africanglobe Report (2012), some African unethical presidents and their political elite are busy amassing fortunes in European and North American countries while the majority of their citizens are living in abject poverty. It is also mind-boggling that these poor African people do not have access to basic public goods or social services such as good health systems, elementary schools, sanitation, clean drinking water, and electricity, yet their presidents own majestic buildings and palaces in foreign countries and in their home countries, respectively (AfricanGlobe 2012; Dibie 2022). It is rather unfortunate that while their citizens are dying of diseases, and sick patients sleeping on the floor of hospitals due to no availability of beds, political leaders travel to receive better or modern healthcare in western developed countries (Chiwanza 2018; Daley 2017). Rather than investing in building good hospitals and equipping them, African presidents do not trust their poorly funded hospitals and travel overseas to use the money, which they are supposed to use for the benefit of all the citizens to seek treatment for their family members and themselves.

According to the World Economic Forum Report (2014) about 30,000 Nigerians spend US$1 billion annually on medical tourism to most countries like Canada, England, France, India, Indonesia, Spain, and Dubai. In addition, Nigerian elites spent 60% of their foreign healthcare payment on four major disease areas: cardiology, orthopedics, renal dialysis issues, and cancer (Adebayo 2020; Obuh 2020; Tseane-Gumbi & Ojakorotu 2022).

According to Anna (2020), African presidents who engage in medical tourism do so because they lack confidence in the health system that they are expected to fund, provide modern equipment, and employ high-quality doctors and nurses. This is the obvious reason why African leaders are the culprits that have created the very bad healthcare systems that exist in their respective countries (Anna 2020; Chiwanza 2018). The lack of the political will by some African political leaders to increase the funding appropriated for their health system has known doubt negatively affected projected progress in the achievement of health goals for the African continent which each president has agreed to accomplish for their respective countries (Chiwanza 2018; WHO 2020; Zane 2017).

Apart from, appropriate funding, it could be argued that technology, human capacity building, and evidence-based approach could reinvigorate or reinvent the African healthcare system as well as effectively discourage medical tourism (Anna 2020; Dibie 2022). By virtue of Africa's good climate coupled with its rich heritage, people, and culture, the technological revolution of the healthcare system will not only discourage African elites from seeking healthcare abroad, but a vibrant health system could also attract patients from other parts of the world to the continent (Anna 2020; Chiwanza 2018). The positive impact these new approaches could have on Africa's GDP, and healthcare systems are unquantifiable (United Nations Development Programme Report 2020; World Economic Forum 2020).

Types of Healthcare Disparities in Africa

The health system is defined as the total national efforts taken in both the public and private sectors as well as nonprofit organizations or nongovernmental organizations (NGOs) to deliver healthcare for all citizens and residents of a country (Besançon et al. 2022; Rajabi et al. 2021).

According to Kraft and Furlong (2021) and the Ministry of Health Nigeria (2021), it is contended that health insurance is a type of scheme that covers the whole or a part of the risk of a person incurring medical expenses. As with other types of insurance, the scheme could be a risk for many individuals. Golden (2021) also defines health insurance as a type of insurance scheme that pays for medical, surgical, prescription drug, and sometimes dental expenses incurred by citizens and permanent residents of the country who are insured. The insurance scheme can reimburse the insured for expenses incurred from illness or injury or pay the care provider directly.

The common health challenges observed while conducting the research for this book are the disparities and lack of access to healthcare in many African countries between people in urban and rural regions. On one hand, there are also major disparities between rich and poor people due to a lack of access to hospitals or health clinics, as well as the inability to afford the payment for treatment. On the other hand, disparities also exist among retired people who do not have family members who could help pay for their healthcare. The challenges of health disparities in healthcare in many African countries are one of the reasons, why life expectancy is exceptionally low. Lack of access to immunization or vaccines and appropriate drugs to treat malaria, hepatitis B, tuberculosis, HIV/AIDs, and most recently COVID-19 has also reduced the life expectancy for many poor people and those living in rural regions in the African continent.

According to Dibie (2022) and the World Health Organization (2023), there is evidence that confirms disparities in the use of health services such as birth assistance by skilled medical personnel, antenatal visits, and birth-given hospitals and clinics in many African countries. In most cases, women in rural areas are twice as unlikely to attend antenatal care or deliver with the assistance of professional skilled healthcare staff.

Previous studies found that there are major disparities in health insurance coverage for women living in rural regions in several African countries. It was also mind-boggling to find out that most of these women did not even know that there was anything called health insurance because whenever they visited local health centers or dispensaries or hospitals in their respective regions, they often paid the cost out of pocket for their treatment (Clausen 2015; Gile et al. 2022; Giles-Vernick 2022). Standford Medicine 2020). Dassah et al. (2018) contend that the disparities among uneducated older women, compared with their male affluent were much higher and more pronounced in several SSA countries. As a result of a wide range of barriers in finance, information sharing, and other geographical factor, access to healthcare in rural settings is beyond imagination. In addition, equitable access by all citizens is expected to be the major premise or goal of a nation's healthcare system, however, in some African countries, people with disabilities often experience greater disparities in the process of seeking primary healthcare than their able counterparts. Dibie (2022) and Haque et al. (2020) argued that disparities in maternal health services in SSA occur due to women living in rural regions not having access to high-quality healthcare services.

Safe Drinking Water and Sanitation

Access to safely managed drinking water and sanitation for all citizens is one of the major predicaments confronting many governments in SSA. Further, providing safe water has been argued to galvanize many benefits (Frii 2019; Nhamo & Muchuru 2019; Skolnik 2008). According to Bain (2020) and Dibie (2022), safe water is a fundamental mechanism for good health and economic and social development in any country. This is because a regular supply of water with better bacteriological quality can reduce the morbidity of various diseases such as dracunculiasis by 78%, schistosomiasis by 77%, and trachoma by 27% (Cairnecross & Valdmines 2006 ; Frii 2019; Skolnick 2008). Despite the crucial relationship between the lack of safe water and health danger, the governments of many African countries have been developing political will in providing the required funding to address this major problem (Emenike et al. 2017; Nhamo & Muchuru 2019). The World Health Organization (2020) estimated that about 50–120 million children lack access to safe water in the African continent.

It has been stated that taking precautionary measures is better than cure (Frii 2019). Sanitation problems facing more than 300 million people in many African countries are leading to many social problems, the spread of diseases, and poverty. It has been argued by many scholars that financial mobilization and increased allocation of funds in the budget to solving sanitation as a priority is an incremental approach to achieving sanitation and hygiene. Rather than building hospitals that are poorly equipped, why can the government adopt precautional measures by funding the establishment of better sanitation systems?

In most developing countries, including those in Africa contaminated water has been linked to the outbreak of cryptosporidiosis among the people living in the rural and some urban communities (Frii 2019; Skolnik 2008; Yasi et al. 2001). Thus, waterborne diseases are a source of ongoing concern in many countries in the African continent.

In most cases, waterborne diseases are in the form of cholera fever, abdominal distress of long duration, diarrhea, and typhoid fever (Frii 2019; Leigland et al. 2016; Nhamo & Muchuru 2019).

Disparities caused by national state and local governments' failure to supply safe water to their citizen have often caused the spread of waterborne diseases that resulted in the death of newborns and children from conditions such as dehydration especially under the extremely hot tropical climate. (Frii 2019; Skolnik 2008). Citizens no longer have faith in the government's ability to deliver safe water, thus, they try to seek alternative means of getting water (Emenike et al. 2017; World Health Organization 2021).

African Traditional Health System

The continent of Africa is endowed with enormous biodiversity resources, and it is estimated to contain between 55 and 45,000 different species of plants (Abd El-Ghani 2017; Mutombo et al. 2023). The availability of these plants creates great potential for the development of traditional medicines as well as modern pharmaceutical drugs (Abd El-Ghani 2017; Sundararajan et al. 2021). Some scholars have argued that the availability of these biodiversity of plants is due to the tropical climate and strong ultraviolet of the tropical sunlight in the continent (Okafor 2013; Sawadogo et al. 2012). The conducive tropical ecosystem also provides numerous pathogenic microbes, including several species of bacteria, fungi, and viruses, suggesting that African plants could accumulate chemo-preventive substances more than plants from the northern hemisphere (Mutombo et al. 2023). On the other hand, Abegaz et al. (1999), and Sawadogo et al. (2012) contend that the African species, *Dorstenia mannii* Hook., a perennial herb growing in the tropical rain forest of Central Africa contained more biological activity than related species around the world (Mutombo et al. 2023). In addition, Nolna et al. (2020), argued that in the past five decades, there has been evident that there exists a plethora of plants with medicinal potential, and it is increasingly being accepted in the world (World Health Organization 2020). Therefore, it could be argued that African traditional medicinal plants might offer potential vibrant molecules in future modern drug discovery and manufacturing all over the world (Mutombo et al. 2023).

Mutombo et al. (2023) and Nolna et al. (2020) contend that African traditional medicine also includes a combination of beliefs, skills, diverse cultures, theories, and indigenous experiences. These knowledge are used not only to establish traditional medicines but also to diagnose, prevent, and treat physical and mental sicknesses. According to Ezekwesili-Ofili and Okaka (2019) and Sundararajan (2021), traditional medical practitioners are also very good psychotherapists, proficient in faith healing (spiritual healing), therapeutic occultism, circumcision of the male and female, tribal marks, treatment of snake bites, treatment of whitlow, removal of tuberculosis lymphadenitis in the neck, cutting the umbilical cord, piercing ear lobes, removal of the uvula, extracting a carious tooth, abdominal surgery, infections, midwifery, and so on.

The World Health Organization (2020) reported that 80% of the emerging world's population relies on traditional medicine for therapy. In some countries such as Ethiopia, Canada, Nigeria, Germany, and China, 70%–90% of the population have used herbal remedies for their primary healthcare (Ezekwesili-Ofili & Okaka 2019). Further, in Ghana, herbal medicine is often one of the alternative approaches to treat any sickness or disease noticed by citizens (Afolabi et al. 2020; Tuasha et al. 2018). Two West African countries, Ghana and Mali, have also established traditional medical directorates as alternative systems of healthcare for their citizens (Ezekwesili-Ofili & Okaka 2019; Sundararajan 2021). On the other hand, traditional medicine is reported to be used by people of all ages in Tanzania (Tambwe 2017). In the Republic of South Africa, it is reported that approximately 80% of the nation's population uses traditional medicine, which is derived from plants (Ezekwesili-Ofili & Okaka 2019; Street & Prinsloo 2013). In addition, it is reported that in Kenya, traditional medical practitioners are the only healthcare people available to treat citizens in some rural regions in the country (World Health Organization 2020). According to Abdul-Aziz et al. (2018), a common practice in countries such as Nigeria, Ghana, Zambia, and Mali, the first choice for approximately 60% of children suffering from high malarial fever is herbal medicines. Furthermore, in Nigeria, the major ethnic groups, for example, Fulani, Hausa, Igbo, and Yoruba have their different traditional health practitioners in addition to the modern medical doctors whom they can visit in the public or private hospitals in the country (Abd El-Ghani 2017; Ekeanyanwu 2011; Tuasha et al. 2023).

The popular use of traditional medicines all over the world and the discovery of vibrant medicine plants in the African continent has galvanized the World Health Organization to encourage its African member states to continue to promote the integration of traditional medicine practice in their current and modern health system (Ezekwesili-Ofili & Okaka 2019; Tuasha et al. 2023; World Health Organization 2020). In its 2020 report, the World Health Organization recognized the importance of traditional medicine as an alternative source of medication that has benefited the African people for many centuries. The World Health Organization has also been providing technical and financial resources in the areas of marketing authorization in 14 countries in the continent, as well as supporting 89 traditional medicine products that met national and international standards (Ezekwesili-Ofili & Okaka 2019; World Health Organization 2020). The most positive outcome is that 43 of the new traditional medicines have been included in the essential list of traditional medications approved for use and for sale to consumers (World Health Organization 2020). The World Health Organization has played a crucial role in encouraging African nations to provide evidence for the high quality, safety, and efficacy of traditional medicines (Abdullahi 2011; Mutombo et al. 2022).

Public Health Practice in Africa

The tropical characteristics of the SSA countries' climate make them vulnerable to the challenges of widespread malaria and widespread pandemics such as COVID-19 incidence (Sherrard-Smith et al. 2020). According to Gatzweiler and Zhu (2018) and Vearey et al. 2019), between 2015 and 2050, over half of the expected global population growth will be in Africa. In addition, it is anticipated that by the year 2050, nearly 60% of the population of the African continent could be expected to reside in urban areas due to employment in the public and private sectors (United Nations 2017). Furthermore, it is estimated that 35%–40% of children and adolescents could be living in Africa (Vearey et al. 2019; United Nations 2017).

In addition, the COVID-19 pandemic crisis has also galvanized countries in many Africa to seek better public health management solutions in addressing the widespread of the disease in order to curtail further transmission of COVID-19 (Massinga Loembé et al. 2020; Brand et al. 2020). The rapid global spread of the COVID-19 virus has augmented the world's vulnerability of citizens to new infectious diseases. In other for African countries to better address and curtail the spread of communicable diseases in the continent, there is an urgent need for the governments, private sector, and other foreign stakeholders to collaborate to adopt a comprehensive public health strategy agenda. The need for trained experts in public health to effectively implement the established policies is also very essential for the success of safety for all the citizens in SSA.

What is Special about each Chapter of this Book?

The book *Transforming Health Care in Africa: A Comparative Analysis* validates the multidimensional approaches to understanding health policies in many African countries. It asserts that health is a human right and a cornerstone for reinvigorating economies in African countries. It consistently argued that the state of citizens' health, and physical and mental well-being is what constitutes a pleasant, meaningful, and productive life. The book not only offers a window into future comparative study of healthcare policies in Africa's countries but seeks to leverage on the globalizing voices that promote or leverage on healthcare accomplishments and challenges.

Chapter 1 introduces the reader to key measures of healthcare delivery, and concepts. Health policy, as used in this book, includes actions that governments in African countries adopt to influence the provision and implementation of healthcare services delivery to all its citizens. It also provides a panoramic overview of health systems in Africa. Most textbooks about comparative health administration in Africa lack these details. Chapter 2 introduces readers to key health theories. It deploys a comprehensive strategy to fill the huge knowledge deficit for the proper understanding of policy inconsistencies, practice misapplications, and outright failure in many instances of healthcare policy. It also explores the basic mechanism of social justice and equity that are related to the provision of healthcare. Chapter 3 discusses the links between healthcare and development in Botswana. It uses data analysis to explain how the health of the citizens of the country tends to be improving even though environmental conditions in some parts of Botswana tend to be incredibly challenging to a large population of the nation.

Chapter 4 examines health policy and challenges in the People's Democratic Republic of Burkina Faso. The chapter also discusses the challenges of morbidity for children, maternal mortality for pregnant women, sanitation, and water challenges as well as shortage of health workers in Burkina Faso. It also explores the links between healthcare and development, health and education, equity, and poverty in Burkina Faso. Chapter 5 provides an analysis of the nature of health policies and the effectiveness of the healthcare delivery system in Cameroon. It also discusses how challenges such as inadequate funding, shortage of skilled healthcare professionals, disparities in healthcare access, and inadequate compensation of health professionals have negatively affected the healthcare delivery system in Cameroon. Chapter 5 also covers how the political conflict between English and French-speaking citizens of Cameroon has affected the healthcare delivery system in the country.

Chapter 6 examines the link between culture, religion, and healthcare in Egypt. It also investigates the nature and impacts of health policies and healthcare services' delivery equitably to all the citizens and residents of Egypt. The cause of disagreement is how can the Government of Egypt promote changes in healthcare behavior in the country. Chapter 7 examines the major health policy initiatives that the Federal Democratic Government of Ethiopia has formulated to improve the nation's healthcare system for all citizens in the country. It also explores some of the major health, and social challenges such as environmental issues, nutrition, communicable diseases, reproductive health, and child health, and unintentional injuries that the government is currently dealing with in the country.

Chapter 8 investigates how citizens' reaction to the ineffective health policies in Ghana has led to citizens in both the urban and rural communities moving from seeking modern medicine for their health treatment to using traditional medicine. These health challenges have also galvanized a preference for self-medication for treatment rather than going to hospitals to seek healthcare from qualified physicians. The aftermath of the National Health Insurance Scheme and the current outcomes of the policy's impact on the citizens and residents of Ghana are analyzed. The recent increased health spending in Ghana has led to an improvement in life expectancy. Chapter 9 explores how communicable diseases such as lower respiratory infection, diarrhea, and vaccine-preventable diseases have been controlled to a positive level in Kenya. The data analysis reveals that the value the Government of Kenya places on the health of its citizens is partially reflected in the proportion of available resources appropriated to the delivery of healthcare in the country.

Chapter 10 examines how cooperative healthcare action has been used to address the health delivery system in Mali. It also reviews how the impact of Malatia groups, conflicts, natural disasters, and other health emergencies has negatively impacted the role of health policy in Mali. The main goal of the chapter is to describe the effects of the current health policy and services as well as identify challenges associated with community-based health schemes in Mali. Chapter 11 explores how different actors in Nigeria work both individually and cooperatively to ensure effective health delivery in the country. It discusses the positive and negative benefits that citizens are deriving from the current healthcare system. It argues that the Nigerian government needs to adopt more pragmatic healthcare policies that could be effectively implemented.

Chapter 12 examines the nature of health policies in Rwanda and how the nation's government has been effective in improving mobility, and mortality rates over the past two decades. It also covers the mechanism that the Government of Rwanda has adopted to achieve effectively, formulated and implemented healthcare policies to accomplish the highest percentage of enrolment into the health insurance system in the African continent. Chapter 13 examines the health system in Sierra Leone. It discusses how the prevention of diseases, respect for the rights of the citizens of the country, and the commitment to developing public health efforts in conjunction with communities have not been effective in Sierra Leone. People living in poverty in the country are at a greater risk of death than their wealthier counterparts, largely because they lack access to public health initiatives like clean water, sanitation, food security, education, and economic opportunities.

Chapter 14 discusses the health policies and physical infrastructure of healthcare delivery in Somalia. It argues that the humanitarian crisis because of the civil war in Somalia for many decades has negatively affected the formulation of policies and effective implementation of the healthcare delivery system in the country. Further, apart from the civil wars in Somalia, the healthcare delivery system in the country is severely affected by inadequate medical products, funding technology in the healthcare delivery system, inadequate health workforce, and ineffective health delivery networks in rural communities. Chapter 15 discusses the nature of health policy and the challenges of healthcare delivery in South Africa. It provided a convincing argument that equitable, affordable, and high-quality health coverage cannot be accomplished in the future without solving the current healthcare disparities predicament in South Africa. Moreover, there are glaring differences even between urban and rural regions that are usually attributed to South Africa's apartheid-derived racial and socioeconomic inequalities.

Chapter 16 provides a description of the nature of health policy and implementation in Sudan. It analyzes the challenges of the healthcare delivery system in the country. It argues that despite the previously well-established healthcare system in the country, the challenges of several years of political instability have prevented Sudan's ability to effectively prevent the spread of communicable and noncommunicable diseases. Chapter 17 examines the nature of healthcare and the effectiveness of the health policies in Tanzania. It also seeks to explain the factors that led the nation's government to adopt various health strategic plans that could reach all households with essential health and social welfare services. It also discusses how many decades of foreign health professionals have driven health research in Tanzania without creating adequate local capacity in the country.

Chapter 18 provides a vivid discussion of the nature of healthcare policy and administration in Uganda. It also discusses the extent to which the government uses healthcare policy and other mechanisms to influence the private sector's decision-making and practices for the purpose of achieving a lesser burden of preventable diseases. It also discusses how government policies in Uganda have not been able to effectively address the disparity in healthcare delivery in both urban and rural regions of the nation. Chapter 19 examines how the nation of Zambia in East Africa has adopted health policies that are modeled along the national health vision of "equity of access, cost-effective, and affordable health services, which is close to the family is possible." It also discusses the notion that in politics in Zambia, financial managers, and medical professionals must be mindful that the healthcare in which the citizens of the country have invested their tax funds should be effectively managed to improve their health.

Chapter 20 investigates the nature of health policies and healthcare delivery as well as the challenges facing health policy implementation in Zimbabwe. This is because the nation's healthcare system and funding mechanism do not recognize the citizens' rights to affordable healthcare and other protected interests. It also discusses how the huge disparities in healthcare that exist in Zimbabwe constitute one of the immoral predicaments in the nation. Chapter 21 examines why African leaders, senior public administrators, and rich citizens prefer to seek their healthcare in England, France, Spain, Portugal, Canada, the United States, India, Singapore, and so on. It discusses how it is mind-boggling that millions of poor African people do not have access to basic public goods or social services such as good health system, elementary schools, sanitation, safely managed drinking water, and electricity, yet their presidents own majestic buildings and palaces in foreign countries and their home countries, respectively. Chapter 21 also discusses why African government leaders cannot comprehend the fact that the effectiveness of the healthcare system in the foreign countries that they go to seek treatment tends to function effectively because they were appropriately funded, maintained, and staffed with visionary health experts. It is, therefore, high time for the injustice in governance, which prevails in many African countries to stop.

Having traveled to more than 37 countries around the world, I can argue with great confidence that this book will help a large group of students, scholars, and practitioners learn about the nature of healthcare delivery and policy in the African continent. Readers are also likely to learn about how some African countries have established breakthrough accomplishments in medical science and technology, as well as successful in implementing vibrant health insurance schemes. Thus, incremental improvement in health delivery systems does not only happen in the richer countries, but it has also taken place in some African nations.

Conclusion

This chapter has examined the major problems of health policy challenges in many African countries. It explores the concept that a good health system should be people-centered at the individual and household levels. However, governments are expected to enact policies to enhance, knowledge, provide and share public goods, infrastructure, access to essential health services and promote strong community involvement to have the sustainable development goals for their respective countries in SSA. The chapter also discusses the nature and key components of a health system in African countries including health-related policies, knowledge, medicines, health facilities, health personnel, and delivery of health services within a framework of leadership, governance, stewardship, and community involvement.

It also presents the argument that while many African countries are making progress in their respective healthcare system, others are still struggling to meet the needs of all their citizens. It also argues that there is a need for many African countries to reinforce their healthcare collaborative governance initiatives with the private sector and nongovernmental organizations with a larger dialogue process. Strategically adopting such an all-stakeholders model could galvanize the health financial systems in many African countries as well as help the nations to get value for their collective investments. This social justice approach could also help many African countries to meet both their MDGs as well as sustainable development goals.

Africa today is lagging far behind in the delivery of quality and modern healthcare while North America, Europe, and Asia countries have the best healthcare systems in the entire world. These regions of the world are on the top of the ladder not because they have more resources than Africa but because of good governance, the role of law, ethical leaders, good innovation, less corruption, better performance management systems, and advanced technology. Therefore, a universal health system for all citizens, state-of-the-art hospitals, technology, highly qualified doctors and nurses, and innovation are the basic things that will push or propel and shape the healthcare system in Africa. In addition, prudent use of scarce resources and economic discipline as well as a transparent leadership style will be very critical for African countries to successfully overcome their current healthcare dilemmas.

References

Abegaz B. M., Bonaventure T., Ngadjui B. T., Bezabith M., and Mdee L. (1999). Novel natural products from marketed plants of eastern and southern Africa. *Pure Applied. Chemistry*, 71(6): 919–926.

Abd El-Ghani M. M. (2017) Traditional medicinal plants in Nigeria: An overview. *Agriculture and Biology Journal of North America*. 7(5): 220–247.

Abdullahi A. A. (2011). Trends and challenges of traditional medicine in Africa. *African Journal of Traditional, Complementary, and Alternative Medicines*, 8(5 Suppl): 115–123. DOI: 10.4313/ajtcam. v8i5S.5. Accessed February 27, 2024.

Adebayo A. (1969). *Nigerian Federal Finance; Its Development, Problems, and Prospects*. New York: Africana Pub. Corporation.

Adebayo B. (2020). Africa's leaders forced to confront healthcare systems they neglected for years. https://cdition.cnn.com/2020/04/10/africa/african-leaders-healthcare-coronavirusintl/ index.html. Accessed March 3, 2024.

Adjei M. (2018). *Poverty in Africa: Causes, Solution, and the Future*. Saarbrucken, Germany: LAP Lambert Academic Publishing.

Afolabi F J., De Beer P., Haafkens J. A (2020). Orthodox or traditional medicine? Private or public healthcare? Exploring treatment pathways for occupational health problems among informal automobile artisans, *Social Science & Medicine*, *265*, 113510, DOI: 10.1016/j. socscimed.2020.113510. Accessed August 20, 2024.

African Development Bank (2020). Annual Report and Financial Report. https://www.afdb. org/en/annual-report-and-financial-report-2020. Accessed August 19, 2024.

African Development Bank (2023). African Economic Outlook 2023. https://www.afdb.org/en/ knowledge/publications/african-economic-outlook. Accessed February 13, 2024.

AfricanGlobe (2012). Africa: Rich Presidents Poor Nations. https://www.africanglobe.net/ africa/africa-rich-presidents-poor-nations/. Accessed November 12, 2020.

Ake C. (1996). *Democracy and Development in Africa*. Washington DC: The Brookings Institutions.

Anna C. (2020). African elite who once sought treatment abroad are grounded. https://apnews. com/article/3fd908519a2a746f965150d8bf1f83ae. Accessed February 6, 2021.

Ansah E.W., Maneen S., Ephraim A. et al. (2024). Politics–evidence conflict in national health policy making in Africa: a scoping review. *Health Research Policy System*, 22 (1): 47–61.

Atake E. H. (2018). Health shocks in Sub-Saharan Africa: are the poor and uninsured households more vulnerable? *Health Economics Review.* 8, 26. DOI: 10.1186/s13561-018-0210-x.

Ayana ID, Demissie WM, Sore AG. (2023). Effect of government revenue on economic growth of sub-Saharan Africa: Does institutional quality matter? *PLoS One* 18(11): e0293847. DOI: 10.1371/journal.pone.0293847.

Ayittey G. (2005). *Africa Unchained: The Blueprint for Africa's Future.* New York: Palgrave Macmillan.

Aziz, M.A., Adnan, M., Khan, A.H. *et al.* (2018). Traditional uses of medicinal plants practiced by the indigenous communities at Mohmand Agency, FATA, Pakistan. *Journal of Ethnobiology and Ethnomedicine,* 14 (2). DOI:10.1186/s13002-017-0204-5.

Bain K. (2020). The challenge to prioritize infant mental health in South Africa. *South African Journal of Psychology.* 50(2):207–217. DOI: 10.1177/0081246319883582.

Bastos de Morais Jean Claude. 2017. "Digital technologies can deliver better healthcare to subSaharan Here's how." World Forum. www.weforum.org/agenda/2017/10/digital-paths-for-better-healthcare-in-sub-saharan-africa. Accessed August 16, 2024.

Besançon S, Sidibé A, Sow DS, Sy O, Ambard J, Yudkin JS, Beran D. (2022). The role of non-governmental organizations in strengthening healthcare systems in low- and middle-income countries: Lessons from Santé Diabète in Mali. *Global Health Action.* 15(1): 2061239. DOI: 10.1080/16549716.2022.2061239.

Brand S. P. C. et al. (2020). Forecasting the scale of the COVID-19 epidemic in Kenya. Preprint at *medRxiv* https://doi.org/10.1101/2020.07.03.20144949. Accessed February 13, 2024.

Brand G., Collins J., Bedi G., Bonnamy J., Barbour L., Ilangakoon C., Schwerdtle P. N. (2020). "I teach it because it is the biggest threat to health": Integrating sustainable healthcare into health professions education. *Medical Teacher,* 43(3): 325–333. DOI: 10.1080/0142159X.2020.1844876.

Cairncross S. and Valdmines V. (2006) Water supply, sanitation, and hygiene promotion. In Jamison D. T., Berman J. G., Measham A.R., et al. ed. *Disease Control Priorities in Developing Countries.* Second Edition. New York: Oxford University Press, p. 784.

Chenery H. B., Syrquin M. (1975). *Patterns of Development, 1957–1970.* London, England: Oxford University Press.

Clausen L. B (2015). Taking on the challenges of health care in Africa. https://www.gsb.stanford.edu/insights/taking-challenges-health-care-africa. Accessed January 27, 2021.

Coccia M. (2019). Theories of development. In Faramand A. (eds) *Global Encyclopedia of Public Administration, Public Policy, and Governance.* Springer, Cham. DOI: 10.1007/978-319-31816-5_9391-1. Accessed February 1, 2024.

Daley B. (2017). African politicians seeking medical help abroad is shameful, and harms health care. https://theconversation.com/african-politicians-seeking-medical-help-abroad-is-shameful-and-harms-health-care. Accessed October 30, 2020.

Dassah E, Aldersey H, McColl MA, Davison C. (2018). Factors affecting access to primary health care services for persons with disabilities in rural areas: a "best-fit" framework synthesis. *Glob Health Res Policy.* 25(3): 36. DOI: 10.1186/s41256-018-0091-x.

Di Muzio M., De Vito C., Tartaglini D., Paolo Villari P. (2017). Knowledge, behaviors, training and attitudes of nurses during preparation and administration of intravenous medications in intensive care units (ICU). A multicenter Italian study. *Applied Nursing Research,* 38(1): 129–133.

Dibie R. (2017). *Business and Government Relations in Africa.* New York: Routledge Press.

Dibie R. (2018). *Women's Empowerment for Sustainability in Africa.* New Castle Upon Tyne, United Kingdom: Cambridge Scholars Publishing.

Dibie R. (2022). Health policy and administration in Nigeria. *The Journal of African Policy Study,* 28(1): 101–139.

Dibie R., and Dibie J. (2017). "Analysis of the paralysis of government leadership in sub-Saharan Africa." *Africa's Public Service Delivery and Performance Review.* 5(1): 150–167.

Dibie R. and Quadri M. O. (2018). Analysis of effectiveness of e-government in the federal government of Nigeria. *Journal of Public Administration and Governance*. 8(3): 75–98.

Edoho F. M., and Dibie R. (2017). Global corporations: Corporate environmental accountability and the future of sustainability. *Global Journal of Science Frontier Research*. XVII (3): pp. 1–11.

Ekeanyanwu C. R. (2011). Traditional medicine in Nigeria: Current status and the future. *Research Journal of Pharmacology*. 5(6): 90–94.

Emenike C. P., Tenebe I. T., Omole D. O., Ngene B. U., Oniemayin B. I., Maxwell O., B. I., Onoka B. I. (2017). Accessing safe drinking water in sub-Saharan Africa: Issues and challenges in South–West Nigeria. *Journal of Sustainable Cities and Society*, 30(1): 263–272.

Esan D. T, Fasoro A. A, Odesanya O. E., Esan T. O., Ojo E. F., & Faeji C. O. (2018). Assessment of self-medication practices and its associated factors among undergraduates of a private university in Nigeria. *Journal of Environment and Public Health*. December 20:5439079. DOI: 10.1155/2018/5439079.

Ezekwesili-Ofili JO and Okaka ANC (2019). *Herbal Medicines in African Traditional Medicine*, Herbal Medicine, Philip F. Builders, IntechOpen. https://www.intechopen.com/books/herbal-medicine/herbal-medicines-in-african-traditional-medicine. Assessed August 20, 2024.

Federal Ministry of Health Nigeria (2021). Nigeria Malaria Indicator Survey. https://dhsprogram.com/pubs/pdf/MIS41/MIS41.pdf. Accessed October 29, 2024.

Ferrell O. C., Fraedrich J., Ferrell L. (2022). Business Ethics: Ethical Decision Making and Cases. 13th Edition. Boston, MA: Cengage Learning.

Friis, R. (2016). *Occupational Health and Safety in the 21st Century*. Burlington, MA: Jones & Bartlett Publishers.

Gatzweiler F, and Zhu Y-G. (2018). *Advancing Health and Wellbeing in the Changing Urban*. New York: Springer Press. http://www.springer.com/gp/book/9789811033636. Accessed April 11, 2021.

Gile P.P., van de Klundert J. & Buljac-Samardzic M. (2022). Human resource management in Ethiopian public hospitals. *BMC Health Service Research*. 22(1): 763–777. DOI: 10.1186/s12913-022-08046-7. Accessed February 9, 2024.

Giles-Vernick T. (2022). Postscript: A pandemic read on African health and environmental histories. *Health & Place*, 77 102846. https://pdf.sciencedirectassets.com/271845/1. Accessed August 18, 2022.

Haddiya, I., Janfi T. and Guedira.M. (2020). Application of the concepts of social responsibility, sustainability, and ethics to healthcare organizations. *Risk Management and Healthcare Policy*. 13, 1029–1033.

Handley SC, Nembhard IM. (2020). Measuring patient-centered care for specific populations: A necessity for improvement. *Patient Experience Journal*. 7(1): 10–12.

Harrison J. (2016). *Essentials of Strategic Planning in Healthcare*. Second Edition. Chicago, IL: Health Administration Press.

Haque M., Isalm T, Rahman A. A., Mckimm J. Abdullah A. and Dhingra S. (2020). Strengthening primary health care to help prevent and control long-term chronic non-communicable diseases in low and middle-income countries. *Risk Management and Healthcare Policy*. 13, 409–426.

Henderson, M., Ryan, T., & Phillips, M. (2019). The challenges of feedback in higher education. Assessment & Evaluation in Higher Education, 44(8), 1237–1252.

Holsinger J. (2018). *Leadership for Public Health: Theory and Practice*. Chicago, IL: Health Administration Press.

Hopkins WG, Marshall SW, Batterham AM, Hanin J. (2009). Progressive statistics for studies in sports medicine and exercise science. *Medical Science Sports Exercise*. 41(1): 3–13.

Hubbard G., and O'Brien A. P. (2021). *Essentials of Economics*, 5th edition. Hoboken, NJ: Pearson Learning.

Human Development Report (2020). https://www.un-ilibrary.org/content/books/9789210055161. Accessed July 2023.

Human Development Report 2021–22 (2022). Uncertain Times, Unsettled Lives: Shaping our Future in a Transforming World. https://hdr.undp.org/content/human-development-report-2021-22. Accessed November 6, 2024.

Industrial Development Report (2020). Industrializing in the digital age. https:// www.unido.org/ resources-publications-industrial-development-report-series/idr2020. Accessed November 6, 2024.

Infoplease (2020). March 2020 Current Events: US News. https://www.infoplease.com/march-2020-current-events-us-news. Accessed June 25, 2023.

Jacobs L, Skocpol T. (2016). *Health Care Reform and American Politics*. Oxford, United Kingdom: Oxford University Press.

Jimenez K, Kulnigg-Dabsch S, Gasche C. (2015). Management of iron deficiency anemia. *Gastroenterology Hepatology (N Y)*. (4): 241–50.

Kraft M and Furlong S. (2021). *Public Policy Analysis*. Washington D.C: Congressional Quarterly Press.

Kwame A., Petrucka P.M. (2024). Effective nursing leadership as a catalyst for person-centered care and positive nursing-patient interactions: evidence from a public Ghanaian hospital. *Discover Health Systems* 3 (50): DOI: 10.1007/s44250-024-00095-5.

Leigland J., Tremolet S., Ikeda J. (2016). *Achieving Universal Access to Water and Sanitation by 2030: The Role of Blended Finance*. Washington, D.C.: World Bank Publication.

Lidetu, H., Hoban, G., Lock-year, O., Belcher, A., Svanhström, V. J., & Darbyshire, I. (2024). Additions to and revisions of the endemic and near-endemic Acanthaceae of Ethiopia. Webbia. *Journal of Plant Taxonomy and Geography* 79(2): 201–225.

Lidetu T., Muluneh E. K., Wassie G. T. (2023). Incidence and predictors of aspiration pneumonia among stroke patients in Western Amhara Region, North-West Ethiopia: A retrospective follow up study. *International Journal of General Medicine* 16(1): 1303–1315.

Longest B. B. (2016). *Health Policymaking in the United States*. Chicago, IL: Health Administration.

Longest B. B. Jr., Darr K. (2014). *Managing Health Services Organization and Systems*. Sixth edition. Baltimore, MD: Health Professions Press.

Mankiw GN. (2014). *Principles of Economics*. Tenth Edition. Boston, MA: Cengage Learning.

Mansouri A. (2024). Healthcare predictions for Africa. https://www.iqvia.com/locations/middle-east-and-africa/blogs/2024/01/2024-healthcare-predictions-for-africa. Accessed August 18, 2024.

Map of Africa (2024). Map showing the Countries in Africa. https://www.google.com/search?client=fire fox-b--d&q=Map+of+ Africa#imgrc=l8cWicpoKmpgTM. Accessed January 25, 2024.

Marks K. L, Martel D. T, Wu C, Basura G. J, Roberts L. E, Schvartz-Leyzac K. C, Shore S. E. (2018). Auditory-somatosensory bimodal stimulation desynchronizes brain circuitry to reduce tinnitus in guinea pigs and humans. *Science Translational Medicine*. 10(422): eaal3175. DOI: 10.1126/scitranslmed.aal3175.

Massinga Loembé M, Tshangela A, Salyer SJ, Varma JK, Ouma AEO, Nkengasong JN. (2020). COVID-19 in Africa: the spread and response. *Nature Medicine.*, 26(7): 999–1003. DOI: 10.1038/s41591-020-0961-x.

Matchaba-Hove T. and Troskie T. (2019). Familily business owners' perception on seeking planning assistance. *International Journal of Economics and Finance Studies*, 11(2): 53–71.

Moyce S. C., Schenker M. (2018). Migrant workers and their occupational health and safety. *Annual Review of Public Health*, 39, 351–365. DOI: 10.1146/annurev-publhealth-040617-013714.

Muchuru, S., Nhamo, G. (2019). Sustaining African water resources under climate change: Emerging adaptation measures from UNFCCC national communications. *African Journal of Science, Technology, Innovation and Development*, 11(2), 181–196.

Mutombo P. N., Kasilo O. M. J., James P.B., Wardle J, Kunle O., Katerere D., Wambebe C., Matsabisa M. G., Rahmatullah M., Nikiema J. B., Mukankubito I., Sheridan R, Sanogo

Nissapatorn V., Sivakorn C., Tripathy S., Goyal R., Dhobi M. (2023). Experiences and challenges of African traditional medicine: Lessons from COVID-19 pandemic. *BMJ Global Health*. 8(8): e010813. DOI: 10.1136/bmjgh-2022-010813.

Mutombo CS, Bakari SA, Ntabaza VN, Nachtergael A, Lumbu JS, Duez P, Kahumba JB. (2022) Perceptions and use of traditional African medicine in Lubumbashi, Haut-Katanga province (DR Congo): A cross-sectional study. *PLoS One*. 2022;17(10): e0276325. DOI: 10.1371/journal.pone.0276325.

Nafziger E. W. (2005). Theories of economic development. In *Economic Development*. Fourth Edition. New York: Cambridge University Press, 123–164.

Nkalu, C. N., & Agu, C. C. (2023). Fiscal Policy and Economic Stabilization Dynamics in Sub-Saharan Africa: A New Evidence from Panel VEC Model and Hodrick-Prescott Filter Cyclical Decomposition. *Sage Open*, 13(2). DOI:10.1177/21582440231178261.

Nolna S. K., Nton R., Mbarga N. F., Mbainda S. (2020). Integration of traditional healers in human African trypanosomiasis case finding in central Africa: A quasi-experimental study. *Tropical Medical Infect Diseases*. 5: 172–187.

Obuh J., Onobun M. Eluwa 0., Azama A. A., Aguele 0. 0. (2020). Medical tourism in Nigeria. *Developing Country Studies*. 10(8): 1–8.

OECD (2023). Africa's development dynamics 2023: investing in sustainable development. https://www.oecd.org/en/publications/africa-s-development-dynamics-2023_3269532b-en.html. Accessed August 18, 2024.

Okafor JC. (2013). *Tropical Plants in Healthcare Delivery in Nigeria: A Guide in the Treatment of Common Ailments and Conditions*. Ibadan, Nigeria: Book Builders Publishers; 2013.

Rajabi M, Ebrahimi P, Aryankhesal A. (2021). Collaboration between the government and nongovernmental organizations in providing health-care services: A systematic review of challenges. *J Educ Health Promotion*. 10: 242. DOI: 10.4103/jehp.jehp_1312_20.

Ratchinsky K. (2016). Cloud today and tomorrow: Why hospitals are tripling the use of cloud services. https://www.healthcareitnews.com/blog/cloud-today-and-tomorrow-why-hospitals-are-tripling-use-cloud-services. Accessed November 7, 2024.

Sama, I.E., et al. (2020), Circulating plasma concentrations of angiotensin-converting enzyme 2 in men and women with heart failure and effects of renin–angiotensin–aldosterone inhibitors. *European Heart Journal*, 41(19): 1810–1817.

Sawadogo B, Gitta SN, Rutebemberwa E, Sawadogo M, Meda N. (2012). Knowledge and beliefs on cervical cancer and practices on cervical cancer screening among women aged 20 to 50 years in Ouagadougou, Burkina Faso, 2012: a cross-sectional study. *Pan African Medical Journal*.;18: 175. DOI: 10.11604/pamj.2014.18.175.3866.

Sherrard-Smith E., Hogan A.B., Hamlet A. Churcher T. S. (2020). The potential public health consequences of COVID-19 on malaria in Africa. *Natural Medicine Journal* 26, 1411–1416.

Shi L. (2019). *Introduction to Health Policy*, Second Edition (Gateway to Healthcare Management). Chicago, IL: Health Administration Press.

Slavin S. (2020). *Microeconomics*. Twelfth Edition. New York: McGraw-Hill.

Skolnik R. (2008). *Essentials of Global Health*. Sudbury, MA: Jones and Bartlett Publishers.

Standford Medicine. (2020). The rise of the data-driven physician. https://med.stanford.edu/content/dam/sm/school/documents/Health-Trends-Report/Stanford%20Medicine%20Health%20Trends%20Report%202020.pdf. Accessed August 17, 2024.

Sundararajan R., Ponticiello M., Lee M. H., Strathdee S. A., Muyindike W., Nansera D., King, R., Fitzgerald D., Mwanga-Amumpaire J. (2021). Traditional healer-delivered point-of-care HIV testing versus referral to clinical facilities for adults of unknown serostatus in rural Uganda: a mixed-methods, cluster-randomised trial. *Lancet Global Health*, 9: e1579–88. https://www.thelancet.com/action/showPdf?pii=S2214-109X%2821%2900366-1. Accessed August 20, 2024.

Street R A., and Prinsloo G. (2013). Commercially important medicinal plants of South Africa: A review. *Journal of Chemistry*. 205048. DOI: 10.1155/2013/205048.

Tambwe M (2017). Tanzania: Traditional medicine has place in health. *Tanzania Daily News* (Dar-es Salaam). https://allafrica.com/stories/201211040038.html. Accessed November 4, 2020.

Tseane-Gumbi L.A., Ojakorotu V. (2022). Medical tourism and African healthcare system: behavioral analysis of the role of Africa leaders. *Gender and Behavior.* 1 (3): 1–9.

Tuasha N., Fekadu S. & Deyno S. (2023). Prevalence of herbal and traditional medicine in Ethiopia: A systematic review and meta-analysis of 20-year studies. *System Review.* 12, 232–243. DOI: 10.1186/s13643-023-02398-9. Accessed February 9, 2024.

Tuasha N., Petros B. & Asfaw Z. (2018). Medicinal plants used by traditional healers to treat malignancies and other human ailments in Dalle District, Sidama Zone, Ethiopia. *Journal Ethnobiology Ethnomedicine.* 14, 15 DOI: 10.1186/s13002-018-0213-z. Accessed August 19, 2024.

United Nations. (2017). World population prospects: the 2017 revision, key findings, and advance tables. Working paper no. ESA/P/WP/248. [internet]. New York: United Nations, Department of Economic and Social Affairs, Population Division. https://esa.un.org/unpd/wpp/Publications/Files/WPP2017. Accessed April 11, 2023.

United Nations Development Programme (2020). UNDP Annual Report 2020. https://www.undp.org/publications/undp-annual-report-2020. Accessed July 23, 2024.

United States International Development (USAID). (2020). Power Africa Annual Report (English). https://www.usaid.gov/powerafrica/document/power-africa-2020-annual-report-english. Accessed May 18, 2023.

Vearey J., Luginaah I., Magitta N. F., Shilla D. J., Oni T. (2019a). Urban health in Africa: A critical global public health priority. *BMC Public Health.* 19(1): 340–350.

Vearey J., Orcutt M., Gostin L., Braham C A., Duigan P. (2019b). Building alliances for the global governance of migration and health. *BMJ* ; 366: 14143 DOI: 10.1136/bmj.l4143. https://www.bmj.com/content/366/bmj.l4143. Accessed August 20, 2024.

Wilensky S. E., Teitelbaum J. B. (2023). *Essentials of Health Policy and Law,* Fifth edition. Burlington, MA: Jones & Bartlett Learning.

World Alas (2020). World Map. https://www.worldatlas.com/aatlas/world.htm. Accessed August 17, 2024.

World Bank. (2020). Access to safe water. http//www.worldbank.org/depweb/English/modules/environ/water/. Accessed May 3, 2020.

World Economic Forum (2014). Global Competitiveness Report 2014–2015. https://www.weforum.org/publications/global-competitiveness-report-2014-2015/. Accessed November 7, 2024.

World Economic Forum (2023). Building resilient healthcare systems in Africa with a focus on outbreaks and epidemics. https://www.weforum.org/agenda/2023/07/building-resilient-healthcare-systems-in-africa-with-a-focus-on-outbreaks-and-epidemics/. Accessed August 19, 2024.

World Health Organization. (2008). *Health Financing Mechanisms: Private Health Insurance.* Geneva: World Health Organization.

World Health Organization. (2014). WHO African Region Expenditure Atlas. https://www.afro.who.int/sites/default/files/2017-06/who-african-region-expenditure-atlas_-november-2014.pdf. Accessed January 29, 2024.

World Health Organization. (2020a). Types of sanitation. https://www.Publichealth.com.ng/the-7-types-of-sanitation/. Accessed April 28, 2023.

World Health Organization (WHO). (2020b). WHO supports scientifically proven traditional medicine. https://www.afro.who.int/news/who-supports-scientifically-proven-traditional-medicine. Accessed February 25, 2024.

World Health Organization. (2021). Universal health coverage (UHC). https://www.who.int/en/newsroom/factsheets/detail/universal-health-coverage-(uhc). Accessed April 19, 2023.

World Health Organization (2023). Ending disease in Africa: vision, strategies and special initiatives, 2023-2030. https://www.afro.who.int/sites/default/files/2023-09/Ending%20disease%20in%20Africa_ENDISA_ENG_0.pdf. Accessed August 17, 2024.

Yamey G, Ogbuoji O., Nonvignon J. (2019) Middle-income countries graduating from health aid: Transforming daunting challenges into smooth transitions. *PLoS Med* 16(6): e1002837. DOI: 10.1371/journal.pmed.1002837.

Yassi A., Kjellstrom T., de Kok T., Guidotti T. L. (2001). Water and sanitation. In *Basic Environmental Health*. New York: Oxford University Press.

Chapter Two

THEORIES OF HEALTHCARE SYSTEMS

Robert Dibie

Introduction

There are many theories that are related to health policies and healthcare service delivery. Many factors often affect a particular healthcare policy initiative that may have little to do with the merit or validity of any enacted health policy. Therefore, theories could help readers and scholars to better understand, the environmental conditions, and events that may escape the detailed explanation and impacts (McGain et al. 2020; Birkland 2016). According to Anderson (2011) and Kraft and Furlong (2024), theories could illustrate vital correlations between important variables as well as explain the significant effects of government actions that often affect the day-to-day lives of all citizens in a country.

Government, private sector, and nongovernmental organizations (NGOs) are essential components of healthcare delivery systems in many African countries. This is because healthcare is very significant in the African continent, and everybody needs it in other to live a better life with less painful stress and injuries. According to Patel and Rushefsky (2015) and Patashnik et al. (2020), the government and the private sectors in many countries around the world provide healthcare to the citizens. Healthcare could be related to preventing disease, illness, or injury, and treating people who are sick (Kraft and Furlong 2024; Grad 2002). Governments of various African countries engage in many activities to influence public and private institutions in making the right decisions in the management and regulation of healthcare systems for all citizens (Janati et al. 2018; Johnson & Stoskopf 2010). Governments also decide how to help their citizens get access to healthcare and other human needs such as water supply, sanitation, and waste remover (Kraft and Furlong (2024). Without these services, the health of human beings will be deplorable in modern societies. Although medicine plays a major part in healthcare-related models, there are other services such as the Food and Drug Administration, the Center for Disease Control and Prevention, and the National Institute of Health in any nation that is critical for facilitating a better health system (Luciano et al. 2019). In addition, all public healthcare delivery services and the production or importation of medicines are regulated and funded by the government. The private companies could also own and operate health facilities, as well as engage in the production or importation of medicines, however, they must obtain a license from the government, as well as comply with health policies that are enacted by the government

(Janati et al. 2018). Without a good source of medicine and medical equipment, doctors, nurses, and nations around the world including African countries will not be able to provide healthcare for their sick citizens (Dibie 2022).

The constitution of the World Health Organization (WHO) stipulates that "the enjoyment of the highest attainable standard of health is one of the fundamental rights of every human being without distinction of race, religion, political belief, economic or social condition" (World Health Organization 2021). Therefore, the right to health or life, liberty, and the pursuit of happiness should not be granted or denied by any African government because they are fundamental, inalienable human rights which all human beings already have (World Health Organization 2021). These human and health rights' principles are sometimes missing or not adequately upheld in many African countries (Oleribe et al. 2020). This is because access to the highest standard of healthcare is not effectively delivered to all citizens respective of their economic status. The disparities in healthcare delivery due to the location of health facilities and affordability for treatment by low-income people living in rural and some urban locations in many African countries have been a major challenge. Furthermore, some scholars contend that the provision of good healthcare to all citizens is a major mechanism for the attainment of peace and security (Gatwiri et al. 2020; World Health Organization 2021).

This chapter examines some theories that explain the processes of how the government of a nation could initiate public policy laws to address health problems. In most cases, government policies on healthcare could include the passage of laws or may entail an executive order such as directing a government agency to implement or enforce the healthcare policies. The theories and concepts in this chapter constitute the instrument for understanding the fundamentals of the practice of medical treatment and the regulation of health. Rather than discussing all public policy theories, this chapter focuses on the most common theories and healthcare models to explain the often-convoluted process that could help readers understand what it takes to deliver good healthcare services and appropriate prevention or precautionary measures in any country. The final section provides an assessment of whether or not health policy theories and concepts help readers or citizens comprehend the dynamics of what it takes to have a better healthcare system in Sub-Saharan countries.

Theories of Healthcare

Evidence-Based Practice

Evidence-based practice (EBP) is a clinical problem-solving approach, involving the collecting and analysis of data, processing the best evidence from well-designed research, and patients' values, and implementing research findings to improve clinical practice and positive patient outcomes (Chrisman et al. 2014; Porter-O'Grady and Malloch 2015). Preffer and Sutton (2006) argued that EBP holds a higher standard in the provision of patients' healthcare. EBP is also defined as a client-centered, question-in-context-driven process of information-seeking, collaboration, and critical reasoning to facilitate defensible healthcare decisions (Bannigan & Moores 2009; Dawes et al.

2005; Hoffmann et al. 2017). This scientific model allows physicians and nurses to critically analyze the research data, approved guidelines, patients, values, and other available resources in order to adopt the most high-quality intervention approach to provide patients with healthcare (Hoffmann et al. 2017).

On the other hand, evidence-based management is defined as the commitment to identifying and utilizing the best theories, scientific evidence, and data available to make decisions. It also involves the commitment to fact-based decision-making, which means being determined to be getting the best evidence and using it to guide actions (Griffin et al. 2017). Unfortunately, sometimes it takes several medical clinics and hospitals many years to adopt a practice or treatment after the first systematic evidence shows it helps patients (Luciano et al. 2019). This is because hospital leaders have to balance two conflicting needs such as (1) adhere to standards and (2) customize for the local context.

According to Karnick (2016) and Luciano et al. (2019), there are four approaches that healthcare leaders could adopt in order to effectively maintain a close relationship to fundamental evidence and standard operating procedures. The four approaches are (1) maintain a health organizations' principles; (2) engage in data-driven decisions; (3) have good physical and human resources and goals; and (4) have preferences (Luciano et al. 2019). Wilson and Austria (2019) contend that evidence-based clinical practice should include the following processes (1) ask questions; (2) acquire the current evidence; (3) review the literature; (4) apply your findings to clinical decision-making; (5) evaluate your outcomes; and (6) disseminate the information. While each of these approaches may have its own opportunities and problems, it is necessary to understand the local context and the people involved in it (Janati et al. 2018). Figure 1 illustrates how to apply EBP in a clinical health environment.

Figure 1 shows the six processes of EBP in clinical healthcare. In order to accomplish a better health outcome medical practitioners or providers will have to (1) ask questions; (2) acquire the current evidence; (3) review the literature; (4) apply your findings to clinical decision-making; (5) evaluate your outcomes; and (6) disseminate the information (Hoffmann et al. 2017; Janati et al. 2018). It should be noted that EBP enables health providers to abandon outdated care delivery practices and choosing effective, scientifically validating new methods to meet individual patient needs (Wilson & Austria 2019). One of the main emphases of this approach is the focus on using evidence from successful clinical trials and other research studies in order to care for patients.

In addition, hospitals exploring EBP must also consider any legal or professional guidelines that may restrict options. Karnick (2016) and Stevens (2013) contend that the move and adoption of standardization and best practices reduce rather than create risks because such new initiatives often replace idiosyncratic or outdated practices and preferences that could be an impediment to outstanding healthcare treatment to patients.

According to Nevo and Slonim-Nevo (2011) and Karnick (2016), the main goal of the evidence-based medicine approach is to provide healthcare for patients by applying the best available evidence from scientific methods that have been successfully used to make

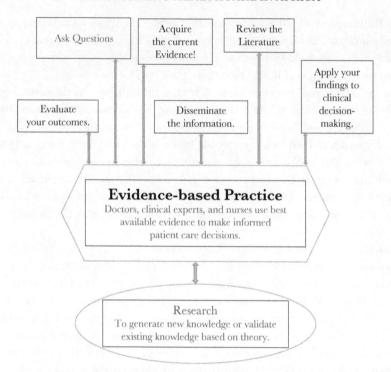

Figure 1: How to Apply EBP in Clinical Health Designed by Dibie R. 2023.

clinical decisions that could lead to positive treatment or outcomes for all sick patents. Thus, EBP holds great promise for moving healthcare to a high level of likelihood of producing the intended health outcome. Almost all of the evidence utilized by doctors, nurses, public health experts, and health administrators originates from research. It should be noted however that EBP expands beyond research because clinicians and doctors who are experts and other healthcare practitioners and their respective patients are also involved in the processes, as shown in Figure 2.

Furthermore, the American Nurses Association (ANA) stipulates that nursing interventions should be practical, methodical decisions based on EBP. Therefore, the utilization of an EBP approach to nursing practice could galvanize very high-quality and cost-efficient patient care in all ramifications (Luciano et al. 2019).

Hospitals that use an evidence-based approach can improve their management effectiveness. This is because an evidence-based hospital doctor is a person who uses all evidence sources in a six-step decision-making process illustrated in Figure 2. It should be noted that the goal of EBP is not about developing a new approach (Janati et al. 2018; Luciano et al. 2019). Its main purpose is to verify and utilize existing knowledge and apply it to clinical practice and decision making in order to achieve positive outcomes for patients.

Apart from the doctors and other clinical experts working in the hospitals, nurses also benefit from using evidence-based nursing. This is because their success in treating their respective patients depends on research and evidence. The bone of contention is that with due diligence to teamwork and the application of EBPs, they could ensure that patients can receive high-quality and cost-effective care. The advantage of adopting EBP in the education curriculum of nurses and doctors in order to better care for patients as well as save lives. An additional benefit is that doctors and nurses who practice evidence-based medicine could also become familiar with clinical trials, research, and writing academic journals and papers in the fields of medicine and nursing (Hanberg 2006; Hoffmann et al. 2017; Stevens 2013; Troseth 2016; Wilson & Austria 2019). There is therefore no doubt that the integration of EBP into the clinical curriculum could positively galvanize successful medical training and practice outcomes in all African countries in the future. It should be noted however that on one hand, practice based on evidence seeks consistency and standardization. On the other hand, innovation is about creating new and different processes and products (Porter-O'Grady & Malloch 2015). Thus, whenever a patient is confronted with difficulties in responding to recommended treatments the doctor or nurse in charge may need to explore other ideas and issues to discover innovative solutions. The bone of contention about EBP is to avoid decisions on untested but strongly held beliefs, what you have done in the past, or uncritical benchmarking of what winners do (Griffin et al. 2017; Hoffmann et al. 2017; Prefer & Sutton 2006).

Resource Dependency Theory

The resource dependency theory was propounded by Pfeffer and Salanciks (1978). Pfeffer and Salanciks (1978) contended that firms that depend on the environment can and do explore multiple strategies to combat these contingencies to become successful. Resource dependence theory (RDT) in healthcare stipulates how the external resources of organizations could affect the behavior of the organization (Davis &. Cobb 2010; Pfeffer and Salanciks 1978).

The theory is also a healthcare-related model because it is needed for survival. RDT proposes that actors lacking in essential resources will seek to establish relationships with other organizations or be dependent on other institutions in order to obtain needed resources to accomplish their strategic goals (Ozcan & Eisenhardt 2009). Thus, theory analyzes how the external resources of organizations affect the behavior of the institution. As a result, the ability of a health company to procure external resources is an important tenet of both its strategic and tactical management of success.

As a result of the nature of this dependency perspective, organizations are viewed as coalitions alerting their structure and patterns of behavior to acquire and maintain needed external resources (Malatesta & Smith 2014). Davis and Cobb (2010), Drees and Heugens (2013), Lomi and Pattison (2006), and Sharif and Yeoh (2014)contend that RDT is a mechanism that has helped to propel NGOs or nonprofit organizations to be more commercialized in recent times in many developed and developing countries. Because of fewer government grants and resources being used for public and social services, competition for contracts between the private and nonprofit sectors has compelled nonprofit organizations to use customer service management techniques to compete for resources to maintain their organization's livelihood (Dibie 2018; Ozcan & Eisenhardt 2009).

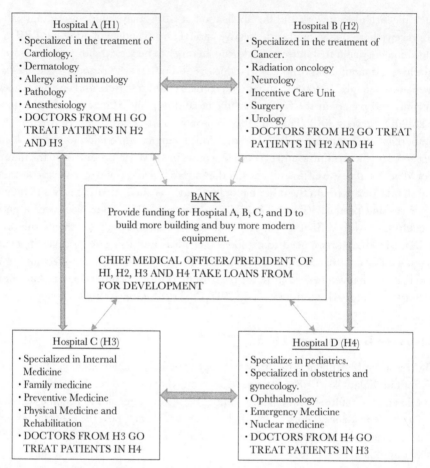

Figure 2: A Model of Four Hospitals and a Bank that Depend on Resources of each other. Designed by Dibie R. (2024).

Resource dependency and institutional theories are the principles of modern management theories that are mostly applied to healthcare and other organizations. This theory is based mainly on organized behavior among the environments. According to Celtekligil (2020) and Malatesta and Smith (2014), acquiring the external resources needed by an organization comes by decreasing the organization's dependence on others and/or by increasing other's dependency on it, that is, modifying an organization's power with other organizations. It should be noted however that the RDT does not just refer to the dependency on resources like employees, capital, and raw materials (Celtekligil 2020). The theory attempts to encourage managers and administrators in the healthcare system of any country to understand that their success could link to strategic customer service management to stimulate positive consumer demand for their goods and services (Janse 2020). Figure 2 shows how four hospitals and a bank could lead to greater success.

Figure 2 illustrates RDT and how the four hospitals and a bank— (five organizations) depend on each other in order to be successful. The resources that each of the five organizations needs ultimately originate from an organization's environment. In addition, the environment (state or nation), to a considerable extent, contains other organizations. Dependence makes it possible in such a way that the resources that one organization needs are thus often in the hands of other organizations. Apart from the fact that resources are a basis of power, legally independent organizations can therefore depend on each other in order to be successful. Therefore, the bank has to give loans to Hospitals 1, 2, 3, and 4 in order to make a profit. Doctors in hospitals 1, 2, 3, and 4 have to cross the border to treat patients in hospitals in their region due to their areas of specialty. In the end, their dependency and relationship are to maximize their humanitarian and profit-making goals. In addition, the theory is important for the health system management of African countries because it discusses how public and private sector organizations are able to collaborate to seek resources, which could enable them to be very successful (Malatesta & Smith 2014).

Multiple Streams Framework

Multiple streams framework is used to explain the interrelationship between public officials (politicians) and the general public that they are supposed to be representing in a democratic country. However, constraints of information, time, and cost often prevent policymakers from analyzing all alternatives and before selecting the best alternative solutions to the general public problems (Dye 2013). According to Rinfret et al. (2023), the multiple streams framework attempts to explain the convoluted nature of the policy-making process. It contends that public policies are not often made in a neat and systemic order. The multiple streams framework could be regarded as a theory in its own right. It illustrates the three different policy streams (1) problem stream, (2) policy stream, and (3) politics stream that are crucial in the policy window that could enhance the policymaking process. Figure 3 shows the relationship between the three streams and the policy window as well as how the streams affect the policy-making process.

According to Rinfret et al. (2023) and John Kingdom (2010), the problem stream tends to identify all sorts of public challenges, problems, and issues facing citizens and residents of a democratic country. It also helps the media and major policy actors to be familiar with the problems facing the citizens (Dye 2013; Peters 2009). Furthermore, the policy stream comprises a mixture of ideas and solutions that compete to get the attention and acceptance of policymakers for use as a tool for solving an identified

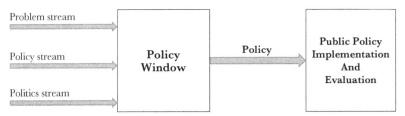

Figure 3: Multiple Streams Framework.
Source: Designed by Dibie R. (2024).

public problem. On the other hand, the political stream deals with all the political aspects and approaches that could be adopted for policymaking. It should be noted that if only two streams come together, it will be very difficult for policymaking to take place (Rinfret et al. 2023). Thus, all three streams must come together for the health policy window to occur. Further, issue network or health policy subsystem are terms sometimes used to describe the network of health policy actors that are collaborating to accomplish set policy goals (Kraft and Furlong 2024).

Dynamics of Public Policy Theories

Public policy is what public officials within the government, and the extent the citizens they represent, choose to do or not to do about public problems (Dye 2013; Kraft & Furlong 2024). Rinfret et al. (2023) contend that public policy is a course of action adopted or created by the government in response to public problems. Public problems refer to conditions that the public widely perceives to be unacceptable and therefore require intervention (Kraft & Furlong 2024; Peters 2018). Problems such as economic development, economic recession, slow small business development, lack of entrepreneurship, environmental degradation, insufficient access to healthcare, consumer safety, energy generation crisis, low agricultural harvest, bad roads, and so on are resolved with public policies (Dibie 2022). According to Pennock (2018), Chrisinger (2017), and Anderson (2011), these public problems can be addressed through government action, private action, or where individuals or corporations take responsibility or a combination of the two (Kraft & Furlong 2024). In a given case, the choice depends on how the public defines the problem and the prevailing societal attitudes about private action in relation to the government's role in solving the problem. A response to a public problem could entail the enactment of public policy or laws or may involve an executive, such as the president, or a legislative action or a governor directing a government agency or ministry to do something to address the problem. Figure 4 shows the public policy-making process in a democratic country.

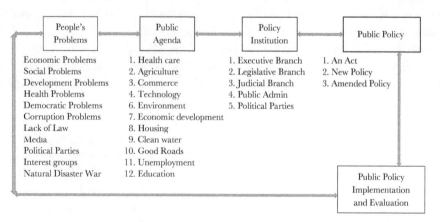

Figure 4: Public Policy Making Process.
Source: Designed by Dibie R. (2024).

According to Thomas Dye (2013), Thomas Dye (2013), Thomas Birkland (2016), and Deborah Stone (2012), exploring the methods of enacting health policy and social welfare policies in many developed democratic countries reveals that there are many theories that could be used to explain how public policies are adopted and implemented. It should be noted that the values that are adopted when we think about public policymaking individually or collectively, have not only shaped the laws that have been enacted but also shaped the policy solutions. For instance, the public choice theory assumes that individuals and organizations seek to maximize their own benefits in politics. The theory also applies economic analysis to the study of public policy (Dye 2013). The public choice theory postulates that all voters, politicians, taxpayers legislators, interest groups, political party members, public administrators, and citizens often seek to maximize their personal benefits in politics as well as in the marketplace at any time (Anderson 2011). In addition, public choice theory scholars underscore the importance of efficiency and tend to support the contracting out and privatization of services' policies of the government (Holzer & Schwester 2016). The game theory presents an argument that rational decision makers are involved in choices that are interdependent. The theory suggests that layers of the game of policymaking must adjust their conduct to reflect not only their own desires and abilities but also their expectations about what other political players might do or exploit (Holzer & Schwester 2016; Lindblom 1979). It should be noted that a player in the game's theory may be a national government, group, political party, individual, nonprofit organization, or NGO, or any citizen's advocate who is capable of taking rational actions that could benefit the general public of a nation.

Another very important theory in the public policy process is the elite theory. The elite theory argues that public policies are not determined by the demands and actions of the people or the masses but rather by the ruling elite whose preferences are carried into effect by public officials or public administrators, government ministries, and agencies' staff (Anderson 2011; Holzer & Schwester 2016). Thus, the theory argues that people are apathetic and ill-informed about public policy. Because people are not well informed about public policy issues, it is the well-informed elites who actually shape mass opinion on policy issues, questions, and solutions more than the general public. This is the reason why public policies are likely to be the preferences of elites rather than the common citizens.

Health Psychology Theories

Health psychology, often referred to as behavioral medicine or medical psychology, is the application of psychological theory to health-related practices (Billington 1933; Ogden 2012). According to Dahlgren and Whitehead (1991), the field of health psychology includes two subfields. Behavioral health focuses on prevention of health problems and illnesses, while behavioral medicine focuses on treatment. In addition, health psychology is concerned with the psychology of a range of health-related behaviors, including nutrition, exercise, healthcare utilization, and medical decision-making. Health psychology also addresses individual and population-level issues across four domains: clinical, public, community, and critical social justice issues (Murray 2008).

Research reveals that the discipline of health psychology developed from the growing recognition of the contribution of psychological processes to health and illness (Sarafino 2002). Further, the theory of health psychology can be practiced in three very important ways: (a) health psychologist try to study treatment and preventive strategies of illness; (b) health psychologist could also encourage or promote healthy behavior through proper maintenance; and (c) health psychologists also attempt to focus on the etiology and corelates of health illness, and dysfunction (Brannon et al. 2014; Sarafino 2002). Some scholars have also contended that interventions during any patient's sickness could also prevent it from escalating to a more serious situation (Skolnik 2008; Johnson & Stoskopf 2010). Therefore, taking precautionary measures could save the life of any sick person. The goal of the health psychology theory is to create an awareness that the impact of a wide range of biological, psychological, and social factors on wellness and chronic illness could be properly treated if the right approach is adopted on time. Braun et al. (2012) and DeStasio et al. (2019) argued that the important features, which are often more broadly considered as the wider determinants of health challenges could galvanize advancement in the field of generic research or the main circumstances that led to any major sickness (Ogden 2012; Sarafino 2002).

It is often typical, to realize that lifestyle, psychological factors, and social factors constitute the causes of heart diseases that could lead to the death of any person (Mason et al. 2015; Norcross 2005). Therefore, it could be argued that health psychology measurement could be taken by specialists to understand patient's behavior and the appropriate psychological processes in health, illness, and healthcare delivery cause or change. Further, health psychology focuses on understanding how people react to, cope with, and recover from sickness. Basically, illnesses that are associated with psychological and behavioral issues include birth defects, stroke, heart disease, COVID-19, infant mortality, HIV/AIDS, cancer, infectious diseases, and many more (Mason et al. 2015; DeStasio et al. 2019). Figure 5 shows the relationship between health and psychological, sociological, and biological courses of illness.

In the past two decades, the new approach to health psychology has been called the biosocial model. The biosocial model views that illness and healthcare are caused by a combination of biological psychology and social factors (Engel 1977; Noar & Ziammerman 2005). According to Mason et al. (2015), psychological, social, and cultural factors could exacerbate a biological predisposition by putting a genetically

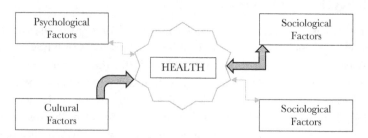

Figure 5: Relationship between Health and Psychological, Sociological, and Biological Causes of Illness. Designed by Dibie R. (2024).

vulnerable person at risk for other behaviors, such as social pressure. Thus, the culture of an environment could incrementally alter an individual's genetic makeup attributes, or lifestyle. Finally, it should be noted that the behavior of patients in adhering to medical recommendations has long been recognized and methods of assessing adherence have been debated and developed, but the role of health professionals in determining patient outcomes has been less adequately assessed (Marteau & Johnston 1986).

Conclusion

This chapter attempts to provide the theories and concepts that are needed to explain health policy issues in nations in the African continent. It explores evidence of how complex the enactments and implementation of health policy could be in developing countries such as those in the African continent. It should be noted that theories could help readers and students to better understand phenomena, conditions, and events that seem to escape explanation or the imagination of what really takes place in the health system of any country. For readers and students to better understand the intricacies of the process, the chapter discusses some models of the policy-making process as well as the theories that could medical doctors, nurses, and other practitioners in the profession to better perform their duties effectively to patients under their care. Therefore, since health policy can and does have very important effects on the lives of every human being, it is paramount that we need theories to help us better understand the dynamics of our economic, social, and political environment that help shape our health system. This chapter also provides a detailed discussion of the complexities of health policies and the official and unofficial actors that are involved in the process of delivering healthcare. The rules of these domestic and foreign official and unofficial healthcare officials and organizations are explained in all the chapters of this book.

References

Anderson E. (2011). *Public Policy Making*. Seventh Edition. Boston, MA: Cengage Learning.

Bannigan K., Moores A. (2009). A model of professional thinking: Integrating reflective practice and evidence-based practice. *Canadian Journal of Occupational Therapy*, 76(5), 342–350.

Baum A., Revenson T. A., Singer J. E. (2012). *Handbook of Health Psychology*. Second Edition. New York: Psychology Press.

Billington C. M. (1933). Mind and body. *British Medical Journal*, 1, 1026.

Baum S. J. (2012). Evidence-based medicine: what's the evidence? *Clinical Cardiology*, 35(5): 259–260.

Birkland T. A. (2016). *An Introduction to the Policy Making Process: Theories, Concepts, and Models of Public Policy Making*. Fourth Edition. New York: Routledge Press.

Brannon L., Updegraff J. A., Feist J. (2014). *Health Psychology: An Introduction to Behavior and Health*. Cengage Learning.

Braun, K. L., Kagawa Singer, M., Holden, A. R., Burhansstipanov, L., Tran, J. H., Seals, B., Corbie-Smith, G., Tsark, J. U., Harjo, L., Foo, M. A., Ramirez, A. (2012). Lay navigator tasks across the cancer care continuum. *Journal of Health Care for the Poor and Underserved*, 23(1), 398–413.

Celtekligil, K. (2020). Resource dependence theory. In H. Dincer & S. Yuskel (Eds.) Strategic outlooks for innovative work behaviors (pp. 131–148). Springer.

Chrisinger, B. W. (2017). Ethical imperatives against item restriction in the Supplemental Nutrition Assistance Program. *Preventive Medicine*, 100, 56–60. doi: 10.1016/j.ypmed.2017.04.009.

Chrisman J., Jordan R., Davis C. (2014). Exploring evidence-based practice research. *Nursing Made Incredibly Easy*, 13(4), 8–12.

Cochran, M. (2011). International perspectives on early childhood education. *Educational Policy*, 25(1), 65–91.

Dahlgren G., Whitehead M. (1991). *Policies and Strategies to Promote Social Equity in Health*. Stockholm: Institute for Future Studies.

Davis G. F., Cobb J. A. (2010). Resource dependence theory: Past and future. *Public Administration Review*, 64(2), 132–140.

Dawes M., Summerskill W., Glasziou P., Caartabellota A., Martin J., Hopayian K., Porzsolt F., Burls A., Osborne J. (2005). Sicily statement on evidence-based practice. *Biomed Central Medical Education*, 5(1), 1–7.

DeStasio K. L., Clithero J. A., Berkman E. T. (2019). Neuroeconomics, health psychology, and the interdisciplinary study of preventative health behavior. *Social Personality Psychology Compass*, 13(10), 1111–12404.

Dibie R. (2022). Health policy and administration in Nigeria. *The Journal of African Policy Studies*, 28(1), 101–139.

Dibie R. (2018). *Business and Government Relations in Africa*. New York: Routledge Press.

Dibie R. & Dibie, J. (2024). Development administration and government performance in Nigeria. *Review of Public Administration and Management Journal*, 21(1): 18–32.

Drees, J. M., & Heugens, P. P. M. A. R. (2013). Synthesizing and extending resource dependence theory: A meta-analysis. Journal of Management, 39(6), 1666–1698.

Dye T. (2013). *Understanding Public Policy*. Fourteenth Edition. Boston, MA: Pearson Learning.

Engel E. L. (1977). The need for a new medical model: A challenge for biomedicine. *Science*, 196, 719–732.

Gatwiri K., Amboko J., Okolla D. (2020). The implications of Neoliberalism on African economies, health outcomes and wellbeing: A conceptual argument. *Social Theory & Health*, 18(2). DOI:10.1057/s41285-019-00111-2.

Grad F. P. (2002). The preamble of the constitution of the World Health Organization. *Bulletin of the World Health Organization*, 80(12), 981–984. World Health Organization. https://apps.who.int/iris/handle/10665/268691. Accessed February 24, 2021.

Griffin R. W., Phillips J. M., Gully S. M. (2017). *Organizational Behavior: Managing People and Organizations*. Boston, MA: Cengage Learning.

Hanberg A. (2006). Bridging the theory–practice gap with evidence-based practice. *The Journal of Continuing Education in Nursing*, 37(6), 248–249.

Hoffmann S., Devleesschauwer B., Aspinall W., Cooke R., Corrigan T., Havelaar A., Angulo F., Gibb H., Kirk M., Lake M., Speybroeck N., Torgerson P., Hald T. (2017). Attribution of global foodborne disease to specific foods: Findings from a World Health Organization structured expert elicitation. *PLoS One*, 12(9), e0183641. DOI: 10.1371/journal.pone.0183641.

Holzer, M., Schwester, R. W. (2016). *Public Administration: An Introduction*. Second Edition. New York: Routledge/Taylor and Francis Press.

Janati A, Hasanpoor E, Hajebrahimi S, Sadeghi-Bazargani H, Khezri A. (2018). An evidence-based framework for evidence-based management in healthcare organizations: A Delphi study. *Ethiopia Journal Health Science*, 28(3):305-314.

Janse B., (2020). Resource dependence theory (RDT). https://www.toolshero.com/management/resources-dependence-theory-rdt/. Accessed January 29, 2024.

Johnson, J., Stoskopf, C. (2010). *Comparative health systems: global perspectives*. Sudbury, MA: Jones and Bartlett Publishers.

Karnick P. M. (2016). Evidence-based practice and nursing theory. *Nursing Science Quarterly*, 29(4), 283–284.

Kingdom J. (2010). *Agendas, Alternatives, and Public Policies*. Second Edition. New York: Pearson Learning Press.

Kraft M., Furlong S. (2024). *Public Policy Analysis*. Washington DC: Congressional Quarterly Press.

Lindblom C. E. (1979). Still muddling, not yet through. *Public Administration Review*, 39 (6), 517–526.

Lomi A. & Pattison P. E. (2006). Manufacturing relations: an empirical study of the organization of production across multiple networks. *Organization Science*, 17(3): 313–332.

Luciano M. M., Aloia T. A., Brett J. F. (2019). 4 Ways to Make Evidence-Based Practice the Norm in Health Care. https://hbr.org/2019/08/4-ways-to-make-evidence-based-practice-the-norm-in-health-care. Accessed February 11, 2024.

Malatesta D., Smith C. R. (2014). Lessons from resource dependence theory for contemporary public and nonprofit management. *Public Administration Review*, 74(1), 14–25.

Marteau, T. M., & Johnston, M. (1986). Determinants of beliefs about illness: a study of parents of children with diabetes, asthma, epilepsy, and no chronic illness. *Journal of Psychosomatic Research*, 30 (6), 673–683.

Mason P. H., Roy A., Spillane J., Singh P. (2015). *Social Historical and Cultural Dimension of Tuberculosis*. Boston, MA: Cambridge University Press.

McGain, F., Muret, J., Lawson, C., Sherman J. D. (2020). Environmental sustainability in anesthesia and critical care. *British Journal of Anesthesia*, 125 (5): 680–692.

Murray, T. (2008). Exploring Epistemic Wisdom: Ethical and Practical Implications of Integral Theory and Methodological Pluralism for Collaboration and Knowledge-Building. Accessed September 1, 2024.

Nevo I., Slonim-Nevo V. (2011). The myth of evidence-based practice: Towards evidence-informed practice. *The British Journal of Social Work*, 41(6), 1176–1197.

Noar S. M., Zimmerman R. S. (2005). Health behavior theory and cumulative knowledge regarding health behaviors: Are we moving in the right direction? *Health Education Research*, 20(3), 275–290.

Norcross J. C. (2005). *Psychotherapy Relationships that Work: Evidence Based Responsiveness*. Second Edition. London: Oxford University Press.

Ogden J. (2012). *Health Psychology: A Textbook*. Fifth Edition. London: Open University Press.

Oleribe O., Ezechi O., Osita-Oleribe P., Olawepo O., Musa A. Z., Omoluabi A., Fertleman M., Salako B. L., Taylor-Robinson S. D. (2020). Public perception of COVID-19 management and response in Nigeria: A cross-sectional survey. *BMJ Open*, 10(10), e041936. DOI: 10.1136/bmjopen-2020-041936.

Ozcan P., Eisenhardt K. M. (2009). Origin of alliance portfolios: Entrepreneurs, network strategies, and firm performance. *Academy of Management Journal*, 52, 246–279.

Patashnik, E. M., Gerber, A. S., Dowling, C. M. (2020). Unhealthy politics: The battle over evidence-based medicine. Accessed August 31, 2024.

Patel, K., Rushefsky, M. E. (2015). *The Politics of Public Health in the United States*. New York: Routledge Press.

Pennock, R., T. (2018). Beyond research ethics: how scientific virtue theory reframes and extends responsible conduct of research. In David Carr (ed.), *Cultivating Moral Character and Virtue in Professional Practice*. New York: Routledge.

Peters, E. (2018). Compassion fatigue in nursing: A concept analysis. 10.1111/nuf.12274. Accessed September 1, 2024.

Peter B. G. (2009). *American Public Policy: Promise and Performance*. Eighth Edition. Washington DC: Congressional Quarterly Press.

Pfeffer J. (1982). *Organizations and Organization Theory*. New York, NY: Pitman Press.

Pfeffer J., Salancik G. R. (1978). *The External Control of Organizations: A Resource Dependence Perspective*. New York: Harper & Row.

Porter-O'Grady T., Malloch K. (2015). *Quantum Leadership: Building Better Partnerships for Sustainable Health*. Fourth Edition. Burlington, MA: Jones & Bartlett Learning.

Preffer, L., Sutton, R. (2006). *Hard facts, dangerous half-truths, and total nonsense profiting from evidence-based management.* Boston, MA: Harvard Business Press.

Prefer J., Sutton R. I. (2006). *Hard-Facts, Dangerous Half-Truths, and Total Nonsense: Profiting from Evidence-Based Management.* Cambridge, MA: Harvard Business School Press.

Rinfret S. R., Schebele D., Pautz M. (2023). *Public Policy: A Concise Introduction.* Second Edition. Thousand Oaks, CA: Sage/CQ Press.

Sarafino, E. P. (2002), *Health psychology: Biopsychosocial interactions.* Fourth Edition, New York: Wiley & Sons.

Sharif P, S. & Yeoh, K. K. (2014). Independent directors' resource provision capability in publicly listed companies in Malaysia. *Corporate Ownership and Control,* 11(3), 113–121. https://ssrn.com/abstract=2822679. Accessed November 8, 2024.

Skolnik, R., (2008). *Essentials of Global Health.* Sudbury, MA: Jones and Bartlett Publisher.

Stevens K. (2013). The impact of evidence-based practice in nursing and the next big ideas. *OJIN: The Online Journal of Issues in Nursing,* 18(2), 2–11.

Stone D. A. (2012). *Policy Paradox: The Art of Political Decision Making.* Third Edition. New York: W. W. Norton & Company.

Troseth M. R. (2016). Evidence-based practice: The key to advancing quality and safety in healthcare. https://www.beckershospitalreview.com/quality/evidence-based-practice-the-key-to-advancing-quality-and-safety-in-healthcare.html. Accessed February 11, 2024.

Wilson B., Austria M. (2019). What is evidence-based practice. https://accelerate.uofuhealth.utah.edu/explore/what-is-evidence-based-practice. Accessed February 11, 2021.

World Health Organization (2021). Universal health coverage (UHC). https://www.who.int/en/news-room/fact-sheets/detail/universal-health-coverage-(uhc). Accessed April 19, 2023.

Chapter Three

HEALTH POLICY AND CHALLENGES IN BOTSWANA

Robert Dibie and Josephine Dibie

Introduction

The chapter on health policy analysis in Botswana explores the dynamic of the types of healthcare policy formulated by the government of the nation. It uses data analysis to explain how the health of the citizens of the country tends to be improving even though environmental conditions in some parts of Botswana tend to be very challenging to a large population of the nation. Unlike many African countries, the chapter focuses on the vision of sustainability and the challenges in Botswana that are inconsistent with those of neighboring countries. The chapter also uses graphics to explain the positive impacts of the new healthcare policies implemented by the nation's government in the past decade. It analyzes the extent to which affordable healthcare policies have expanded treatment options for rural and urban residents of Botswana simultaneously. Further, the chapter describes the condition of health promotion infrastructure, investment in health promotion, human resource training, and collaboration between public and private healthcare providers to improve health delivery in the country. Infrastructure and services for health promotion in Botswana are provided by the government through educational institutions, faith-based organizations, nongovernmental organizations, general medical practitioners, and mining companies complementing the efforts of the Ministry of Health. The research for this chapter involves the administration of a survey and content analysis of government reports, academic journals, and World Health Organization reports. A review of government gazette documents was conducted to trace health policy evolutionary developments and their impact on the general lives of the people of Botswana. The research findings reveal that limited resources such as transport and financial resources are a major challenge to health and education promotion activities across the country. Health educators are limited when it comes to traveling to rural communities in Botswana. Some health policy recommendations that could help to enhance the effectiveness of healthcare delivery in the country are also provided.

Brief History

Botswana is a democratic country in the southeastern part of Africa. It has a border with South Africa, Zimbabwe, Zambia, and Namibia. Botswana is almost engulfed by the Kalahari Desert, thereby making the country a sparsely populated nation with little agricultural activity (Dibie 2018). Botswana had a population of 2.6 million, with a gross domestic product (GDP) of US$20.3 billion in 2022 (World Bank 2022). The nation continues to depend on the export of diamonds as its major source of foreign revenue. In 2022, diamonds contributed more than 90% of total exports and are a major source of fiscal revenues (World Bank 2022).

The Tswana people originally resided in the region, which is now called Botswana before the fourteenth century (History of Botswana 2020; Chan et al. 2019). In addition, the San and Khoi ethnic groups were among the original inhabitants of the now Republic of Botswana and the Republic of South Africa (de Kadt & Lieberman 2020). It should be noted that the Tswana, Bantu, and Khoi people were hunter-gatherers. The Tswana people were believed to be descendants of King Mogale, a farmer in a region that is now called Magaliesberg Mountain in the northern part of the Republic of South Africa (History of Botswana 2020). Further, the people from the Khoe-Kwadi, Kx'a, and Tuu ethnic groups are believed to have lived in the region called Botswana (BBC 2024; Chan et al. 2019; Evan 2022; Nick 2017). In the nineteenth century, the various ethnic groups that lived in the area known as Botswana were made up of more than eight Chiefdoms whose peoples shared a common language and history and coexisted in relative peace (BBC 2024; Chan et al. 2019; de Kadt & Lieberman 2020). The various ethnic groups traded ivory and skins with the Europeans in exchange for guns and were Christianized by missionaries (Evans 2019; History of South Africa Online 2023; History of Botswana 2020).

As more ethnic groups crossed the river Limpopo to settle in the region now called Botswana in the nineteenth century, hostilities began to escalate between the Shona people and the Ndebele tribes who were migrating into the territory from Kalahari Desert (Evans 2019, History of South Africa Online 2023; History of Botswana 2020). To prevent the Dutch and Germans from further exploring the southeastern region, in 1885, the British Government declared the Bechuanaland under its protection (Acemoglu et al. 2001; Colclough & McCarthy 1980), but the northern territory remained a part of the Bechuanaland Protectorate and its name was changed to the Republic of Botswana after independence in 1967. The southern territory was declared British Bechuanaland and later renamed the Cape Colony or the Northwest Province of South Africa (Africa Botswana 2017; South Africa History Online 2022; Woodward 2019). In addition, during the same period, part of the Matabele Kingdom that was called the Tati Concession Land was governed by the British Bechuanaland Protectorate administration that was previously annexed in 1911 (South Africa History Online 2022, Wikipedia. 2020).

According to Africa Botswana (2017), Nick (2017), and Wikipedia (2020), three traditional leaders from the various ethnic groups in the Bechuanaland presented a request for protection and frustration about the desire for the Dutch and German settlers to annex their farmland. Most of the British traders and organizations operating in the Protectorate also lobbied to support the request of the traditional leaders (Wikipedia 2020). The protection request was approved by the British colonial administration in 1885 and the Bechuanaland Protectorate was declared (Africa Botswana 2017; Botswana 2023; Nick 2017).

The following historical events later happened after the 1885 declaration of the Bechuanaland. In 1867, the European gold prospectors started exploring the Protectorate for gold, found gold, and mining began. About a few decades later, the diamond was also found in the Bechuanaland Protectorate (Evan 2017; South Africa History Online 2022). More than two centuries later, Botswana has become one of the world's largest producers of diamonds, a trade that has transformed the nation into a middle-income country (Colclough & McCarthy 1980; Kenneth 1992). According to Eawcus and Tilbury (2000) and Evan (2017), the British colonial administration did not establish any major economic development until the discovery of diamonds in the 1970s by the Belgium company called De Beers Diamond Consortium. After the discovery of diamonds, there were negotiations between the Government of Botswana and the De Beer Diamond Consortium on how to share the diamond natural resource.

The initial agreement stipulated that the Government of Botswana would receive 25% of the rough stones extracted, while De Beers would have 75%. A new agreement stated that Botswana would immediately receive a 30% share, and its share would rise to 50% within a decade (Eligon 2023). Despite the reluctance of the British colonial administration to enhance development trade, mining, and visionary political leadership after independence has made Botswana a progressive country (Africa Botswana. 2017; South Africa History Online 2022). As of 2023, Botswana is regarded as the world's largest diamond producer. Some of the nation's leaders are however wary of the Dutch disease trap of over-dependence on only one industry or product (Dibie 2018). The revenue derived from diamond and other agricultural exports has raised the economy to the middle-income level (Dibie 2018; History of Botswana 2020).

Following a series of events and negotiations in the Bechuanaland Protectorate, the British Government accepted a proposal to establish a new constitution in 1960. In 1966, the British colonial administration accepted the new proposal for a new self-government democracy system led by the Indigenous black people of Botswana (Eawcus & Tilbury 2000; Nick 2017). Therefore, in 1965, the nation's capital city was changed from Mafeking in South Africa to a newly built city called Gaborone (History of Botswana 2020). A new constitution was written and approved in 1965 after which the first general election of the new nation was conducted, and the Botswana Democratic Party leader Sertse Khama won. In 1965, Seretse Khama was appointed as the Prime Minister of the Republic of Botswana. On September 30, 1966, the nation became officially independent from Britain (Dibie 2018; Ewans 2017; Nick 2017; History of Botswana 2020).

According to British Broadcasting Corporation (2023), Botswana (2023); Colclough & McCarthy. (1980), and Wikipedia (2020), the Botswana Democratic Party has been in power since the first democratic elections in 1966 and continues to draw support from a wide range of the Botswana population. After President Seretse Khama, Ketumile Masire served as Botswana's second president in July 1980 and continued a tradition of good governance. He voluntarily retired from office in 1998 and was succeeded by President Festus Mogae. Mr. Mogae finished his second term in 2008 handing over power to the incumbent President Ian Khama. Mokggweetsi Eric Keabetwe Masisi was elected the fifth president of Botswana in April 2018. All the former presidents of the country came from the same political party (BBC 2023; Botswana 2023; Colclough & McCarthy 1980; Wikipedia 2020). Unlike many other African countries, since its independence, the Republic of Botswana has maintained a thriving democracy, clean government, an up-right judiciary, peace and stability, and a well-managed economy (Dibie 2018; GlobalEdge 2014).

Botswana currently depends on mining and exporting diamonds for about 90% of its foreign currency earnings. Tourism accounts for 12% of its GDP, and the agriculture sector contributes 2.8% of its GDP (Botswana Ministry of Health and Wellness 2020).

Healthcare Challenges

The government of the Republic of Botswana has formulated several health policies and National Health Strategic Plans since it became an independent country. The main goal of these policies is to incrementally achieve universal health coverage for its citizens. The health policies require the government to provide health services to the citizens of Botswana regardless of their ability to pay. The slogan of the National Health Policy of Botswana is "towards a healthier Botswana" (Republic of Botswana Ministry of Health 2013). This slogan postulates that the provision of health services in the country is not just for curing the sick but also to promote healthy lifestyles, prevent diseases, and provide better environmental conditions for every person living in the country (Republic of Botswana Ministry of Health and Wellness 2018).

Despite the well-crafted goals of the health policies enacted by the Government of Botswana, equality of healthcare and service delivery utilization remain a major challenge because of inadequately skilled health professionals, especially in rural healthcare facilities. In addition, some scholars argue that Botswana faces a new set of challenges to its universal health coverage because of the brain drain of specialist physicians who could provide advanced training for health professionals who just graduated from medical school. A lack of adequate workforce to improve the quality of healthcare for complicated medical conditions in public hospitals in the country could be detrimental to the high-quality healthcare delivery system in the country (Global Health 2020).

In addition, the implementation of these health policies required the citizens to pay user fees, an approach that conflicted with the 1970 user-fee policy. Some patients who were aware of this policy and implementation conflict refused to pay the user fee (Pagiwa et al. 2022). Further, due to insufficient staff, implementation practices, poorly administered revenue collection practice, lack of resources to collect fees and corruption, the current user-fee practice could result in worse health outcomes and higher healthcare cost in the future if the Government of Botswana does not overhaul mandatory pre-repayment methods (Hulton 2004; Khulumai et al. 1999; Mbogo & McGill 2016; Pagiwa et al. 2022; Ministry of Health and Wellness Botswana 2016). Olusola Ogunseye (2020) contends that another challenge for the Government of Botswana is its financing which is bedeviled by inequity, inefficiency, fragmentation, and uncertainty in the sustainability of the government funding system (Kamrany and Gray 2014; Ogunseye 2020).

Other healthcare challenges for the Republic of Botswana include the HIV/ AIDS pandemic in 2004. Botswana was once known to have the world's highest rate of HIV/AIDS infection (BBC 2023, United Nations Report 2022). The disparities in the spread of HIV/AIDS in the country led the government to collaborate with its international partners to adopt one of Africa's most advanced treatment programs for HIV/AIDS. As of current times, the majority of the medications to treat HIV/ AIDS and COVID-19 are readily available all over the country (BBC 2023, World Health Organization 2022). The tremendous effort of the Government of Botswana to combat the HIV/AIDS pandemic as well as its ability to effectively distribute free anti-HIV/AIDS drugs to all its citizens and residents of the country has drastically decreased the spread of the disease (Center for Disease Control 2021; Seloiliwe & Kealeboga 2022). The Republic of Botswana is the first African country to provide free antiretroviral treatment to all its citizens and residents infected by the HIV/AIDS pandemic (Center for Disease Control 2021; Pathak 2019). The Botswana Ministry of Health and Wellness is also confronted with major challenges in influencing the behavior of private providers (Keetile et al. 2023; Seloiliwe & Kealeboga 2022). The private healthcare sector has grown over the past three decades in diversity, but the limited health policy implementation has failed to adequately influence the quality of services that the sector provides in the country. Over the past three decades, the lack of oversight in ensuring national priorities in the private healthcare sector in Botswana has been a major predicament (Ncube et al. 2020). The private medical sector allows the affluent residents of the country to eat their cake and have it. Unfortunately, the market failure factors that often occur in private healthcare hospitals require major intervention by the Botswana Ministry of Health and Wellness however, needed regulation seems not to be forthcoming. In addition to the lack of genuine regulation of the private sector, there are major disparities between the quality of healthcare provided by the private sector compared to the public sector hospitals and clinics (BBC 2023; Pathak 2019). The disparity is because the private sector healthcare typically caters to the affluent or rich residents of Botswana, while the public healthcare facilities predominantly provide treatments to the poor or middle social economic groups in the country (Ogunseye 2020). There are also disparities in how physical resources are distributed around the country. There is a positive correlation between physical access to services and limited or adequate delivery of services as well as governance of public hospitals. Pathak (2019) contends that a lack of autonomy in the proper management of public hospitals limits the ability of specialist doctors and administrators to freely adopt evidence-based performance or best practices in the respective hospitals.

Types of Health Policies

The health system in the Republic of Botswana has been incrementally improved over the past three decades. The formulation and implementation of good policies have resulted in several new health infrastructures across the country. New health policies have made it possible for citizens of the country to access hospitals or health clinics within five miles of distance (Botswana Ministry of Health 2013; UNICEF 2018). In addition,

Botswana's National Development Plans 2017–2027 include new policy initiatives to galvanize health promotion and universal health coverage. promotion of mental health, prevention of noncommunicable diseases, and strengthening household food security and nutrition among other goals (Botswana Ministry of Health and Wellness 2019). Below are some of the major health policies that the Government of Botswana has enacted over the past three decades.

National Health Policy for Botswana of 1995: The goal of this policy is to guide the development of the health sector in the country. Since the policy was formulated and implemented in Botswana, there have been a lot of changes in the epidemiological sector, socioeconomic, demographic arrangements, and health technology. This policy also encompasses all the social determinants that impact the health system in the country (Republic of Botswana Ministry of Health and Wellness 1995).

Legislation Relevant to Nutrition 2005: This regulation makes provision for the control of stocking, distributing, selling, or marketing in Botswana of any food for infants and young children as defined by regulation 2. The regulation provides for the designation of monitors for purposes of control and defines their functions and power. The regulation also lays down rules relative to the labeling and advertising of food for infants and young children and makes provisions with respect to education in the field of the feeding of infants and young children (the Republic of Botswana Ministry of Health and Wellness 2011).

Health Sector Policy Strategy or Plan with Nutrition Component enacted in 2010: A strategy for Changing the Health Sector for Healthy Botswana 2010–2020. The goal of this policy is to develop policies and regulations related to public health as well as to improve access and utilization of quality prevention, promotion, and rehabilitation services. This policy ended in 2020 (Republic of Botswana Ministry of Health and Wellness; 2010).

Legislation Relevant to Nutrition 2010: Policy on Food Salt Regulations 2010– Current. This policy states that no person in Botswana shall manufacture, sell, import, or distribute any food-grade salt that is not iodate except under and in accordance with terms and conditions specified under regulation 6 (5). This policy is still current (Republic of Botswana Ministry of Health and Wellness 2010).

National Health Policy enacted in 2011: Health Sector Policy or Plan with Nutrition Component 2011–2021. The goal of this policy is to increase affordable healthy food and promote healthy eating habits and increased physical activity to reduce malnutrition as well as prevent chronic diseases such as diabetes, cardiovascular disease, osteoporosis, and so on. among residents and citizens of Botswana. This policy ended in 2021 (Republic of Botswana Ministry of Health and Wellness 2011).

Public Health Act enacted in 2013: The goal of this policy is to improve public and private sector engagements, as well as enhance joint planning synergies in the implementation of established policies and accountability in health management and leadership in Botswana (Republic of Botswana Ministry of Health 2013).

Botswana Multisectoral Strategy Act 2018: The goal of this policy is to prevent and control noncommunicable diseases in Botswana and reduce the risk factors through awareness, promotion of healthy lifestyles, and creation of enabling environments. The implementation started in 2018 and was scheduled to end in 2023 (Republic of Botswana Ministry of Health 2013).

The Botswana health improvement case shows that without effective public policies, the government and administration are rudderless. Botswana's universal healthcare policy has benefited most of its citizens (Tsima et al. 2022; Wikipedia 2024) as the policy covers 95% of the nation's population. It could be argued that successful policies could enhance successful government and administration (Dibie 2022).

Nature of Health Administration

The Republic of Botswana uses a decentralized model in the management of its health system. The Ministry of Health and Wellness of Botswana is the main institution that enforces the national health policies, ACTs, and strategies of the nation (Government of Botswana Ministry of Health and Wellness 2023). The nation has about 104 clinics with beds, 195 clinics without beds, and 338 health posts. Unlike many other African countries, Botswana has established an effective 844 mobile stops (World Health Organization 2017). Primary healthcare delivery services are also part of hospital operations in the country (Wikipedia 2024).

In respect of the administration of the health system in Botswana, the nation is divided into 27 districts. According to the National Health Policy of 2011, the major function of the Ministry of Health and Wellness is the implementation of health policies, strategies, and goals. It is also responsible for health policy development initiatives and delivery all over the country. The districts and their local administration are mandated to ensure the delivery of primary healthcare services through medical posts, clinics, primary hospitals, and district hospitals that administer care to the rural regions (World Health Organization 2017). In addition, each district has a healthcare team whose function includes the supervision of several public health disease prevention initiatives in their respective regions. There are several faith-based and nongovernmental healthcare organizations in Botswana that also provide similar healthcare services to their public sector counterparts in the country.

The Botswana Ministry of Health and Wellness is responsible for monitoring and regulating private hospitals and clinics (Tepera et al. 2018; UNICEF 2018; Republic of Botswana Ministry of Health and Wellness 2005; World Health Organization 2017). Accreditation is granted to both public and private professionals by the professional council as stipulated by the Dental, Medical, and Pharmacy Act, as well as the Nurses and Midwives Act of the Government of Botswana (UNICEF 2018; World Health Organization 2014–2020 Report). One other responsibility of the Botswana Ministry of Health and Wellness is the registration of private hospitals and clinics in the country.

In Botswana, the private health sector comprises not-for-profit and for-profit hospitals and clinics including pharmacies and medical laboratories (Tapera et al. 2017). There are three main Medical Aid Schemes that play a significant role in financing private healthcare (World Health Organization 2014–2020 report). Other key players in the healthcare delivery system in Botswana include international agencies such as World Health Organization (WHO), the United Nations Children's Fund (UNICEF), United

Nations Development Program (UNDP); Center for Disease Control (CDC), United States Agency for International Development (USAID), donor agencies, and other countries through bilateral and multilateral partnerships (Government of Botswana Ministry of Health and Wellness 2023; Ogunseye 2020).

According to scholars, institutions in Botswana that regulate health professions face the challenge of capacity building (Kealeboga et al. 2022; Mabunda et al. 2023; Mamalelala et al. 2022) that creates difficulty in implementing health regulation in Botswana. Lack of knowledge of legislation by managers in Botswana also tremendously negatively affects the healthcare delivery system in the country by limiting their ability to enforce or adhere to the mandates of the National Health Policies in the country (Ogunseye 2020; Mabunda et al. 2023). Further, there seems to be no health policy in the country that deals with the accreditation of government hospitals and clinics (British Broadcasting Corporation 2022; Seitio-Kgokgwe et al. 2016). Unfortunately, this means that the Government of Botswana could build hospitals and clinics of any standard without considering high quality and best practices in healthcare delivery. Another challenge in the administration of healthcare in the country is the shortage of health workers in some rural districts. It has been reported that during the serious stages of the HIV/AIDs and COVID-19 pandemics, nurses were made to operate in health specialist areas due to shortage of medical doctors. On some occasions, clinics and health posts in rural regions had to close because there were no doctors or nurses to operate such health facilities due to shortage of health workers even though there were patients on admission (Country Report 2023; Mabunda et al. 2023; World Health Organization 2021).

Data Analysis and Discussion

The purpose of this chapter is to analyze the effectiveness of the health policy in Botswana. The data used were derived from both primary and secondary sources. The secondary research methods adopted include the review of the Government of Botswana Ministry of Health and Wellness, African Development Bank, the World Health Organization reports, the United Nations Human Development Index annual report, the Center for Disease Control, and the United States Agency for International Development, academic as well as professional journal articles.

The primary research involves the administration of a questionnaire to 160 respondents. One hundred and thirty-three respondents returned their completed questionnaire. The respondents were 51.6% male and 48.4% female. Sixty-two percent of the respondents had visited a hospital or clinic to receive treatment at least twice a year, and 38% had visited a hospital or clinic 2–4 times recently to receive treatment. Data were analyzed using SPSS to determine the effectiveness and challenges facing the health policy and quality of the healthcare delivery system in Botswana.

Table 1 shows data on the nature of healthcare delivery and policy in Botswana. The questionnaire data reveal that 74.4% of the respondents indicated that the lack of appropriate funding for the healthcare system in the country is an issue because the Government of Botswana has been appropriating only an average of 6% of its GDP

Table 1 The Nature of Healthcare Delivery and Policy in Botswana

Questions	Strongly Agree	Agree	Neutral	Strongly Disagree	Disagree	Agree %	Disagree %
1 Healthcare provided by doctors in my city is highly commendable	15	48	31	7	32	63 / 47%	39 / 29.3%
2 Most hospitals in my country do not have modem equipment	13	61	11	6	42	74 / 55.6%	48 / 36%
3 I can afford my Healthcare treatment and medication costs without the government subsidies.	15	43	23	15	37	58 / 43.5%	52 / 39.1%
4 Most rural public hospitals in my country do not have specialist doctors and nurses.	13	59	14	18	29	72 / 54%	47 / 35.3%
5 Government pay of low salaries to doctors and nurses has encouraged their migration to foreign countries.	17	56	13	17	30	73 / 55%	47 / 35.3%
6 Patients' medical treatment outcomes in hospitals in the rural regions of my country are very high	12	38	29	13	41	50 / 7.6%	54 / 40.6%
7 Government promotes equity in the delivery of healthcare to underserved citizens in the country.	9	31	20	13	60	40 / 30%	100 / 75%
8 Political leaders and rich citizens of my country prefer to seek healthcare services in foreign nations.	47	51	5	11	24	98 / 73.6%	35 / 26.3%
9 Government is effectively regulating medical professional licensing and disciplinary boards	11	39	24	19	40	50 / 37.6%	59 / 75.2%
10 Hospitals and health centers in my city have constant electricity.	24	52	8	21	28	76 / 57%	49 / 37%
11 Lack of appropriate funding of the healthcare system in my country.	5	23	6	27	72	28 / 21%	99 / 74.4%
Mean						46.5%	42.6%

Source: Derived from field research in Botswana in 2024.

per capita for healthcare. In 2020, the Government of Botswana provided 68.1% of the health finance, while the private sector provided 24%, and donors 7.9% (Ogunseye 2020). Seventy-five percent of the respondents disagree that the Government of Botswana promotes equity in the delivery of healthcare to underserved citizens in the country. This is not surprising because the public sector tends to serve the lower-income citizens and residents of the country while only the rich can afford private and better healthcare services from private hospitals. Approximately, 73.6% of the respondents agree that political leaders and rich citizens of Botswana prefer to seek healthcare services in foreign nations. The result also indicates that 57% of the respondents agreed that public hospitals in which they live have constant electricity, while 55.6% agree that most hospitals in the country do not have modem equipment.

It is noteworthy that 74.2% of respondents indicated that the Government of Botswana is not effectively regulating medical professional licensing and disciplinary boards. Fifty-five percent of them reported that the low salary paid by the Government of Botswana to doctors and nurses is fueling their migration to foreign countries that offer better working conditions and wages. Further, only 37.6% of the respondents reported that patients' medical treatment outcomes in hospitals in the rural regions of the country are very high, while 40.6% disagree that the rural districts' healthcare delivery systems are lower than those of both the urban and private hospitals in the country. Fifty-four percent of the respondents indicated that most rural public hospitals in the country do not have specialist doctors and nurses. On the other hand, 35.3% of the respondents reported that hospitals and clinics in rural districts do not have specialist doctors and nurses. While 43.5% of the respondents indicated that they could afford to pay healthcare treatment and medication costs without government subsidies, 39.1% reported that they could not pay their healthcare costs without government subsidy through the government universal healthcare coverage scheme. It is also noteworthy that 47% of the respondents indicated that healthcare provided by doctors in their respective cities was highly commendable, while 29.3% reported that the health services that they had received from the doctors in public hospitals in the city they live in are not commendable.

Table 2 shows the analysis of secondary data with respect to the healthcare system in Botswana. There is a consensus that because most adults in Botswana were infected with the HIV/AIDS pandemic, the country's healthcare system is more focused on preventing the spread of the disease. The United Nations Human Development Index (2022), British Broadcasting Corporation (2023), and World Health Organization report (2022) indicate that 20.3% of people 15–49 years old are infected with the disease. Further, the Central for Disease Control (2021) and the United States Agency for International Development (2022) reported that the major causes of death in Botswana are HIV/AIDS, lower respiratory infections, ischemic heart disease, stroke, diabetes, neonatal disorder, road injury as well as tuberculosis.

The Government of Botswana currently spends an average of 6.19% of its GDP to finance the public healthcare system in the country. The number of physicians/doctors per 1,000 people was 0.3 in 2018), while the number of nurses and midwives per 1,000 people was 5.0 in 2018 (World Bank Indicators 2023). Furthermore, 99.1% of births

Table 2 Economic and Health Indicators in Botswana

No.	Major Indicators in Botswana	Explanation
1	Population	2.6 million (2022)
2	Gross domestic product (GDP) PPP	US$20.3 billion (2022)
3	Current health expenditure (% of GDP)	6.1% (2020)
4	Physicians/doctors per 1,000 people	0.3 (2018)
5	Nurses and midwives per 1,000 people	5.0 (2018)
6	Hospital beds (per 1,000 people)	1.8 (2018)
7	Birth attended by skilled health personnel	100% (2017)
8	People using basic drinking water (% of population)	80.% (2022)
9	Population using safe managed drinking water service	Urban 73%; Rural 528% (2022)
10	People using safely managed sanitation services (% of the population)	24% (2022)
11	People practicing open defecation	Urban 1%; Rural 5%
12	Unimproved sanitation access	36.6%
13	Common disease	HIV/AIDS, lower respiratory infections, ischemic heart disease, stroke, diabetes, neonatal disorders, tuberculosis, road injuries, diarrheal diseases, interpersonal violence
14	Life expectancy in 2020 at birth	61 years (2021)
15	Life expectancy in 2019 at birth for females	64 years (2021)
16	Life expectancy in 20 I9 at birth for males	59 years (2021)
17	Mortality rate for female adults (per 1,000 people)	290 (2021)
	Mortality rate for male adults (per 1,000 people)	400 (2021)
18	Mortality rate for infants (per 1,000 people)	28 (2021)
19	Mortality rate for male adults (per 1,000 people)	249
20	Tuberculosis incidence (per 100,000 people	229 (2022)
21	Poverty head count ratio at $2.15 a day (% of the population)	45.3%
22	Population in multidimensional headcount poverty (%)	17.2%
23	Multidimensional poverty handout ratio (% of total population)	25.73% (2002)
24	Infants lacking immunization for measles (% of one-year-old)	90% (2002)
25	Malaria incidence (per 1,000 people at risk)	192.8 (2021)
26	HIV/AIDS prevalence adults (% ages 15–49)	18.6 (2021)
27	Access to electricity (% of population)	73.7% (2021)

Sources: World Bank Indicator 2023; United Nations Human Development Index 2022.

were attended to by skilled health professionals (United Nations Human Development Programme 2020). The population of Botswana that has access to clean water is 73% in the urban area, and 52% in the rural area 2022 (United Nations Human Development Index Report 2022; World Bank Indicators 2023). However, 80% of the nation's population is still using basic drinking water services. It has been reported that some rural districts as well as sections of Gaborone, the capital city of Botswana's tap water are unsafe and should be avoided. It is also recommended that tap water in the nation should be boiled before drinking (Country Report 2023). As previously discussed, diarrhea is one of the major causes of death in Botswana. Thus, there have been occasions when the incidence of diarrhea had spread due to heavy rainfall (Country Report 2023; World Health Organization 2022). In addition, people who have access to improved sanitation in Botswana constitute 63.4% of the population, while citizens and residents of the country who do not have access to improved sanitation access constitute 24% of the population in 2022 (World Bank Indicators 2023). In the bigger cities of the country, there are modern toilets although a few numbers of latrines are still in use. Despite the improvement people practicing open defecation in the urban cities, 1%, while those engaging in the same practice 5% in the rural areas of Botswana (World Bank Indicators 2023).

The life expectancy at birth in 2021 in Botswana was 59 years for males, while the life expectancy at birth for females was 64 years in the same year (World Bank Indicators 2023). Further, the mortality rate for female adults per 1,000 people was 290 in 2021, while the mortality rate for male adults per 1,000 people was 400 (World Bank Indicators 2023; Nation Human Development Index Report 2022).

According to the African Development Bank (2022), and the United Nations Human Development Index Report (2022), the Botswana economy grew from 8.7% in 2020 to 11.9% in 2021 due to the decline in the COVID-19 pandemic. During the same period, the diamond market also improved (African Development Bank 2022; World Bank 2021; United Nations Human Development Index 2022). It should be noted that public hospitals in Botswana are still struggling with a lack of experienced doctors and nurses. In addition to these challenges, some government hospitals and clinics do not have enough beds to accommodate patients who are admitted. Therefore, it could be argued that appropriate health workforce, facilities, and modem equipment should be the cornerstone of the Government of Botswana's healthcare system in the future.

Conclusion

This chapter has examined the effectiveness of health policies in the Republic of Botswana. It argued that although Botswana's healthcare system has improved from what it used to be several decades ago, the nation's health delivery system still faces considerable challenges. There continues to be the political will and the Government of Botswana's commitment to universal health coverage for all its citizens. Further, there is major growth in the regional healthcare hub. The strong financial standing from diamond mining has also galvanized the economy as well as the health industrial sector.

Unlike in the past, the public healthcare system is beginning to contract services to private hospitals in the country (Mabunda et al. 2023; Ogunseye 2020).

For the Republic of Botswana to accomplish its healthcare delivery aspirations, it must provide exemplary stewardship of institutional resources to foster the long-term sustainability of health delivery. The crucial approach should include aligning the nation's physical, technological, and human resources through comprehensive financial, budget, and sustainable information technology plans, along with building well-equipped modern hospitals and clinics to address the current disparities in healthcare delivery in the rural districts in the country. There is also the need to bridge the gap between government and private sector spending by formulating innovative national health insurance. It is paramount for private hospitals, nongovernmental organizations, and the government to start working together to improve the public health system in the country.

To achieve Botswana's healthcare goal of equitable access to healthcare by all citizens, there is an urgent need for pragmatic stewardship of resources to ensure the long-term sustainability of healthcare resources as well as success. There is no doubt that the Government of Botswana has the obligation to use operational practices that reflect sound stewardship, efficiency, and sustainability while affirming that its efforts are mainly for the common good of all the citizens and residents of the country.

Finally, the analysis of health policy in Botswana reveals that shortage of medical doctors and nurses has often negatively affected the delivery of high-quality healthcare in the country. Moving forward will require a strategic doing plan that could attract as well as retain both domestic and foreign health practitioners. Part of this new plan should include better salary and conditions of service. There is no doubt that Botswana's weak regulatory services and supervisory practices have negatively affected the coordination of the communication system between the Ministry of Health and Wellness and the public hospitals. Thus, a need for information and technology in Botswana's health system delivery. An enhanced telemedicine strategy could galvanize a high-standard evidence-based healthcare system in the country. Telemedicine could also enhance the ability of doctors to remotely diagnose and treat patients in rural regions of the country by means of telecommunication technology. It is paramount that the Ministry of Health and Wellness in Botswana continues to listen and learn from its stakeholders in all aspects of its mission and operations. The new vision of the health management of Botswana should be ethics, equity, high-quality, evidence-based care, innovation, retention of skilled doctors and nurses, partnership with the private sector, and patient satisfaction. Providing an avenue for this new vision would propel better engagement and ethical leadership in the health system of Botswana.

References

Acemoglu D., Johnson S., Robinson J. (2001). An African success story: Botswana. https://economics.mit.edu/sites/default/files/publications/An%20African%20Success%20Story%20Botswana.pdf Accessed September 2, 2024.

Africa Botswana (2017). *Q-Files: The Great Illustrated Encyclopedia*. Orpheus Books Limited. https://www.q-files.com/history/africa. Accessed September 3, 2024.

African Development Bank (2022). Botswana and African Development Bank. https://www.afdb.org/en/countries/southern-africa/botswana/botswana-and-the-afdb. Accessed January 30, 2024.

Botswana (2023). History of Botswana. www.thuto.org. Accessed January 15, 2024.

British Broadcasting Corporation (2022). Botswana country profile. https://www.bbc.com/news/world-africa-13040376. Accessed September 2, 2024.

British Broadcasting Corporation News (2023). Botswana country profile. https://www.bbc.com/news/world-africa-13040376. Accessed January 18, 2024.

Center for Disease Control (2021). *CDC Botswana* conducts TB and HIV research. https://bw.usembassy.gov/centers-for-disease-control/. Accessed September 2, 2024.

Chan E. K. F., Timmermann A., Baldi B. F. et al. (2019). Human origins in a Southern African palaeo-wetland and first migrations. *Nature*, 575, 185–189.

Colclough C., McCarthy S. (1980). *The Political Economy of Botswana: A Study of Growth and Income Distribution*. London: Oxford University Press.

Country Report (2023). What is healthcare in Botswana like? https://www.countryreports.org/country/Botswana/health.htm. Accessed January 26, 2024.

de Kadt D., Lieberman E. S. (2020). Nuanced accountability: voter responses to service delivery in Southern Africa. *British Journal of Political Science*, 50(1): 185–215.

Dibie R. (2022). Healthcare policy and administration in Nigeria: A critical analysis. *The Journal of African Policy Studies*, 28(1): 101–139.

Dibie R. (2018). *Business and Government Relations in Africa*. New York: Routledge Press.

Eawcus P., Tilbury A. (2000). *Botswana: The Road to Independents*. Gaborone, Botswana: Pula Press.

Eligon J. (2023). Botswana and De Beers Sign Deal to Continue Rich Diamond Partnership. *New York Times*. https://www.nytimes.com/2023/07/01/world/africa/botswana-de-beers-diamond-deal.html. Accessed July 18, 2023.

Evans A. B. (2019). A brief history of Botswana. https://www.thoughtco.com/brief-history-of-botswana-43607. Accessed June 30, 2019.

Evan P. (2022). *Climate Politics and the Power of Religion*. Bloomington, IN: Indiana University.

GlobalEdge (2014). Botswana profile. globalEdge.msu.edu and Export.Gov. Accessed February 10, 2024.

Global Health (2020). Building a healthy future: Medical education in Botswana. Children Hospital of Philadelphia. https.chop.edu/news/building-healthy-future-medical-education-botswana. Accessed July 21, 2023.

Government of Botswana Ministry of Health and Wellness (2023). https://www.moh.gov.bw/. Accessed February 29, 2024.

History of Botswana (2020). http://www.botswanaembassy.org/page/history-of-botswana #:~:text=After%2080%20years%20as%20a,until%20his%20death%20in%201980. Accessed June 20, 2023.

History of South Africa Online (2023). The social and political history of South Africa from prehistory to the present day. https://www.sahistory.org.za/. Accessed September 2, 2024.

Hulton G. (2004). *Charting the Path to the World Bank's No Blanket Policy on User-Fees in Health and Education, and Reflection on the Future*. London: DFID Health System Resources Center.

Kamrany N., Gray J. (2014). Botswana: An African Model for Progress and Prosperity. http://www.huffingtonpost.com/make-m-Kamrany/botswana-economic-growth_b_2069226.html. Accessed February 11, 2023.

Kealeboga K. M., Khutjwe J. V., Seloilwe E. S. (2022). Nurses and Covide-19 response in Botswana. *Journal of Nursing Scholarship*, 55(1): 149–152.

Keetile, M., Ndlovu, K., Setshegetso, N. *et al.* (2023). Prevalence and correlates of tobacco use in Botswana: evidence from the 2014 Botswana STEPwise survey. *BMC Public Health* 23, 40. doi: 10.1186/s12889-022-14879-y

Kenneth G. (1992). Interpreting the exceptionality of Botswana. *Journal of Modern African Studies*, 30(1): 69–95.

Khulumai P., Moalosi G., Keetile M. (1999). *An Evaluation of the Revenue Collection System in Botswana: Health Financing Study.* Gaborone: Ministry of Health and Wellness.

Mabunda S., Durbach A., Chitha W., Moaletsane O., Angell B., Joshi R. (2023). How were return-of-service schemes developed and implemented in Botswana, Eswatini and Lesotho? *Healthcare,* 11(10): 1512–1523.

Mamalelala T. T., Mokone D. J., Obeng-Adu F. (2022). Health-related reasons patients transfer from a clinic or health post to the Emergency Department in a District Hospital in Botswana. *Africa Journal of Emergency Medicine,* 12(4):339-343.

Mbogo B. A., McGill D. (2016). Perspectives on financing population-based healthcare towards universal health coverage among employed individuals in Ghanzi district, Botswana: A quantitative study. *BMC Health Service Research,* 16(1): 413–425.

Ministry of Health, Botswana (2016). *Health Accounts 2013–2014.* Gaborone: Government Press.

Ncube B., Mars M., Scott R. E. (2020). The need for telemedicine strategy for Botswana? A scoping review and situational assessment. *BMC Health Service Research,* 20(1): 794–807.

Nick H. (2017). *The Statement's Yearbook 2016: The Politics, Culture, and Economies of the World.* New York: Springer.

Ogunseye O. O. (2020). Analysis of the health financing structure of Botswana. *Health Systems and Policy Research,* 7(3–5): 1–5.

Pagiwa V., Shiell A., Barraclough S., Seitio-Kgokgwe O. (2022). A review of the user fees policy for primary healthcare consultations in Botswana: Problems with effective planning, implementation, and evaluation. *International Journal of Health Policy Management,* 11(10): 2228–2235.

Pathak N. (2019). Public health infrastructure in Botswana. https://www.jliedu.com/blog/publichealth-infrastructure-botswana/. Accessed July 28, 2023.

Republic of Botswana Ministry of Health. (2013). National Health Quality Standards. https://www.moh.gov.bw/Publications/standards/Volume_1_ED.pdf. Accessed September 2, 2024.

Republic of Botswana Ministry of Health and Wellness (2020). https://www.gov.bw/ministries/ministry-health-and-wellness. Accessed March 1, 2024.

Republic of Botswana Ministry of Health and Wellness (2018). *Noncommunicable Disease Policy.* Gaborone, Botswana: Government Press.

Republic of Botswana Ministry of Health and Wellness (2011). *National Health Policy.* Gaborone, Botswana: Government Printers.

Republic of Botswana Ministry of Health and Wellness (2010). *Health Sector Policy Strategy or Plan with Nutrition Component Enacted 2010–2020.* Gaborone, Botswana: Government Printers.

Republic of Botswana Ministry of Health and Wellness (1995). *National Health Policy for Botswana of 1995-Current.* Gaborone, Botswana: Government Printers.

Tapera R., Manyala E., Erick P., Maswabi T. M., Tumoyagae T., Letsholo B., Mbongwe B. (2017) Knowledge and Attitudes towards Cervical Cancer Screening amongst University of Botswana Female Students. *Asian Pacific Journal of Cancer Prevention,* 18(9): 2445–2450. doi: 10.22034/APJCP.2017.18.9.2445.

Tsima B. M., Setlhare V., Nkomazana O. (2022). Developing the Botswana primary care guideline: An integrated, symptom-based primary care guideline for the adult patient in a resource-limited setting. *Journal of Multidisciplinary Healthcare,* 1(1): 347–354.

Seitio-Kgokgwe, O., Gauld, R. D. C., Hill, P. C., Barnett, P. (2016). Analysing the Stewardship Function in Botswana's Health System: Reflecting on the Past, Looking to the Future. *International Journal of Health Policy and Management,* 5(12): 705–713.

Seloiliwe E. S., Kealeboga K. M. (2022). A coordinated health policy in response to COVID-19: A case of Botswana. *Journal of Nursing Scholarship,* 1(1): 1–4.

South Africa History Online (2022). Botswana. https://www.sahistory.org.za/place/botswan. Accessed July 17, 2023.

UNICEF (2018). Botswana Budget Health Brief. https://www.unicef.org/Botswana/media/296/file/Health-Budget-Brief-2018.pdf. Accessed January 22, 2024.

United Nations. (2022). United Nations Annual Results Report Botswana. https://botswana.un.org/en/254214-2022-united-nations-annual-results-report-botswana?afd_azwaf_tok. Accessed September 2, 2024.

United Nations (2020). Human Development Report 2020. https://www.un-ilibrary.org/content/books/9789210055161. Accessed September 3, 2024.

United Nations Human Development Report (2022). Botswana's second Voluntary National Review Report. https://www.undp.org/botswana/publications/botswana-2022-voluntary-national-review-report Accessed November 8, 2024.

United States Agency for International Development (USAID) (2022). Botswana. https://bw.usembassy.gov/t he-united-states-agency-for-international-development/. Accessed November 8, 2024.

Wikipedia (2024). Health in Botswana. https://en.wikipedia.org/wiki/Health_in_Botswana. Accessed September 2, 2024.

Wikipedia (2020). History of Botswana. https://en.wikipedia.org/wiki/HistoryofBotswana. Accessed July 15, 2023.

Woodward A. (2019). New study pinpoints: The ancestral homeland of all human alive today. *ScienceAlert.com.* Accessed July 30, 2023.

World Bank Indicators (2023). Botswana Data. https://data.worldbank.org/indicator/SI.POV.MDIM?locations=BW-XM. Accessed February 29, 2024.

World Bank (2022). The World Bank in Botswana. https://www.worldbank.org/en/country/botswana/overview. Accessed July 28, 2023.

World Bank (2021). World Development Report 2021: Data for better lives. https://www.worldbank.org/en/publication/wdr2021. Accessed September 3, 2024.

World Health Organization (2022). Botswana: World Health Organization covid-19. https://www.who.int. Accessed July 21, 2023.

World Health Organization. (2021). Botswana country report. https://www.who.int/about/accountability/results/who-results-report-2020-2021/country-profile/2021/botswana. Accessed January 26, 2024.

World Health Organization (2017). Comprehensive analysis profile: Botswana. https://www.ah.afro.who.int/profiles_information/index.php/Botswana:index/. Accessed July 25, 2023.

World Health Organization (2014–2020). WHO country cooperation strategy 2014–2020: Botswana. www.afro.who.int/sites/default/files/2017-05/ccs-bwa-en.pdf.

Chapter Four

HEALTH POLICY AND CHALLENGES IN BURKINA FASO

Mariam Konaté, Robert Dibie, and Hassimi Traore

Introduction

This chapter examines health policy and challenges in the People's Democratic Republic of Burkina Faso. It argues that despite the substantial progress in health delivery that has taken place in the country in the past three decades, the nation is confronted with major barriers to expanding healthcare coverage to all its citizens as defined by the sustainable development goal (section 6). The chapter discusses various aspects of communicable and non-communicable diseases as well as shortage of health workers in Burkina Faso. It also examines the challenges of morbidity for children, maternal mortality for pregnant women, and sanitation and water challenges in Burkina Faso. The goal of this chapter is to fill the gap in the literature, by providing an extensive discussion of health policy successes and challenges in Burkina Faso. The nature of health policy implementation in the country reveals that there has not been political will among previous and current leaders of Burkina Faso on how to effectively improve healthcare delivery in both the rural and urban regions in the country. Therefore, it is paramount that all stakeholders in the country must recognize the major health system challenges, and effective vibrant solutions on how to solve the health disparity and lack of accessibility problems. This is because while many low-income people in the rural and congested urban regions of Burkina Faso do not have access to affordable healthcare, there continues to be tremendous growth in the population of the country. In addition, high growth rate of consumption, inferior quality of life, and lack of access to improved sanitation, and safe water also constitute mechanisms for the spread of communicable diseases. These predicaments could be regarded as a time bomb for a major health disaster in Burkina Faso in the near future. The chapter provides some health policy recommendations on how to address these healthcare delivery problems in Burkina Faso.

Brief History

The People's Republic of Burkina Faso is a French-speaking country in sub-Sahara Africa. The nation was formerly called the Republic of Upper Volta until 1984 when it was changed to Burkina Faso. The nation achieved its independence from France in 1960. It had a population of about 19.8 million people in 2020 (United Nations Human

Development Index 2021; World Factbook 2020). The Republic of Burkina Faso is a landlocked country that is located in the southern part of the Sahara Desert in West Africa. It has boundaries with the Republic of Benin to the east, Ghana and Togo to the south, Mali to the north, the Niger Republic to the east, and Côte d'Ivoire to the Southwest. According to the World Bank Indicators (2023) Burkina Faso's gross domestic.

The product was US$18.82 billion in 2022. The country's GDP per capita was estimated to be about US$830 in 2022 (World Bank Indicators 2023; World Factbook 2022). The People's Republic of Burkina Faso joined the African Union on May 25, 1963. In addition, Burkina Faso exported 61 tons of gold worth about US$3.5 billion in 2020, and 67 tons of the same mineral was estimated to be US$544 million in revenue in 2021 (International Trade Administration). The Government of Burkina Faso also adopted a semi-presidential system after independence. The type of government adopted is called semi-presidential system of democracy. A prime minister is elected as the head of government, while the president is the ceremonial head of state. On one hand, Burkina Faso's constitution also authorizes the president and prime minister to execute executive powers. On the other hand, the legislative power of the country is vested in both the government and parliament.

The history of the People's Republic of Burkina Faso reveals that Captain Thomas Sankara became the Head of State after a military coup on August 4, 1983 (Harsch 2014). Captain Sankara later changed his title from Captain to President Thomas Sankara and on August 2, 1984. Further, he changed the nation's name from Upper Volta to Burkina Faso. Some of President Sankara's major healthcare accomplishment includes mass vaccination of over 2.5 million children and measures to prevent the spread of measles, meningitis, and yellow fever (Omar 2007). Unlike previous leaders of Burkina Faso, President Sankara introduced new initiatives for his government to build medical dispensaries in every village in the country (California Newsreel 2000; Harsch 2014; Omar 2007). During his administration as President, Sankara also introduced many socioeconomic initiatives such as infrastructure development, such as building schools. According to Harsch (2014) and Omar (2007), Sankara's public health initiatives spill over into the building of a vibrant network of hospitals in the country. In addition to Sankara's public health initiatives, he planted over 10 million trees to reduce the impact of environmental conditions and desertification in the country. President Sankara also enacted a policy to ban the traditional practice of female genital mutilation in Burkina Faso (California Newsreel 2000; Harsch 2014). He also outlaws forced marriage of girl child in the country (Ajayi, et al. 2023). In addition, his administration constructed roads and railway networks all over Burkina Faso. He also redistributed farming land and promoted nationwide literacy and agrarian self sufficiency. economic culture in the country.

Healthcare Challenges

Research reveals that the People's Republic of Burkina Faso has been facing different dimensions of humanitarian and health crises in the past three decades as a result of insecurity, violence, and criminal actions by various military groups from within the country, and surrounding nations (USAID 2020; United Nations Human Development Report 2021; World Health Organization 2020a; 2020b). This humanitarian crisis has made majority of the people living in some rural and urban regions of the country to flee from their homes. The displacement of a sizable percentage of the population of the country has also resulted in the aftermath of a lack of health services and accessibility of hospitals (Kouanda et al. 2014; Ridde & Yameogo 2018; World Health Organization 2020a).

According to Ayeleke et al. (2018) and Meda et al. (2020), for a nation to have a good healthcare system leadership and strategic management, experts are needed to ensure high-quality performance health delivery to the citizens. The lack of optimal performance in the healthcare system in Burkina Faso has been due to the challenges of an adequate health workforce that are spread across the country (Meda et al. 2020). The World Health Organization (2019) and Meda et al. (2020) argued that good health facilities, regulation, and health management workforce could strengthen the health delivery system in developing countries like Burkina Faso where resources might be scarce.

One other major challenge that is facing Burkina Faso's health system includes the shortage of healthcare specialists and disparities in healthcare delivery. These major challenges in the provision of healthcare for the citizens and residents of the country have also created an uneven distribution of medical personnel between rural and urban regions in Burkina Faso (Sween-Cadieux et al. 2019; Zombre et al. 2017). In an effort to address these predicaments in a landlocked nation with limited financial and human resources, the government of Burkina Faso adopted a new policy for the recruitment of doctors and nurses to work in rural health facilities in the country (Meda et al. 2019; SweenCadieux et al. 2019).

In the past decade, there has been a high rate of morbidity due to malaria as well as HIV/AIDS and COVID-19 in most urban regions of the country (Public Policy Plus 2020). In addition, there has been a lack of basic hygiene and sanitation facilities in districts in the country. Furthermore, Burkina has been reported to have some challenges in the administration of vaccination efforts for children in the country (Ajayi et al. 2023; Bocourun et al. 2018; Kiendrebeogo et al. 2022). Because lack of adequate public relations campaigns to create awareness of immunization services for the children in the country the knowledge and concerns of the affected citizens of the country are often ignored or not put into consideration (Kiendrebeogo et al. 2022). There are times when the immunization processes are inadequate due to delays in the delivery of vaccines. These challenges often result in situations where children are not completely vaccinated (Kiendrebeogo et al. 2022).

Skrip et al. (2020) contend that Burkina Faso was among the first countries in sub-Saharan Africa to report the incidence of COVID-19. Although the nation instituted several measures, it has reported the highest number of deaths in West Africa. The reason for this shortfall of an effective health system has been linked to constraints in the inadequate supply of medical equipment, low financing, and infrastructure capacity for isolation and treatment (African Center for Strategic Studies 2020; Gilbert et al. 2020). Furthermore, these healthcare delivery challenges have been at odds with health policies to strategically enhance presumptive COVID-19 cases in precautionary regions and healthcare centers in the country. Because of the vulnerabilities of Burkina Faso's security system caused by mounting insurgent armed groups, the provision of quality healthcare services has been severely hindered. Compounded with this crisis is the low financing and the inability of the nation to invest in mechanisms of intervention in reducing the morbidity and mortality associated with respiratory and viral communicable diseases (Maclean & Marks 2020; World Health Organization 2020b; Skrip et al. 2020).

In an effort to address the health challenges in Burkina Faso, the national government enacted a free-of-charge health policy for children under five years old in 2016 (Quedraogo et al. 2020). Pregnant women in the country were also entitled to the free-of-charge healthcare policy in Burkina Faso. The purpose of free-of-charge healthcare has been to improve maternal and child health in the country (Ministry of Health of Burkina Faso 2022). In addition, one of the major goals was also to reduce charges and increase access to treatment that could eliminate or reduce malaria morbidity in the country. The nation also has an established test and treatment health policy (Ministry of Health of Burkina Faso 2022). It has also been reported that the implementation of the free healthcare policy has significantly increased the number of citizens evaluated and treated compared to when the policy was established (Quedraogo et al. 2020). Despite this progress in the healthcare system, there are major impediments and disparities in the access to healthcare in rural districts due to long-distance travel to hospitals and medical centers in Burkina Faso.

The health policy mandating restrictive vital opening to avoid vaccine wastage has been identified as one of the causes of the lack of timely immunization of only 80% of the eligible children in Burkina Faso (Ministry of Health of Burkina Faso 2022; Bocourun et al. 2018). The barriers identified above have prevented the nation from achieving its goal of increasing immunization or vaccination coverage in some districts in the country. Thus, scholars argued that vaccination coverage and quality continue to be a predicament in the country (Kiendrebeogo et al. 2022; Ministry of Health of Burkina Faso 2022; World Health Organization/UNICEF 2019).

According to the International Reference Center (IRC) Report (2020), some of the major healthcare challenges in Burkina Faso are the inability of the citizens and residents of the country. to have access to basic sanitation, water, and hygiene. It has been reported that 54 % of the population of the country has no access to basic safe and managed water. In addition, basic sanitation is only available to 23% of the nation's population, while 48% of the citizens in Burkina Faso engage in open defecation (Ministry of Health of Burkina Faso 2022). Therefore, the ability of Burkina Faso to accomplish the sustainable development goals by 2030 is further constraint by poor sanitation, water, and hygiene because untreated human defecation matters often make their way into the food chain and environmental habitat that are consumed by the citizens of the country (World Health Organization/UNICEF 2019).

The People's Democratic Government of Burkina Faso has made substantial progress in the provision drinking safe and managed drinking water, and urban sanitation since it formulated its National Water Supply and Sanitation Program in 2006 (International

Reference Center (IRC) report 2020; World Health Organization/UNICEF 2019). In spite of these new policy initiatives and partnerships with foreign donors, there still are other healthcare challenges that the nation needs to address. Further, to compound these predicaments, there are increasing relationship between poor sanitation, water, drought, and communicable diseases in the country. The increase in the nation's population constitutes another set of challenges of shortage of hospitals and health facilities in the country.

Healthcare Administration

The administration of healthcare in Burkina Faso is divided into three major areas. The *first level* is the central administration or the Ministry of Health of Burkina Faso. The central administration is made up of the minister's cabinet. This group is responsible for enacting and ensuring the implementation of all health policies in the country (Ministry of Health of Burkina Faso 2022). The second health administration sector is called the intermediate level.

The *intermediate level* is made up of regional health administrators who supervise health operations in more than 75 health districts in Burkina Faso. This group also includes district health management team health administrators who are responsible for ensuring the delivery of health services and programs in the regions.

The *third level* of health administration is at the community level. At this level, healthcare is provided by community-based organizations and civil society organizations that are licensed by the Government of Burkina Faso (Ministry of Health of Burkina Faso 2022). The senior health administrators at the community level also ensure that the necessary drugs and equipment are distributed to all healthcare centers as mandated by the central administration (Ministry of Health of Burkina Faso 2022); Strategic Health Purchasing in Burkina Faso policy brief (2021).

Types of Health Policy

There are many reasons why people engage in certain health behaviors in Burkina Faso. The nation's Ministry of Health has formulated several health policies to encourage changes in those behaviors. One of the mechanisms that the government of Burkina Faso has adopted is health policies. Below are selected national policies and laws that regulate or support healthy actions and practices for disease control, early detection, control, and the management of health facilities in Burkina Faso. Below are selected health policies that have been formulated and implemented in the People's Democratic Republic of Burkina Faso.

Community-Based Health Insurance Policy enacted in 2004: These are voluntary schemes that provide health coverage to informal sector workers and organized communities. Members ship fees are pooled to meet the cost of healthcare services for beneficiaries (Parmar et al. 2014).

Delegated Credits—Subsidy Policy enacted in 2006: The goal of the tax-financed grants is to provide public hospitals and clinics with guaranteed access to health services for the general population (Ministry of Health Burkina Faso 2012a; Ridde et al. 2011).

Transfer to Municipalities Policy enacted in 2010: The objective of the tax-financed grants is to provide municipalities with public hospitals and clinics with their district-appropriated budgets. Funds are used for infrastructure improvements and new equipment. Intergovernmental transfers for the health sector have increased over the past 13 years (Bargain et al. 2023; Cashin & Gatome-Munyua 2022).

Performance-Based Financing of Health enacted in 2011: This policy mandated the engagement of health providers in performance contracts to increase both the quantity and the quality of health service delivery in the country (Ministry of Health Burkina Faso 2012b).

National Free Healthcare Program for Pregnant Women and Children under Five Years Old (GRATUITÉ) enacted in 2016: This policy provides tax-financed user fees for free primary and hospital care for women and children under five years old at public hospitals and clinics and some accredited private facilities (Strategic Health Purchasing in Burkina Faso Policy Brief 2021).

Caisse Nationale d' Assurance Maladie Universelle (CNAMU) enacted in 2018: The CNAMU agency was established by the Government of Burkina Faso to ensure the transition of the management of health reimbursement from the Ministry of Health with the goal of promoting health effectiveness through CNAMU (Cashin & Gatome-Munyua 2022).

Universal Health Coverage (RAMU) enacted in 2020: This mandatory national health insurance scheme is intended to be the future vehicle for Universal Health Coverage for all in Burkina Faso. RAMU was officially launched in late 2020 to provide access to health services for the poor (Ministry of Health Burkina Faso 2022).

The "Gratuité" Health Policy enacted in 2016: This health policy provides free healthcare for pregnant women all over the country as well as children under five. The coverage of women's health also included screening and treatment for cervical cancer (Kiendrebeogo et al. 2022). However, because of the increased budget deficits and the decline in the quality of publicly subsidized health services. The government of Burkina Faso decided to stop the free healthcare service policy and introduce a new user fees health policy in 1990 (McPake et al. 1993; Ridde & Yameogo 2018). It should be noted however that the elimination of user fees policy started incrementally in the country in 2008 with major donations from international nongovernmental organizations (NGOs) (Ridde 2015).

Health Policy enacted in 2020: The health policy of 2020 mandated free women's family planning in all the regions of the country (Kiendrebeogo et al. 2022; Ministry of Health of Burkina Faso 2021). The goals of the 2016 and 2020 health policies, respectively, was to reduce the burden of maternal and infant mortality and morbidity rates in the country (Kiendrebeogo et al. 2022). Further, the intention of the Ministry of Health of Burkina Faso was to eliminate user fees to increase access to healthcare services for women and children under five years of age. With the Gratuité health policy provisions, the Government of Burkina Faso takes full responsibility for the payment of maternal health services for women and children of age five (Kiendrebeogo et al. 2022). Specifically, the Gratuité policy covers all health services for children as defined in the integrated management of childhood illness provisions. The policy covers all pregnant women's healthcare services such as antenatal and postnatal care, child deliveries, emergency, obstetric care, and cesarean sections (Cashin & Gatome-Munyua 2022). In addition, the health policy covers the treatment of obstetric fistulas and screening for pre-cancerous cervical lesions and breast cancer are covered for all women (Ridde 2015; Kiendrebeogo et al. 2022).

Data Analysis and Discussion

The respondents for this health policy analysis research in Burkina Faso include 273 (questionnaires) and 300 (interviewed) citizens and residents of the nation. The majority of the respondents are employed in both the public and private sectors in the country. A few of the respondents also worked for NGOs, and some multinational corporations. In addition, 126 of (46.2%) of the respondents were men, while the remaining 147 (53.8%) were female. Ten percent of the questionnaire respondents hold master's degrees. Another 12% earned a bachelor's degree, while 38% of them hold a high-school diploma. Further, 23% of the respondents had less than a high-school education. It was interesting to note that 62.6% of the respondents were single and young adults while 22% were married. A total of 45% of the interviewed respondents were employed in either a public or private organization. However, 55% partially work in the retail sector or are farmers. Fifty-three percent of the questionnaire respondents indicated that they had visited the hospital at least once or twice every year for treatment, while 25.6% stated that they had gone to see their doctor for three or four times due to complicated health issues. Among these respondents, 57.5% stated that the condition of the hospitals or health they had visited was good. However, only 36% of those who have visited health centers or hospitals indicated that the healthcare they received was poor. Table 1 is utilized to analyze the respondents' responses to the research questions.

Table 1 analyzes the patients' experience of the healthcare they received from hospitals and clinics in Burkina Faso. Sixty-nine percent of the respondents indicated that healthcare provided by doctors in the city is highly commendable. While 20% of the survey respondents stated that the doctors in the city where they received treatment did not practice good customer service and could not be praised for their unprofessional practice.

On one hand, 58% of the respondents also stated that the hospitals and health centers in their respective cities could not be rated as particularly good. On the other hand, 58% of the respondents also indicate that the government is effectively regulating medical professional licensing and disciplinary boards' competences and skills of medical practitioners in their city's hospitals. Fifty-four percent of the survey respondents stated that they could afford to pay for healthcare treatment and medication costs without government subsidies. However, 35% indicated that they cannot afford to pay for their treatment.

Table 1 The Nature of Healthcare Delivery and Policy in Burkina Faso

	Questions	Strongly Agree	Agree	Neutral	Strongly Disagree	Disagree	Agree %	Disagree %
1	Healthcare provided by doctors in my city is highly commendable	34	152	31	12	42	186 / **69%**	54 / **20%**
2	Most hospitals in my country do not have modern equipment	26	57	61	39	90	83 / **31%**	129 / **49%**
3	I can afford my Healthcare treatment and medication costs without government subsidies.	54	95	40	24	60	149 / **54%**	84 / **35%**
4	Most rural public hospitals in my country do not have specialist doctors and nurses.	107	94	42	2	13	201 / **79%**	13 / **5%**
5	Government pay of low salaries to doctors and nurses has encouraged their migration to foreign countries.	106	99	31	12	24	205 / **75%**	36 / **13%**
6	Lack of effective health policy implementation or regulations	96	91	35	14	30	187 / **70%**	44 / **17%**
7	Government promotes equity in the delivery of healthcare to underserved citizens in the country.	36	89	5	26	69	125 / **47%**	95 / **35%**
8	Political leaders and rich citizens of my country prefer to seek healthcare services in foreign nations.	133	83	30	9	17	216 / **86%**	26 / **10%**
9	Government is effectively regulating medical professional licensing and disciplinary boards	49	108	60	11	45	157 / **58%**	56 / **21%**
10	Hospitals and health centers in my city have constant electricity.	27	66	70	30	66	93 / **36%**	96 / **37%**
11	Lack of appropriate funding for the healthcare system in my country.	109	86	41	7	28	195 / **72%**	35 / **13%**
12	Corruption and unethical behavior of political and administrative leaders in government	149	79	31	2	9	228 / **84%**	11 / **4%**
	Mean						63.4	21.6%

Source: Derived from Field research in Burkina Faso in 2023 and 2024.

Eighty-six percent of the respondents stated that political leaders and rich citizens of my country prefer to seek healthcare services in foreign nations. While 84% of the questionnaire respondents also indicated that corruption and unethical behavior of political and administrative leaders in government constitute the reason that there is no political will to support the improvement of the nation's health system. On one hand, 36% of the respondents reported that hospitals and health centers in their city or town do not have constant electricity. On the other hand, 37% disagree that there is constant electricity in the hospitals in the city or town where they reside.

Lack of appropriate funding for the healthcare system in my country was reported by 72% of the respondents as the major reason Burkina Faso's healthcare delivery is not operating effectively. However, 13% of the respondents disagree. Another set of reasons why the health system in the country is not operating effectively was confirmed by 79% of the respondents to be lack of specialist doctors and nurses in most rural public hospitals in my country. Further, 75% of the respondents indicated that the low salary payment to doctors and nurses has encouraged their migration to foreign countries. Only 13% of the respondents disagreed that may not be the reason for health workforce migration to foreign countries.

The questionnaire respondents have mixed feelings about the condition of government hospitals and clinics in Burkina Faso. While 31% of the respondents agree that most of the hospitals and clinics do not have modern equipment and buildings are dilapidated, only 49% of the respondents disagreed that the condition of public healthcare facilities was not in bad shape. In addition, 56% of the respondents indicated that the public hospitals in the country do not have modern buildings, and the wards are not kept exceptionally clean.

In respect of the Government of Burkina Faso promoting equity in the delivery of healthcare to the underserved population of the country, 47% agreed while 35% disagree that the government has taken drastic steps to solve the disparity in access to healthcare between urban and rural districts in the country. On the other hand, 69% of the respondents indicate that the healthcare provided by doctors in their respective cities or towns is highly commendable. Healthcare provided by doctors in my city is highly commendable for their hospitality and customer services, only 20% of the questionnaire respondents disagreed the doctors and nurses who treated them behaved professionally and should be commended. The mean of the questionnaire respondents who agree that the healthcare system in Burkina Faso is effective is 63.4%, while the mean of those who disagree is 21.6%.

Table 2 data were derived from secondary sources to analyze the effectiveness of health policies and the healthcare delivery system in Burkina Faso. According to the World Bank Indicators (2022), and the United Nations Human Development Index (2021), the Government of Burkina Faso appropriates 6.72% of its GDP to finance the public healthcare system in the country in 2022. The amount that the Government of Burkina Faso has been budgeting for its health sector in the past few years is far below the 15% of GDP that all the African Union leaders agreed to at the 2001 Abuja Declaration submit. This shortage of the health budget will help to explain the current healthcare challenges in the country.

Table 2 Economics and Health Indicators in Burkina Faso

No.	Major Indicators in Cameroon	Explanation
1	Population	22.6 million (2022)
2	Gross domestic product (GDP)	US$18.82 billion (2022)
3	Gross domestic product (GDP) per capita	US$830 (2022)
4	Current health expenditure (% of GDP)	6.72% (2020)
5	Physicians/doctors per 10,000 people	0.1 (2019)
	Nurses and midwives per 10,000 people	0.9 (2019)
6	Hospital beds (per 1,000 people)	0.4 (2010)
7	Birth attended by skilled health workers (%)	80% (2015)
8	Population using least basic drinking water source % of population	50% urban; 35 rural (2022)
9	Sanitation facility access % of the population	Urban 12%; rural 9% (2022)
10	People practicing open defecation (% of the population)	34% (2022)
11	Common disease	(1) Malaria; (2) lower respiratory infections; (3) neonatal disorders; (4) diarrheal diseases; (5) ischemic heart disease; (6) tuberculosis; (7) congenital defects; (8) stroke; (9) meningitis
14	Life expectancy at birth 2020	59 years (2021)
15	Life expectancy in 2022 at birth for females	61 years (2021)
16	Life expectancy in 2022 at birth for males	57 years (2021)
17	Mortality rate for female adults (per 1,000 people)	246 (2021)
19	Mortality rate for male adults (per 1,000 people)	324 (2021)
	Mortality rate for infants (per 1,000 people)	52 (2021)
20	Tuberculosis incidence (per 100,000 people)	44 (2022)
21	Population living below income poverty line PPP $2.15 a day	31.2% (2018)
22	Poverty head count ratio at national poverty line (% of population)	41.4% (2018)
23	Multidimensional poverty index	83.3% (2021)
24	Infants' immunization measles (children 12–23 months old)	88% (2022)
25	Malaria incidence (per 1,000 people at risk)	376.8 (2021)
26	HIV/AIDS prevalence adults (% ages 15–49)	0.6% (2021)

Source: World Bank Indicators (2022). United Nations Human Development Index (2021); World Health Organization (2022a).

Conclusion

This chapter has examined the nature of healthcare and the major challenges in Burkina Faso. It also explored many of the health policies that have been enacted by the People's Democratic Republic of Burkina Faso government in the past three decades. The chapter attempts to close the gap in the literature on healthcare delivery and policy in both Africa and Burkina Faso, respectively. It specifically provided coverage beyond just discussing the role of donors in the delivery of healthcare in the country and major challenges, but effectively investigated the progressive efforts that the government of Burkina Faso has made in the mix of all the political, environmental, cultural, financial, and religious turbulence in the country.

Despite the progress accomplished thus far in health policies and implementation by the government of Burkina Faso, this study finding reveals that the nation is still struggling with healthcare-related resources such as medical equipment, qualified doctors, and nurses as well as very few functional hospitals or health centers in the rural regions in the country. Some of these challenges has been contrary to the health policies that has been enacted by the government of the country. As a result of these major healthcare capacity predicaments, it is recommended that the government invest in health measures that could help to reduce the high morbidity and mortality in most urban and rural regions in the country. An effective public health department or agency and a more vibrant public relations relation system to effectively communicate to all the citizens of the country especially those in the rural regions. An effective public relations campaign could help to promote precautionary health behavior in the country.

Further, it is paramount for the government to establish urgent policy solutions for the open medication problems in the country. The overwhelming high percentage of the citizens of the country do not have access to safely managed drinking water, modem sanitation, and hygienic toilets are serious health predicament. Thus, efforts to build public latrine structures in appropriate locations around the country could promote a better healthier environment.

Finally, apart from increasing the budget for the health system in the country, the Government of Burkina Faso needs to make more efforts to build more health facilities closer to the population of the country that is living in rural and remote villages or regions. There is also an urgent need to equip the health facilities in the country with modern medical equipment and technology. No nation can operate a good health system without highly qualified doctors, nurses, and other medical staff. Therefore, it is paramount for the Government of Burkina Faso to introduce new health policies for the training of more nurses and doctors in the country. There are two benefits for these new policies: (1) the policy can bestow trust and encourage more citizens to use the health services provided in the country; (2) the policy could also enhance the quality of primary healthcare in both the urban and rural regions all over the country; (3) the policy will also help to address the current challenges of the relationship between supply and demand factors and effective health coverage in the country. One other area that needs immediate action from the government of Burkina Faso is how to recruit and retain high-quality doctors and nurses. Some of the appropriate solutions include health policies that would provide health workers incentive programs: (1) scholarships for nurses and doctors to complete their medical training; (2) Salary bonus to work in a rural community for at least 3 years after graduation; (3). Provide accommodation and car allowance; and (4) better retirement benefits.

References

Ajayi, K. F., Dao, A., Koussoube, M. E. J. (2023). The Effects of Childcare on Women and Children: Evidence from a Randomized Evaluation in Burkina Faso. https://documents. worldbank.org/en/publication/documents-reports/documentdetail/099454207262315093/. Accessed September 3, 2024.

Ayeleke R. O., Dunham A., North N., Wallis K. (2018). The concept of leadership in the health care sector. Leadership, Suleyman Davut Goker, https://www.intechopen.com/books/leadership/theconcept-of-leadership-in-the-health-care sector. Accessed November 16, 2023.

Bargain O., Caldeira E., Vincent R. (2023). Shine a (night)light: Decentralization and economic development in Burkina Faso. ODI Working Paper. London: ODI www.odi.org/en/publications/shine-a-nightlight-decentralisation-and-economic-development-in-burkina-faso/. Accessed February 17, 2024.

Bocourun F. Y., Grimm M., Hartwig R. (2018). The health care burden in rural Burkina Faso: Consequences and implications for insurance design. *SSM Population Health*, 6, 309–316.

California Newsreel (2000). Sankara the right man. http://newsreel.org/nav/title.asp?tc-CN0205. Accessed November 13, 2023.

Cashin C, Gatome-Munyua A. (2022). The strategic health purchasing progress tracking framework: a practical approach to describing, assessing, and improving strategic purchasing for universal health coverage. *Health System Reform*, 8(2), e2051794. doi:10.1080/23288604.2022.2051794.

Gilbert M., Pullaano G., Pinotti F., Valdano E., Poletto C., Boelle P. Y., et al. (2020). Preparedness and vulnerability of African countries against importations of COVID-19: A modeling study. *Lancet*, 395(10227), 871–877.

GlobalEdge (2021). Burkina Faso: Introduction. https:/globalcdge.msu.edu/countries/burkina-faso/. Accessed January 16, 2024.

Harsch E. (2014). Resurrecting Thomas Sankara. https://www.thomassankar.1.net/resum;:cting-thomasankara/?lan=en. Accessed November 15, 2023.

International Reference Center (IRC) report (2020). Burkina Faso; Emergency watchlist. https:/www.rescue.org/site/default/files/documentl4343/ircemeruencywatchlist2020c.pdf. Accessed November 20, 2023.

Kiendrebeogo J. A., Tapsoba C., Kafando Y., Kabore I., Sory O., Yameogo S. P. (2022). The Landscape of strategic health purchasing for universal health coverage in Burkina Faso: Insights from five major health financing schemes. *Health System Reform*, 8(2), 20–49.

Kouanda S., Yameogo W. M., Ridde V., Sombie I., Baya B., Bicaba A., Traore A., Sondo B. (2014). An exploratory analysis of the regionalization policy for the recruitment of health workers in Burkina Faso. *Human Resources for Health*, 12(supplement 1), 1–8.

Maclean R., Marks S., (2020). African countries have no ventilators: That's only part of the problem. *New York Times*, (May 18), 1–2.

Meda Z. C., Ilboundo B., Hien H., Kabore S., Karama R., Nitiema A., Outtara O., Konate I., et al. (2020). International Research Journal of Public and Environmental Health. https:i/www.ioumalis.-;ues.org/IRJPEH. Accessed November 15, 2023.

Meda M. B., Baguiya A., Ridde V., Ouedraogo H. G., Dumont A., Kouanda S. (2019). Out-of pocket payments in the context of a free maternal health care policy in Burkina Faso: A national cross-sectional survey. *Health Economic Review*, (9–11), 1–14.

Mcpake B., Hanson K., Mills A. (1993). Community financing of healthcare in Africa: An evaluation of the Bamako initiative. *Social Science Medicine*, 36(11), 1383–1395.
Ministry of Health of Burkina Faso (2022). Think Well. Retro information on graduate scheme. GDS Bulletin; no. 6. January to December 2021. Ouagadougou (BF): Thinkwell Global https://thinkwell.globahvpcontcnt/upkiads i20..,2i04/Bulletin-GDS N%C2'%B06 05042022 English.pdf. Accessed June 26, 2023.
Ministry of Health Burkina Faso (2012a). *Burkina Faso: Make Maternal Carefree for All Women in Ouagadougou*. Burkina Faso: Ministry of Health Publication.
Ministry of Health Burkina Faso (2012b). *Performance-Based Financing of Health in Burkina Faso*. Ouagadougou, Burkina Faso: Ministry of Health Publication.
Ministry of Health Burkina Faso (2007). *Burkina Faso: Make Maternal Carefree for All Women in Ouagadougou*. Burkina Faso: Ministry of Health Publication.
Omar F. (2007). Commemorating Thomas Sankara. http://www.zcommunicaiions.org/commemorating-thomassankara-by-farid-omar. Accessed November 14, 2021.
Parmar D., De Allegri M., Savadogo G., Sauerborn R. (2014). Do community-based health insurance schemes fulfil the promise of equity? A study from Burkina Faso. *Health Policy and Planning*, 29(1), 76–84.
Public Policy Plus (2020). Burkina Faso: Overview, better policy for better health. https://www.healthpolicyplus.com/BurkinaFaso.cfm. Accessed February 15, 2024.
Quedraogo M., Rouamba T., Samadoulougou S., Samadoulougou S. (2020). Effect of free healthcare policy for children under five on the incidence of reported malaria cases in Burkina Faso by Bayesian modelling: Not only the ears but the health of the hippopotamus. *International Journal of Environmental Research and Public Health*, 17(417), 1–23.
Ridde V., Yameogo P. (2018). How Burkina Faso used evidence in deciding to launch its policy of free healthcare for children under five and women in 2016. *Palgrave Communications*, 4(1). DOI: 10.1057/s41599-018-0173-x. Accessed January 26, 2024.
Ridde V. (2015). From institutionalization of user fees to their abolition in West Africa: A story of pilot projects and public policies. *BMC Health Services Research*, 15(Suppl 3), S6. DOI: I0.1186/1472-6963-15-S3-S6.
Ridde V., Richard F., Bicaba A., Queuille L., Conombo G. (2011). The national subsidy for deliveries and emergency obstetric care in Burkina Faso. *Health Policy Plan*, 26(Suppl 2), 30–40. DOI: 10.1093/heapol/czr060.
Skrip L., Derra K., Kaboré M., Noori N., Gansané A., Valéa I., Tinto H., Brice B. W., Gordon M. V., Hagedorn B., Hien H., Althouse B. M., Wenger E. A., Ouédraogo A. L. (2020). Clinical management and mortality among COVID-19 cases in sub-Saharan Africa: A retrospective study from Burkina Faso and simulated case analysis. *International Journal of Infectious Diseases*, 101, 194–200.
Strategic health purchasing in Burkina Faso policy brief (2021). https://span:.africa.\vp-contentfuploadsi 2021/06/SPARC_policy_Brief_BURK.INA_FASO_LS.pdf. Accessed April 10, 2023.
Mc Sween-Cadieux E., Dagenais C., Somé D. T., Ridde V. (2019). A health knowledge brokering intervention in a district of Burkina Faso: A qualitative retrospective implementation analysis. *PLoS One*, Jul 26; 14(7), e0220105. doi: 10.1371/journal.pone.0220105. PMID: 31349363; PMCID: PMC6660220.
United Nations Human Development Report (2021). Burkina Faso. https://www.undp.orgJjordan/publications/undp-human-development-repon-2020. Accessed August 25, 2023.
United States Agency for International Development (USAID) (2020). Burkina Faso: Water and Sanitation Profile. https://www.usaid.gov. Accessed May 15, 2023.
United Nations Development Programmme (2020). *Human Development Report 2020: Sustainability and Equity*. UNDP, New York: United Nations Press.
World Bank Indicator (2023). Burkina Faso. https://data.worldbank.org/indicator/SH.IMM. MEAS?locations=BF. Accessed February 17, 2024.

World Bank Indicators (2022) Explore databases. https://databank.worldbank.org/. Accessed August 29, 2024.

World Factbook (2020). Burkina Faso. https://www.cia.gov/the-world-factbook/about/cover-gallery/2020-cover/. Accessed September 3, 2024.

World Health Organization (2020a). Burkina Faso. Health? https//www.who.intihealth-cluster-wuntrii,burkina-faso,/en. Accessed January 30, 2024.

World Health Organization (2020b). *Coronavirus Disease (COVID-19): Weekly Epidemiological Update*. Geneva: World Health Organization Publication.

World Health Organization/UNICEF (2019). Burkina Faso: Global data on Water Supply, Sanitation and Hygiene (WASH). https://washdata.org!data. Accessed May 17, 2021.

Zombre D., De Allegri M., Riddle V. (2017). Immediate and sustained effects of user fee exemption on healthcare utilization among children under five in Burkina Faso: A controlled interruption time-series analysis. *Social Science & Medicine*, 179, 27–25.

Chapter Five

ANALYSIS OF HEALTHCARE POLICY IN CAMEROON

Robert Dibie, Peter Ngwafu, and Emmanuel Okonmah

Introduction

This chapter attempts to examine citizens' perceptions of the nature of health policies and the effectiveness of the healthcare delivery system in Cameroon. Healthcare administration in Cameroon is organized at the national, regional, and district levels with the Ministry of Public Health responsible for overseeing the healthcare system, and assisted by several agencies, including the National Health Insurance Fund, the National AIDS Control Committee, performance-based financing, a voucher system, private health insurance, and a mutual health organization. All these entities are expected to work together to implement policies and programs to improve the well-being of Cameroonians. This chapter argues that while there has been some improvement in healthcare administration in Cameroon over the past several decades, challenges persist. Such challenges include inadequate funding, a shortage of skilled healthcare professionals, disparities in healthcare access, and inadequate compensation system for healthcare and professionals, the other major health system challenges in the century include mismanagement of funds allocated for critical health programs and the political conflict between English and French-speaking citizens of the country.

The research findings reveal that the political instability between English- and French-speaking citizens in Cameroon has negatively impacted the health system in the country. The disparity in funding of healthcare services between the above two groups has also negatively affected the development of healthcare standards and the effective implementation of health policies in the country. Although the disparity between rural and urban healthcare delivery systems has been acknowledged for more than two decades, the government and healthcare leaders have done little to improve access to affordable healthcare services in the country. Some health policy recommendation is provided that could help the government to engage in a peaceful win–win conflict resolution process to bring the conflict between the English- and French-speaking groups dispute. The resolution of the existing conflict could also minimize the disparities in funding healthcare institutions, improve modern healthcare awareness, and minimize gender inequality in the provision of health services to all its citizens.

Brief History

The Republic of Cameroon is a country in Central Africa. The nation has boundaries with Nigeria in the west, the Central African Republic in the east, the Republic of Chad in the north, the Republic of Congo, the Democratic Republic of Equatorial Guinea, and the Gabon Republic to the South. The Atlantic Ocean and the Bight of Biafra are in the southern part of Cameroon (Dibie 2018; Government of Cameroon 2015). The Republic of Cameroon has a population of approximately 29.3 million people in 2022 (Global Edge 2023; British Broadcasting Corporation 2023).

African ethnic groups initially settled in the Cameroon region over 150,000 years ago. The archaeological evidence of human settlement dates from around 30,000 years ago at Shum Laka (Lavachery 2001). Further, the Bamenda highlands that are in the western part of Cameroon are reported to be the possible original settlement of the Bantu people of Africa (Cornelissen 2003). Over the past 150 decades, the Bantu culture and language have spread from Cameroon to Central, East, and Southern Africa (Lavachery et al. 2010). Before Europeans arrived in the Cameroon region, the northern part of the territory was highly influenced by the Islamic kingdoms around the Lake Chad basin and the Sahel Savanah (Ityavyar 1987; Lavachery 2001).

Western European explorers and traders started visiting the Cameroon region in the fifteenth century after the Bantu people had inhabited the region for more than 15,000 years (Awasom 1998; Trillo & Hudgens 1999; Wikipedia 2023). The Portuguese were the first group of Europeans that arrived at the Cameroon coast in the fifteenth century. The Portuguese were initially interested in the Rio dos Camaroes River because of the abundant ghost shrimps that were found there (Cornelissen 2003; Lavachery et al. 2010). Eventually, the European interest escalated to the slave trade of the Bantu people of Cameroon (Ardener 1962; Ityavyar 1987). On the other hand, the southern regions of Cameroon were divided into kingdoms that were mostly ruled by Kings and Chieftains (Government of Cameroon 2015; Ityavyar 1987).

Between November 15, 1884, and February 26, 1885, Otto von Bismarck, the first Chancellor of Germany, organized a Berlin Conference following instructions from King Leopold II (Chamberlain 2014; Crowe 1942). At the Berlin conference, European powers decided to divide the African continent into spheres of influence for themselves. During World War I, Britain and France defeated German explorers living in the Cameroon region in 1919. This outcome of World War I, galvanized Britain, and France to occupy the region now called Cameroon. Further, the governments of the United Kingdom and France signed a League of Nations Agreement in 1919 (Ardener 1962). According to Yanou and Foyam (2008), Cameroon was divided under the London Declaration, and France was granted 80% of the country, while Britain received only 20% of the original land size of Cameroon (BBC News 2023; Yanou & Foyam 2008). In addition, the mandate or agreement merged the British-Cameroon colonial administration to Nigeria. On the other hand, the French-Cameroon colonial administration was administered from Yaounde, Cameroon's current national capital city (Ardener 1962; Nzim 2014).

After many deliberations, it was decided that a referendum should be conducted to determine whether the English-speaking British-Cameroon citizens in Southern

Cameroon should join the French Cameroon people to form a new federation. The results of the referendum were announced on February 12, 1960. The vote from the referendum revealed that the British Southern Cameroons had voted for unification with the French Republic of Cameroon. The outcome of the positive vote was later referred to as "reunification" (Ardener 1962; Delancey et al. 2004).

Subsequently, a conference was organized in Foumban by the British-Cameroon and French Cameroon political leaders. At the conference that took place on July 16–21, 1961, John Ngu Foncha represented the English Southern Cameroon people while Ahidjo represented the French-Cameron delegation (Johnson 1970). The agreement reached at the conference called for a federal structure granting former British Cameroons—now West Cameroon—authority over certain issues and procedural rights. Further, Buea City became the capital of British West Cameroon while Yaounde was also chosen to be the new federal capital and East Cameroon's capital city. According to Ardener (1962) and Delancey et al. (2010), both parties did not get what they desired. It has been reported that Ahidjo had wanted a unitary or more centralized state, while on the other hand, the English-speaking West Cameroon people wanted more federal system of government and protections (Mackenzie 1983). Furthermore, the new federal system of government and constitution was adopted on August 14, 1961. Subsequently, Ahmadou Ahidjo was elected the first president of the Federal Republic of Cameroon. While John Foncha was also elected the prime minister of West Cameroon and vice president of the Federal Republic of Cameroon (Ardener 1962; Awasom 1998; Delancey et al. 2010; Nzim 2014).

As a result of the outcome of a 1970 national referendum, Cameroon switched from a federal to a unitary state and became known as the United Republic of Cameroon (British Broadcasting Corporation 2023). In 1982, the former Prime Minister after John Foncha, Paul Biya, succeeded Ahidjo, as President of the country. Ahidjo resigned, only to flee the country the following year after Paul Biya accused him of masterminding a coup (Yanou & Foyam 2008, Trillo & Hudgens 1999). Paul Biya was elected President in 1984 and changed the name of the country to the Republic of Cameroon (BBC New 2023). He has served as the leader of Cameroon for more than four decades. Since 1984, the Government of Cameroon has been operated like a monarchy or a dictatorship whereby the chief of state is the president, and the head of government, and there are no term limits (Delancey et al. 2010; Dibie 2018).

Healthcare Challenges

Before Cameroon became an independent nation the western region of the country that was under the British colonial administration had a well-developed health system that was mostly located in the urban and coastal regions (Ityavyar 1987; Nzim 2014). This British colonial approach to healthcare delivery created disparities in the region because people living in rural areas did not have access to modern healthcare and had to depend on traditional medicine for treatment. There were also religious health clinics that were established to supplement the colonial administration's health system. As of 1960, 47% of the hospitals in the British Cameroon region were Christian mission-operated. Further, by 1946, the British colonial government had established a University College with academic departments such as dental technology, dental hygienists, internal medicine, pharmacy, and medical laboratory (Chapnkem 2019; Egbe 2014).

The World Health Organization report (1963) indicated that in 1960 when Cameroon became an independent nation, there were 2,184 nurses and nursing assistants, 159 doctors, 46 pharmacists, and 45 midwives serving a population of over 5.12 million people (Population Pyramids 2022). During the same period in 1960, there were 72 dispensaries, 58 health centers, and 4 hospitals in Cameroon (Government of Cameroon 2001). In addition, it has also been reported that between 1870 and 1936 while the British administration funded 77% of Black African investment in Africa, the French only funded 5.2% in the African continent (Coquery-Vidrovitch 1985; Delancey et al. 2010).

The Government of Cameroon's Ministry of Health Sector Strategy 2016–2027 reported that the health insurance coverage policy that the government passed in December 2012 was intended to be a mechanism for low-income citizens of the country to have access to healthcare. However, the economic challenges in Cameroon have led to low budget appropriations in the health sector in Cameroon. Another challenge is that of revenue collection to finance the healthcare system in the country. Only about 90% of the citizens who work in the informal sector in the country do not pay taxes (Agbor-Tabi 1984; Cheno et al. 2021; Ondoa 2018). Another set of challenges include the fact that most of the citizens of Cameroon spend about 68% of their annual income on healthcare. Thus, those low-income citizens who cannot afford the out-of-pocket expenses face the risk of a high mortality rate (Cheno et al. 2021; Government of Cameroon Ministry of Health Sector Strategy 2016–2027; Nguefack et al. 2016; Ntembe et al. 2021). Furthermore, most of the uneducated and low-income populations of Cameroon do not understand or are not aware of the importance of health insurance. It has also been argued that the government of the country has not done an excellent job of increasing awareness of the benefits of the health insurance schemes in Cameroon (Cheno et al. 2021). On the other hand, while the Abuja Declaration that the Government of Cameroon co-signed mandated at least 15% of government budget allocation annually for healthcare, the nation has only appropriated a budget of 5%–5.5% or less over the past few years (Government of Cameroon Ministry of Health Sector Strategy 2016). According to Ojongo (2019), the poor or low-income residents of Cameroon have also developed different methods to finance their respective healthcare costs.

Apart from the low funding of the health sector in Cameroon, the Ministry of Health has not been effective in preventing the duplication of health resources and waste in spending due to a lack of appropriate monitoring to maximize the use of public funds. Other challenges that the Ministry of Health in Cameroon faces include ineffective regulations or implementation of policies, low political will, poor management, and the lack of good health infrastructure, as well as basic equipment (Government of Cameroon Ministry of Health Sector Strategy 2016–2027; Government of Cameroon Ministry of Health Sector Strategy 2001 & 2015).

According to Cannata et al. (2022) and Ray et al. (2017), most of the district health centers in Cameroon are not capable of effectively treating disabled patients who suffer problems such as infectious diseases and neurological disabilities. In addition, many district health clinics in the country do not provide treatment for hemiparesis, hemiplegia, and monoplegia because of vehicle accidents or previous inappropriate medical treatment by non-specialist doctors (Cannata et al. 2022; Foti et al. 2016). Also, while the healthcare system in any country is supposed to promote equity among its citizens, the situation in Cameroon is that there is a lack of empathy for a reimbursement system for healthcare for the nation's poor or disabled citizens (Cannata et al. 2022; Country Report 2023; Ray et al. 2017).

During the period of Structural Adjustment programs (SAP) in the 1980s and early 1990s, Cameroon's healthcare system had a significant shortage of medical doctors and nurses. After the economic crisis created by SAP, the nation continues to experience human resources impediments such as a lack of well-trained healthcare specialists and a lack of financial resources to support the policy-making process. These challenges also negatively led to a very weak governance system in the country that could effectively formulate and implement health policies (Saidu et al. 2023). The reform that took place in the 1990s also escalated the suspension of the recruitment of a vibrant healthcare workforce as well as the lack of development in the health infrastructure (Saidu et al. 2023; Tandi et al. 2015).

The medical informational technology system is not effectively practiced in Cameroon. The lack of telemedicine is particularly worse in rural districts, as well as communities where there have been English-speaking and French-speaking citizens' conflicts in Cameroon (Ngo-Bibaa 2020). In addition, one of the barriers to having access to information computer technology in Cameroon is the cost. It has been argued that low-income people who earn less than the minimum wage in the country cannot afford to have access to telemedicine services nor afford to pay for an internet connection (Government of Cameroon Ministry of Health 2020; Ngo-Bibaa 2020). This is happening despite the fact that telemedicine or digital health technology has enormous potential for faster evidence-based healthcare in Cameroon, as well as improving the quality and accessibility of healthcare service delivery to the poor Cameroon population that cannot afford the cost (Association of Cameroonian Physicians in the Americas 2020; Awondo 2020; Pamen & Yepndo 2017). As the population of Cameroon is increasing to about 30 million people it may not be possible for the government of the nation to take care of such a massive population with limited hospitals and clinics (Ako et al. 2015; Ateghang-Awankem & Atanga 2022; Witter et al. 2017).

Health Policies

The Government of Cameroon, just like those of many developing countries, tends to perceive its citizens' health as a mechanism for promoting human rights and social justice (Government of Cameroon Ministry of Public Health 2012 & 2015). Because of the government's value for human rights and the unprecedented era of communicable and noncommunicable diseases that have plagued the nation in the past three decades, there continue to be various forms of health policies that have been enacted but not effectively implemented. Below are some of the major health policies that have been formulated but partially implemented by the Republic of Cameroon Government.

Universal Health Coverage Policy of 2012: This policy was enacted by the Republic of Cameroon Government on December 12, 2012. The main goal of universal health coverage is to ensure that all the citizens and residents of Cameroon have access to the preventive, curative, palliative rehabilitation, and health promotion services they need. The policy mandates that the implementation of healthcare services should be made to have sufficient quality to be efficient without the cost being a burden to citizens and residents of Cameroon no matter their income levels. (Government of Cameroon Ministry of Health 2011 & 2012).

The 2015–2017 Triennial Emergency Plan Policy: The purpose of this policy was to foster the construction and rehabilitation of referral hospitals in all regions in Cameroon as well as the development of basic social infrastructure in the country. The policy was also enacted to provide innovative health financing initiatives such as performance-based financing, health cheques, obstetric kits, values for results, and so on (Government of Cameroon Ministry of Health 2015).

The 2016–2027 Health Sector Strategy Policy: was enacted to accelerate the development of human capital for growth and sustainable development in line with the indications and recommendations of the DESP. The policy was also formulated to complement the United Nations' sustainable development goals by accelerating the implementation of the new universal health coverage in the country (Government of Cameroon Ministry of Health 2016; Kamgnia 2006).

The 2020–2024 National Digital Health Strategic Plan Policy: The goal of this policy is to ensure that by 2024 digital health could galvanize better universal health coverage in Cameroon through informed decision making at central, intermediate, and peripheral levels of the health system in the country. The policy will constitute a new mechanism for improving the quality of health services and the accessibility of health services in all districts and financial endeavors in Cameroon (Government of Cameroon Ministry of Health 2020).

Vision 2035 Policy of 2009: The Vision 2035 policy was formulated to make Cameroon an emerging country by 2035 (Government of Cameroon, Ministry of Economy, Planning and Regional Development 2009). Therefore, the goal of Vision 2035 was based on the Republic of Cameroon Government's intention to accomplish the reduction of poverty at socially acceptable levels. It was also anticipated that Vision 2035 could help Cameroon to become a middle-income country by 2035 (Climate Change Radar 2009; United Nations. 2021).

Health Administration

The Government of Cameroon's Minister of Public Health is responsible for implementing all health policies enacted by the National Parliament. The Ministry of Public Health is regarded as a specialized technical body that comprised an executive board, the permanent secretariat, and two advisory boards, namely the Steering Committee and the Scientific Council (Ndoungue et al. 2022; Saidu et al. 2022). This administration of the health system in the Republic of Cameroon is divided into three levels. To further complicate the health administration system in the country, the public health facilities in Cameroon are also organized into the following seven groups (1) general hospitals, (2) central hospitals, (3) regional hospitals; (4) district hospitals; (5) district medical centers, (6) integrated health centers; and (7) ambulatory health centers (Ojongo 2019).

First, the *central level* covers all the administrative activities that take place at the headquarters of the Ministry of Public Health in Yaoundé. Its functions include the enactment or formulation of health policies, and strategies, as well as the coordination of how health policies are implemented and regulated all over the country (Ministry of Public Health in Cameroon 2020).

The second level is called the intermediate health sector. This sector is represented by 10 regional delegations of public health management boards that coordinate health activities in the different provincial administrative groups. The regional delegation board also provides technical support to health districts (Ministry of Public Health in Cameroon 2020).

Third is *the peripheral level*. This level provides healthcare services in all the districts around the country. There are 189 health districts and 5,284 health areas in the country. Each health district comprised a health center that serves as the first point of contact for patients. The health districts also have one hospital that could refer sick citizens to higher-level health centers. The *district health office* and administrators coordinate and supervise all public healthcare centers. According to the Republic of Cameroon's 2020–2024 National Digital Health Strategic Plan (2020), the Government of Cameroon has about 2,282 clinics and 146 district hospitals spread all over the country. Most of the district hospitals are managed by medical doctors and registered nurses. It has also been a widespread practice for medical doctors who are deployed to district hospitals to be general practice specialists (Ngo-Bibaa 2020). Unfortunately, the ratio of nurse to patient is 1 to 4,260 patients. On the other hand, the ratio of doctors to patients is 1 to 15,939 patients. This high ratio of doctor-to-patient predicament has also resulted in high mortality rates in districts around Cameroon (Ngo-Bibaa 2020; Republic of Cameroon 2020–2024 National Digital Health Strategic Plan 2020).

There are three health sectors in Cameroon. The sectors include (a) public; (b) private; and (c) traditional sectors (Republic of Cameroon 2020–2024 National Digital Health Strategic Plan 2020). These private health centers, hospitals, and clinics are operated by religious organizations, nongovernmental organizations as well as traditional health institutions in Cameroon (Ojongo 2019; Sieleunou et al. 2021). The nature of healthcare implementation of multiple schemes is unnecessarily constrained by the lack of clarity on the responsibilities of the different administrative structures in the Ministry of Health.

Data Analysis and Discussion

The objective of this chapter is to examine citizens' perceptions of the nature of health policies and the effectiveness of the healthcare delivery system in Cameroon. The data used for the analysis of healthcare policy effectiveness were derived from both primary and secondary research methods. The primary research involves the administration of a questionnaire to 150 respondents. One hundred and twenty-eight which is 85.3% of respondents returned their completed questionnaire. The questionnaire respondents constitute 55% men and 45% women. In addition, 59% of the respondents had visited a hospital or clinic to receive treatment at least twice a year. Another 41% had also visited a hospital or healthcare clinic between 2 and 4 times within a year time to receive treatment. Data were analyzed using SPSS to determine the effectiveness of healthcare delivery, and challenges facing the implementation of health policy in the Republic of Cameroon. The secondary research methods adopted include content analysis of the Government of Cameroon Ministry of Health's Public Health reports, World Bank, Development Initiatives report, the World Health Organization reports, United Nations Human Development Index annual report, Center for Disease Control, Country Report, and United States Agency for International Development, academic as well as professional journals articles.

Table 1 analyzes the nature of health challenges and how effective the healthcare policies enacted by the Government of Cameroon have been. The result of the questionnaire reveals that 76% of the respondents agree that the lack of effective health policy implementation or regulations is a major challenge to effective healthcare delivery in the country. Another 72.6% of the respondents reported that political leaders and rich citizens of the country prefer to seek healthcare services in foreign nations. Further, 72% of the questionnaire respondents agree that corruption and unethical behavior of political and senior administrative leaders in government is one of the reasons why the health delivery system in Cameroon is not amazingly effective. On one hand, 74.2% of the respondents indicated that healthcare provided by doctors in some cities is highly commendable, while only 22.6% of the citizens agreed that some doctors' practices in the country are not highly commendable. On the other hand, 69.5% of the questionnaire respondents also agree that most hospitals in Cameroon do not have modern equipment. In addition, 65% of the respondents confirmed that the lack of appropriate funding for the healthcare system in Cameroon is a major challenge to the poor health delivery system in the country.

In addition, 65.6% of the respondents disagree that hospitals and health centers in their cities have constant electricity. While only 32% of the respondents who mostly live in urban cities agree that the hospitals in their cities constantly have electricity. With respect to the affordability of healthcare in Cameroon, 63.3% of the respondents disagree that they can afford their healthcare treatment and medication costs without government subsidies. In addition, 57% of the respondents agree that most rural public hospitals in Cameroon do not have specialist doctors and nurses, while 32.8% of the respondents acknowledge that they have received healthcare treatment from some specialist doctors in their rural districts. Another major challenge in the health system in Cameroon is the retention of health workforce personnel.

Sixty-four percent of the respondents agree that the Government of Cameroon's payment of low salaries to doctors and nurses has encouraged their migration to foreign countries. Meanwhile, 62.8% of the respondents disagree that the Government of Cameroon promotes equity in the delivery of healthcare to underserved citizens in the country. Furthermore, 61.7% of the respondents also disagree that the Government of Cameroon is effectively regulating medical professional licensing and disciplinary boards. The mean of agree, in terms of low health delivery system, is 51.8%, while the disagree is 48.6%. Thus, the general perception of the citizens of Cameroon is that the healthcare system in the country is not effective.

Table 1 The Nature of Healthcare Delivery and Policy in Cameroon

Questions	Strongly Agree	Agree	Neutral	Strongly Disagree	Disagree	Agree %	Disagree %
1 Healthcare provided by doctors in my city is highly commendable	7	22	4	35	60	29 22.6%	95 74.2%
2 Most hospitals in my country do not have modern equipment	27	62	9	13	17	89 69.5%	30 23.4%
3 I can afford my healthcare treatment and medication costs without government subsidies.	11	25	11	32	49	36 28.1%	81 63.3%
4 Most rural public hospitals in my country do not have specialist doctors and nurses.	35	48	3	12	30	73 57%	42 32.8%
5 Government pay of low salaries to doctors and nurses has encouraged their migration to foreign countries.	26	56	4	15	27	82 64%	42 32.8%
6 Lack of effective health policy implementation or regulations	38	59	6	12	13	97 76%	25 19.5%
7 Government promotes equity in the delivery of healthcare to underserved citizens in the country.	9	31	8	13	67	40 31.2%	80 62.8%
8 Political leaders and rich citizens of my country prefer to seek healthcare services in foreign nations.	24	69	3	2	30	93 72.6%	32 25%
9 Government is effectively regulating medical professional licensing and disciplinary boards	11	29	9	18	61	40 31.3%	79 61.7%
10 Hospitals and health centers in my city have constant electricity.	12	29	3	33	51	41 32%	84 65.6%
11 Lack of appropriate funding for the healthcare system in my country.	27	56	3	14	28	83 65%	42 32.8%
12 Corruption and unethical behavior of political and administrative leaders in government	24	68	5	5	27	92 72%	32 25%
Mean						51.8%	48.6%

Source: Derived from field research in Nigeria in 2023 and 2024.

Table 2 Economics and Health Indicators in Cameroon

No.	Major Indicators in Cameroon	Explanation
1	Population	29.3 million (2022)
2	Gross domestic product (GDP)	US$45.3 billion (2021)
3	GDP per capita	US$1,666.93 (2021)
4	Current health expenditure (% of GDP)	4.7%
5	Nurses and midwives per 10,000 people	0.4 (2018)
6	Physicians/doctors per 10,000 people	0.1 (2018)
7	Birth attended by skilled health workers (%)	69%
8	Drinking water source % of population	94.1 Urban; 51.9 rural (2022)
9	Access to safe clean water	70 Urban; 47 rural regions (2022)
10	Population with managed drinking water service 30 minutes from their residents	Urban 15%; rural 18%
11	Sanitation facility access % of the population	61.7% Urban; 26.8 rural
12	Common disease	HIV/AIDS, malaria, respiratory infections, neonatal disorders, tuberculosis, diarrheal diseases
13	Life expectancy at birth	59.3 years (2022)
14	Life expectancy at birth for females	64 years (2022)
15	Life expectancy at birth for males	60 years (2022)
16	Mortality rate for female adults (per 1,000 people)	281 (2021)
17	Mortality rate for infants (per 1,000 people)	50.1 (2021)
18	Mortality rate for male adults (per 1,000 people)	318 (2021)
19	Tuberculosis incidence (per 100,000 people)	186.0
20	Population living below income poverty line PPP $2.15 a day	23.8 (2022)
21	Population in multidimensional head count poverty (%)	45.3% (2022)
22	Contribution deprivation in health to multidimensional poverty index	23.2% (2021)
23	Infants lacking immunization for measles (5 of one and older)	40% (2022)
24	Malaria incidence (per 1,000 people at risk)	247 (2022)
25	HIV/AIDS prevalence adults (% ages 15–49)	3.6% (2022)

Source: World Bank Indicators (2022); United Nations Human Development Index (2021); World Health Organization (2023a).

Table 2 data were derived from secondary sources to analyze the effectiveness of health policies and the healthcare delivery system in Cameroon. According to the World Health Organization report (2023a) and the United Nations Human Development Index (2021), the Government of Cameroon appropriates between 4.7% and 5.5% of its GDP to finance the public healthcare system in the country in the past few years. In 2020, the Government of Cameroon also spent 3.77% of its GDP on healthcare (World Bank 2022). The amount that the Government of Cameroon has been budgeting for its health sector in the past few years is far below the 15% of GDP that all the African Union leaders agreed to at the 2001 Abuja Declaration submit. This shortage of the health budget will help to explain the current healthcare challenges in the country.

In 2018, the physician/doctor ratio per 1,000 people was 0.1, while the ratio of nurses and midwives per 1,000 people was 0.4 in 2018 (World Bank Indicators 2022; World Health Organization Report 2023b). Further, the drinking water source for the population in the urban areas is 94.1%, however, those in the rural areas of Cameroon only have 51.9% access to drinking water. In addition, only 70% of the population in urban areas in Cameroon had access to safe drinking water in 2022, while only 47% of the residents in the rural districts had access to safe drinking water. It is interesting to note that 6% of the nation's population still engages in open defecation (Word Bank Indicator 2022; United Nations Human Development Index 2023). Furthermore, the percentage of the Cameroon population that has access to sanitation facilities is reported to be 61.7% in the urban cities and 26.8% in the rural districts of the country (World Bank Indicators 2022; World Health Organization Report 2023b). The poorest population that lives in both the urban and rural regions of Cameroon are more likely to engage in the practice of open defecation (British Broadcasting Corporation 2023). The overall life expectancy in 2021 was 60.3 years, while the life expectancy at birth for females in 2022 was 63 years, and that for males was 59 years, in 2022 (British Broadcasting Corporation 2023).

Conclusion

This chapter has attempted to analyze the health policies and administration of healthcare in Cameroon. It argues that despite the Cameroon government's national health insurance, performance-based financing, voucher system, private health insurance, and mutual health organization, the nation continues to experience a low rate of health infrastructure, and a shortage of health professionals due to political conflict between English- and French-speaking citizens of the country. The citizens of Cameroon continue to receive, inadequate social services. The lack of a vibrant government institution and leadership has negatively affected its healthcare system. Furthermore, the political instability between the French- and English-speaking parts of the country has negatively affected the healthcare system in the country. The old and ineffective President Paul Biya seems not to have the leadership capacity to lead the country toward accomplishing the nation's strategic plan goals that have, so far, been poorly implemented. Condoling the corruption of his cronies in the nation's government has negatively affected the health delivery system in Cameroon. Furthermore, low-income citizens who cannot afford out-of-pocket expenses continue to face the risk of high mortality rates. Therefore, it could be more effective to consolidate economic growth policies with poverty reduction strategies in Cameroon. Moving forward toward sustainable development in the country requires reviewing policies that could enhance the disposable income of poor citizens, especially those living in the rural regions.

The data analysis of the healthcare policy and delivery system in Cameroon after independence in 1960, reveals that the different financing models adopted by the Government are convoluted and not assigned with set objectives. This is due to the French colonial administration model that was adopted by the current Government of Cameroon. Moving forward, the Government of Cameroon should adopt a new governance arrangement with a comprehensive oversight mandate that could ensure compliance with health insurance purchase regulations and accountability laws. The Ministry of Public Health also needs to establish a new health administration mechanism that could promote visibility, continuity, and consistency in all sectors of healthcare.

This analysis also reveals that currently there are inadequate healthcare workers in different geographical locations of the country. This disparity in the distribution of health workers between different geographical districts in Cameroon could be resolved by providing long-distance consultancy and clinical help using digital healthcare or telemedicine. It is recommended that the Government of Cameroon should provide more access to digital healthcare by developing information computer technology that is aligned with digital health infrastructure all over the Country. Such an inclusive information technology initiative could complement the universal health coverage policy that was enacted in 2022. It should be noted that inclusive fiscal and monetary policies are needed to stimulate the promotion of economic growth and share prosperity for all the citizens of Cameroon.

The occurrence of different disease profiles and epidemiological patterns and the shortage of public health workforce across the geographical regions of Cameroon make it exceedingly difficult to manage a strategy that is designed to minimize the spread of communicable diseases. To address these challenges in the future, better assessment and indicators of the health system capacity such as adequate medical personnel, infrastructure, or pandemic preparedness, need to be developed and properly implemented. There is no doubt that the amount of financial and physical resources dedicated to public health in the country needs to increase tremendously. Furthermore, the level of access to job market information and telemedicine in Cameroon in general is exceptionally low among the extremely digitally poor people. There is also the need to reinvigorate the health administration capacity-building processes to enhance policy implementation processes. To that end, the pathway to healthcare delivery success in Cameroon will depend on the capacity of the government to galvanize the training of the health workforce as well as incentives to retain them in the country. Therefore, revisiting how to increase government spending on healthcare through appropriate budget reallocation and increased domestic resources appropriation could be a much better mechanism to address the healthcare challenges currently faced by the government.

References

Agbor-Tabi P. (1984). Bilateral Assistance in Africa. The Case of Cameroon (Ph. D. Thesis) Laham: University Press of America.

Ako S., Fokoua S., Sinou M., & Leke R. (2015). Reproductive health in Cameroon. Retrieved from http://www.gfmer.ch/Endo/Reprod_health/Cameroon/Net_Reproduction_Cameroun. htm. Accessed September 29, 2024.

Ardener E. (1962). The political history of Cameroon. *Royal Institute of International Affairs*, 18(8): 341–350.

Ateghang-Awankem B. I., Atanga N. S. (2022). Digital health in low resource setting: Overview of telehealth market in Cameroon. *Journal of Quality in Health Care & Economics*, 5(1): 1–10.

Awasom N. F. (1998). Colonial background to the development of autonomist tendencies in Anglophone Cameroon, 1946–1961. *Journal of Third Word Studies*, 15(1): 163–183.

Awondo P. (2020). Public health and digital communication in Cameroon in the time of COVID-19. https://blogs.ucl.ac.uk/assa/2020/08/11/public-health-and-digital-communication-in-cameroon-in-the-time-of-covid-19/. Accessed August 11, 2023.

British Broadcasting Corporation (2023). Republic of Cameroon facts. https://www.bbc.com/news/world-africa-13146029. Accessed August 8, 2023.

Cannata G., Douryang M., Ljoka C., Glordani L., Monticone M., Foti C. (2022). The burden of disability in Africa and Cameroon: A call for optimizing the education in physical and rehabilitation Medicine.

Chamberlain M. (2014). *The Scramble for Africa.* (Fourth Edition). London: Longman.

Chapnkem W. (2019). Perception of Access to Healthcare in Cameroon by Women of Childbearing Age. Ph.D. Dissertation. Walden University. https://scholarworks.Waldenu.edu/cgi/viewcontent.cgi?article=8260&context=dissertations. Accessed August 8, 2023.

Cheno R. W., Tchabo W., Tchamy J. (2021). Willingness to join and pay for community-based health insurance and associate determinants among urban households of Cameroon: Case of Douala, and Yaounde. *Heliyyon*, 7(1): 1–10.

Climate Change Radar (2009). Cameroon Vision 2035. https://climate-laws.org/document/cameroon-vision-2035_a4ed. Accessed August 13, 2023.

Coquery - Vidrovitch C. (1985). The colonial economy of the former French, Belgium, and Portuguese zones, 1914–1935. In *General History of Africa Volume 7: Africa under Colonial Domination 1880–1935.* (First Edition), vol. 1–8, vol.7, 351–381. Calverton, Maryland, USA: UNESCO & Heinemann Publication.

Cornelissen E. (2003). On microlithic quartz industries at the end of the Pleistocene in Central Africa: The evidence from Shum Laka (North-West Cameroon). *African Archaeological Review*, 20(1): 1–24.

Country Report (2023). What is healthcare in Cameroon like? https://www.countryreports.or/country/cmarron/health.htm. Accessed August 16, 2023.

Crowe S. E. (1942). *The Berlin Conference West African Conference 1884–1885.* New York: Longman Green Press.

Delancey, J. O. L, Ashton-miller J. A. (2004). Pathophysiology of adult urinary incontinence. State of the art: Pathophysiology, 126(1S23). https://www.gastrojournal.org/article/S0016-5085(03)01775-X/fulltext. Accessed November 8, 2024.

Delancey M. D., Mbuh R. N., Delancey M. W. (2010). *Historical Dictionary of the Republic of Cameroon.* Laham: The Rowman & Littlefield Publishing Group Inc.

Dibie R. (2018). *Business and Government Relations in Africa.* New York: Routledge – Tylor and Francis Press.

Egbe M. E. (2014). Country report: Healthcare system of Cameroon: Socio-economic characteristics; historical context; organizational & financial aspects; major public health programs & challenges; strength and weaknesses. https://www.researchgate.net/publication/236166490.

Foti C., Azeufack Y. N., Sobze M. S., Albensi C., Guetiya R. W., Mindjomo R. et al. (2016). Characterizing disability and perception of rehabilitation in the health districts of Dschang, Cameroon. *Edorin Journal of Disability and Rehabilitation*, 2(1): 70–77.

Global Edge (2023). Cameroon history. https://globaledge.msu.edu/countries/cameroon. Accessed July 30, 2023.

Government of Cameroon (2020). *National Digital Health Strategic Plan Policy 2020–2024.* Yaoundé, Cameroon: Government Press.

Government of Cameroon (2016). *Ministry of Health Sector Strategy 2016–2027.* Yaoundé, Cameroon: Government Press.

Government of Cameroon Ministry of Public Health (2015). *Triennial Emergency Plan Policy 2015–2017.* Yaoundé, Cameroon: Government Press.

Government of Cameroon Ministry of Health Sector (2017). Government of Cameroon Ministry of Health Sector Strategy 2016–2027. https://p4h.world/en/documents/health-sector-strategy-2016-2027-minsante/Accessed November 8, 2024.

Government of Cameroon Ministry of Public Health (2012). *Universal Health Coverage Policy.* Yaoundé, Cameroon: Government Press.

Government of Cameroon (2009). *Ministry of Economy, Planning and Regional Development: Vision 2035.* Yaoundé, Cameroon: Government Press.

Government of Cameroon (2001). *Ministry of Health Sector Strategy 2001–2015.* Yaoundé, Cameroon: Government Press.

Ityavyar D. A. (1987). Background to the development of health services in Nigeria. *Social Sciences & Medicine,* 24(6): 487–499.

Johnson W. R. (1970). *The Cameroon Federation: Political Integration in a Fragmented Society.* Princeton: Princeton University Press.

Kamgnia B. (2006). Use of health care services in Cameroon. *International Journal of Applied Econometrics and Quantitative Studies,* 3(1): 53–64.

Lavachery P., MacEachern S., Bouimon T., Mbida M. C. (2010). *Komé - Kribi: Rescue Archaeology Along the Chad-Cameroon Oil Pipeline, 1999–2004.* Frankfurt am Main: Africa Magna Verlag. ISBN 978-3937248141.

Lavachery P. (2001). The Holocene archaeological sequence of Shum Laka Rock Shelter (Grasslands, Western Cameroon). *African Archaeological Review,* 18(4): 213–247.

Mackenzie J. (1983). *The Partition of Africa: And European Imperialism 1880–1990.* New York: Routledge Press.

Ministry of Public Health in Cameroon (2020). https://countdown.lstmed.ac.uk/about-countdown/the-partners/ministry-of-public-health-cameroon. Accessed August 10, 2023.

Ministry of Public Health, Cameroon (2015). International Initiative for Impact Evaluation: Health Strategy for Post 2015. https://www.3ieimpact.org/about-us/members/ministry-public-health-cameroon.

Ministry of Public Health Cameroon (2012). Department of Human Resources. General census report of health personnel. Yaounde, Government of Cameroon.

Ministry of Public Health Cameroon (2011). National policies on human resources for health, Yaounde, Government of Cameroon.

Ndoungue V. F., Tiwoda C., Gnigninanjourna O., Bataliack S., Mbondji E., Labat A. (2022). National health observatory: A tool to strengthen the health information system for evidence-based decision making and health policy formulation in Cameroon. *Health Policy Open,* 3(1): 1–6.

Ngo Bibaa L. O. (2020). Primary health care beyond COVID-19: Dealing with the pandemic in Cameroon. *BJGP Open,* 4(4): 1–4. https://bjgpopen.org/content/4/4/bjgpopen20X101113/tab-article-info. Accessed August 9, 2023.

Nguefack H. L. N., Gwet H., Desmonde S., Oukem-Boyer O. O. M., Nkenfou C., Téjiokem M., Alioum A. (2016). Estimating mother-to-child HIV transmission rates in Cameroon in 2011: A computer simulation approach. *BMC Infectious Diseases,* 16(1): 1–11.

Ntembe A., Tawah R., Faux E. (2021). Redistributive effects of healthcare out-of-pocket payment in Cameroon. *International Journal of Equity Health,* 20(1): 227–238.

Nzim N. N. (2014). Health sector Strategy and economic development in Cameroon: History, challenges, and perspectives. Thesis, Georgia State University, DOI: 10.57709/5556286.

Ojongo N. (2019). Healthcare financing in rural Cameroon. *Societies,* 9(77): 1–12.

Ondoa H. A. (2018). Education and labor supply inequality in the informal sector: The case of Cameroon. *Labour History,* 1(1): 1–13.

Pamen E. P. E., Yepndo C. G. D. (2017). Implication of digitalization of individuals' well-being in Cameroon. About this result. https://www.imf.org/-/media. Accessed August 11, 2023.

Population Pyramids (2022). Cameroon: Population Pyramids of the World from 1950 to 2100. https://www.populationpyramid.net/cameroon/1960/. Accessed August 9, 2023.

Ray M., Wallace L., Mbuagbaw L., Cockburn L., (2017). Functioning and disability in recent research from Cameroon: A narrative synthesis. *Pan African Medical Journal*, 27(1): 73–84.

Republic of Cameroon (2020). National Digital Health Strategic Plan (2020)s 2020–2024. https://www.scribd.com/document/517791182/000-Cameroun-National-Strategic-Plan-Digital-Health. Accessed October 30, 2024.

Saidu, Y., Gu, J., Ngenge, B.M. et al. (2023). Assessment of immunization data management practices in Cameroon: unveiling potential barriers to immunization data quality. *BMC Health Service Research* 23, 1033. https://doi.org/10.1186/s12913-023-09965-9. Accessed September 3, 2024.

Saidu Y., Bachaire H., Frambo A., Talongwa R., Mbanga C., Nassiuma Z. R., Wiwa O. (2022). Health policy making process in Cameroon: A case for the utilization of the target policy profile. https://gatesopenresearch.org/articles/6-68. Assessed August 10, 2023.

Sieleunou I., Tamga D. M., Tankwa J. M., Munteh A. P., Tchatchouang E. V. L. (2021). Strategic health purchasing progress mapping in Cameroon: A scoping review. *Health System & Reform*, 7(1): 1–14.

Tandi T. E., Cho Y., Akam A. J., Afoh C. O., Ryu S. H., Choi M. S., Kim K., Choi J. W. (2015). Cameroon public health sector: Shortage and inequalities in geographic distribution of health personnel. *International Journal of Equity Health*, 12(1): 14–43.

Trillo R., Hudgens J. (1999). *West Africa: The Rough Guide*. (Third Edition). London, England: Rough Guide Limited Press.

United Nations Human Development Index (2023). Human Development Report 2023-24. https://hdr.undp.org/content/human-development-report-2023-24. Accessed September 4, 2024.

United Nations (2021). United Nations Sustainable Development Cooperation Framework for Cameroon 2022–226. https://cameroon.un.org/en/166184-united-nations-sustainable-development-cooperation-framework-cameroon-2022-2026. Accessed August 12, 2023.

United Nations Human Development Programme (2021). hde.undp.org/2021-report. Accessed August 16, 2023.

World Bank indicators (2022). Cameroon. https://data.worldbank.org/indicator/NY.GDP.MKTP.CD?locations=CM.

World Health Organization (2023a). Cameroon country profile. https://www.who.int/data/gho/data/countries/country-details/GHO/cameroon?countryProfileId=79e4cda0-11b1-4806-9c63-d40904289ced. Accessed August 16, 2023.

World Health Organization (2023b) Cameroon Statistics. https://www.who.int/data/gho/data/countries/country-details/GHO/cameroon?countryProfileId=79e4cda0-11b1-4806-9c63-d40904289ced. Accessed August 8, 2023.

World Health Organization. (1963). The work of WHO, 1963: annual report of the Director-General to the World Health Assembly and to the United Nations. https://iris.who.int/handle/10665/85765. Accessed September 4, 2024.

Wikipedia (2023). History of Cameroon. https://www.wikipedia.org/wiki/historyofcameroon/main. Accessed August 6, 2023.

Witter S., Govender V., Ravindran S., Yates R. (2017). Minding the gaps: Health financing, universal health coverage and gender. *Health Policy Plan*, 32(1): 4–12.

Yanou M., Foyam J. (2008). Trade unions, labor contracts and industrial peace: The case of tole tea estate. *Revue Africaine des Sciences Juridiques FSJP UYII*, 5(1): 25–32.

Chapter Six

HEALTH POLICY AND ADMINISTRATION IN EGYPT

Robert Dibie and Charles Ubah

Introduction

The Arab Republic of Egypt continues to incrementally formulate national healthcare policies to ensure universal health insurance for all citizens across the nation. The intention of universal health insurance or health sector reform is to ensure a basic package of health services. This chapter investigates the nature and impacts of health policies and healthcare services delivery equitably to all the citizens and residents of Egypt. It argues that the extent to which health policies in Egypt could reduce the direct pathological effects of various chemicals, physical, and biological agents of diseases that are prevalent communicable and noncommunicable diseases could reduce healthcare challenges in the country. Therefore, health policies should not be limited to hospital care and practitioners' issues. It must cover how to manage the deficiencies in the treatment of wastewater, poor sanitation systems, the disposal of untreated sewage, inadequate operations, and maintenance of treatment plants that often result in serious health risks to citizens of the country. Questionnaires and interviews were used to collect data for this research. Secondary research methods were used to determine the effectiveness of health policies in Egypt. The research reveals that although the government of Egypt has adopted several health policies in the past three decades, there are challenges in the investment of more funds in health care because of the continued increase in the population of the nation. In addition, there tends to be more pressure on existing hospital infrastructure in Egypt. There is also a need for the government to update the training of skilled health professionals, including updating healthcare technology in the country. There is also much to do to close the gap between the level of access to quality healthcare in both the rural and urban regions of Egypt. The current challenges facing the health delivery system in Egypt require policies that could create a balance between the citizens' healthcare needs, risks, and benefits. In addition, developing modern information systems could play a significant role in training and enforcing effective and better healthcare delivery systems in the country.

Brief History

The Arab Republic of Egypt is in the northeastern part of the African continent. The nation currently has a population of 107.5 million people (World Health Organization 2022). It has a common border with the Republic of Sudan to the south, and Libya to the west. The major natural resources in Egypt include petroleum, natural gas, iron ore, phosphates, manganese, limestone, gypsum, talc, asbestos, lead, rare earth elements, and zinc (World Factbook 2023). Further, the Arab Republic of Egypt shares a border with the Mediterranean Sea in the northwest and the Red Sea in the northeast. The Arab Republic of Egypt is the most populous country in North Africa, and the Arab world, as well as the third-most populated nation in the African continent, after Nigeria and Ethiopia. Egypt is also regarded as the 15th-most populated country in the world (Embassy of the Arab Republic of Egypt 2021).

The first period of Egyptian history, which ended in 2181 BC is called the Old Kingdom. During the first period of Egypt's history, the pharaoh-built pyramids (Midant-Reynes 1992). However, the first pyramid (the step pyramid) was built by Zoser by about 2665 BC. There were other pyramids that were built by the following pharaohs Sneferu and Khufu (Bard & Shaw 2000; Lambert 2020). Some history scholars reported that by 1281 BC, the Egyptian kingdom had split into parts due to weakness and civil wars between the rival monarchies in surrounding regions (Midant-Reynes 1992). The prehistory of Egypt: from the first Egyptians to the first Kings is called the First Intermediate Period and it lasted until 2055 BC (Lambert 2020). Further, Mentuhotep II succeeded in reuniting Egypt, and he founded the Middle Kingdom. The Middle Kingdom lasted until 1650 BC. It was a great period of art and literature in Egypt. Furthermore, the pharaohs conducted successful military campaigns, and more pyramids were built. However, the Middle Kingdom was followed by the Second Intermediate Period (Midant-Reynes 1992).

The French army under the command of Napoleon defeated the Egyptians at the Battle of the Pyramids in 1798. Within a brief period, the British and Ottoman forces defeated the French army and forced them to surrender. Despite this defeat, the French expedition led to a renewed interest in Ancient Egypt in Europe (Lambert 2020; Office of the Historian 2020). There became a power struggle after the French army was defeated and Napoleon left. Eventually, the Albanian army under the command of Mohammed Ali became the leader of Egypt. During Mohammed Ali's Kingship, he tried to modernize Egypt and built factories and shipyards. However, he died in 1849 (Daly 1998; Lambert 2020). After the death of Mohammed Ali, Khedive Ismail became the Leader of Egypt and continued the policy to modernize and kingdom of Egypt by building railways and post offices (Botman 1991; Lambert 2020). To fund his modernization initiatives in Egypt Khedive Ismail had to borrow funds from some European leaders. After the Suez Canal construction was completed and could not pay his debt to the European lenders, Khedive was forced to sell his shares in the Suez Canal to the British in 1875 to avoid bankruptcy (British Broadcasting Corporation 2019; Hopwood et al. 2023). After the death of Khedive Ismail, his son Tewfik took over the Kingship of Egypt in 1879. Because of the inability of the Egyptian kingdom to pay their debt and concerns about the British investment in the construction of the Suez Canal, the British Government sent their troops to occupy Egypt (Botman 1991; Daly 1998; Midant-Reynes 1992). However, Tewfik Khedive was kept as a puppet ruler, and he reported to the British command in Egypt. After the death of Tewfik Khedive, the British colonial administration appointed a successor called Fuad King of Egypt, and in 1935, Fuad King of Egypt was followed by his son Farouk (Office of the Historian 2020).

After a couple of years in 1919, Egypt was officially made a British colony (Lambert 2020). Although the Egyptian citizens resented British rule over them and constantly engaged in anti-British riots, the British colonial administration prevailed and continued to control the nation's affairs such as communication, foreign affairs, and the legal system (Botman 1991; Hopwood et al. 2023). Furthermore, the German troops invaded Egypt in 1992, however, they were defeated by the British army. Unfortunately, the Egypt citizens continue to be desperate to have full control of their nation's governance and continue to engage in various anti-British riots. Because of the despicable anti-British constant riot, the British troops decided to withdraw from Egypt in 1947 (Lambert 2020; Office of the Historian 2020). After, the withdrawal of the British army in 1948 from Egypt, the nation's political situation escalated by another war with the nation of Israel. The Egyptian people were defeated, and King Farouk abdicated due to an internal military coup, and the leader of the 1952 military coup General Naguib became the new leader of the country (Midant-Reynes 1992; Wikipedia 2023). Unfortunately, General Naguib was replaced by Gamal Abdel Nasser in 1954, and two years later in 1956, he nationalized the Suez Canal (Midant-Reynes 1992; Wikipedia 2023).

As a result of the Egyptian Revolution of 1919 and World War II, the kingdom of Egypt was established as an independent nation, however, the British Government continued to control its defense, foreign affairs, and other initiatives that were of their interest (Botman 1991; British Broadcasting Corporation 2019; Memphis Tour 2023). According to the British Broadcasting Corporation Report (2019), the British colonial occupation and administration ended in 1954 based on the Anglo-Egyptian Agreement of 1954 (Lambert 2020). Thus, a more independent Egypt was established in 1953 after the total withdrawal of the United Kingdom from the administration of the nation as well as the Suez Canal. In addition, President Gamal Abdel Nasser, the first Indigenous candidate of Egypt, was elected in 1956 and led the country from 1956 to 1970 (Bard & Shaw 2000; Memphis Tour 2023). After President Nasser's term was over Anwar Sadat was elected as the second Egyptian President from 1970 to 1981. During President Sadat's term in office, he adopted some socialist philosophy and associated Egypt with the then Soviet Union. He also enhanced the healthcare delivery system and education in the nation (Botman 1991).

After the sudden death of President Anwar Sadat by assassination in 1981, Hosni Mubarak became the next president of Egypt. President Mubarak's authoritarian style of leadership among other factors led to the Egyptian revolution of 2011. Subsequently, President Mohamed Morsi was elected to replace Mubarak, but another political dispute resulted in another military coup in 2013. Unfortunately, the coup plotters jailed President Morsi, and another election was held in 2014. Abdel Fattah El-Sisi was elected the new president of Egypt. General Sisi was one of the military officers who planned the coup that toppled President Morsi's presidency (Daly 1998; Lambert 2020; Office of the Historian 2020; Memphis Tour 2023; Wikipedia 2023).

Because of the political agitation that occurred in the country in June 2013, the Arab Republic of Egypt has transformed its political system to effectively address the demands of its citizens. This innovative approach has galvanized both economic and political stability in the past two decades. It will be recalled that in May 2014, more than 25 million Egypt citizens braved the extreme heat and instigated men and women, as well as youths to refuse allegiance to terrorism to elect a new civilian President, Abdel Fattah El-Sisi. However, after, a month, President El-Sisi was sworn into office on June 8, 2014. The new president has now transformed the political climate toward security, stability, and opportunity for all and reestablished Egypt's regional and global leadership role (Embassy of the Arab Republic of Egypt 2021; Office of the Historian 2020). Currently, the Arab Republic is confronted with many healthcare and economic development challenges. The nation's population is growing amazingly fast, and there seems to be a lack of enough farmland for the citizens of the country to engage in farming. There are also great disparities in the delivery of healthcare in rural regions of the country where most of the low-income population reside (Daly 1998; Memphis Tour 2023; Wikipedia 2023).

Healthcare Challenges

The Egyptian health system faces multiple challenges in improving and ensuring the health and well-being of the Egyptian people. The system faces not only the burden of combating illnesses associated with poverty and lack of education, but also respond to emerging diseases and illnesses associated with modern, urban lifestyles. Emerging access to global communications and commerce is raising the expectations of the population for more and better care and advanced healthcare technology.

The population of Egypt is growing at the rate of 2.5% per annum and as of 2020, the nation's total residents is reported to be 107. 5 million people (World Health Organization Indicator 2022; World Factbook 2020). Thus, the demand for education services, healthcare, and physical infrastructure continues to grow incrementally every year (Ahmed 2021; Mathauer et al. 2019). In addition, some scholars have argued that because of the increase in population in Egypt almost 95% of the population lives on 4% of the nation's land. This increase in the population has often led to pollution and traffic jams on highways along the Nile River Delta (Mathauer et al. 2022). This increase in population challenges has also spillover into a shortage of clean drinking water (Columbia University Public Health Report 2022; Mathauer et al. 2022; Salama 2022).

The nation is also faced with major noncommunicable diseases such as cancer, diabetes, cardiovascular diseases, stroke, kidney diseases, ischemic heart diseases, hypertensive heart diseases, and so on. It is also reported that about 15% of the population of Egypt that are over the age of 20 years old have diabetes, while 32% of the population of the country also suffers from obesity (World Health Organization Indicator 2022). Another 25% of the population of Egypt also suffers from hypertension (World Health Organization Indicator 2022). These noncommunicable diseases have been associated with more vibrant urbanization as well as rising life expectations, and access to more disposable income.

The Government of Egypt has made efforts to increase healthcare access but has often faced many challenges. Moreover, the nation's limited hospital space and beds is a major predicament. The current ratio of hospital beds to people is exceptionally low by international standards, as well as the required health workers' number to take care of people who are admitted to the hospital (Oxford Business Group 2022; USAID 2020;

World Factbook 2020). It has also been reported that the physician density in Egypt is about 0.75 in urban regions and 0.81 per 1,000 people in the rural districts and the nurse density is about 14.8 per 10,000 population (Oxford Business Group 2022; World Factbook 2020). Further, evidence shows that the Arab Republic of Egypt has not closed the gap between access to quality healthcare and appropriate level of provision as well as delivery services in the urban and rural districts in the northern part of the country (Oxford Business Group 2022).

According to Gericke et al. (2018), the public health system in Egypt is confronted with so many challenges. The healthcare delivery predicaments in the country include disparity in access to healthcare between the rich and poor, as well as the urban and rural population of the country (Khalifa et al. 2022; Salama 2022). In addition, the health system is underfunded by the government. Khalifa et al. (2022) contend that under-investment and inefficiencies are associated with the fact that citizens' out-of-pocket payments have been about 62% of the current health expenditure in the past decade. Furthermore, government spending represents only 29% compared to 43% in lower-middle-income countries (Khalifa et al. 2022; Olassa 2020; Thelwell 2020).

There is a consensus in the literature that the quality of healthcare delivery is exceptionally low in rural regions because every sick population in the district must travel to Cairo (Oxford Business Group 2022; World Factbook 2021). Cairo is also reported to have a bigger share of the nation's medical doctors while the rural regions or governorates that are far from the bigger cities are short of physicians. To compound the healthcare challenges most regional hospitals, lack modern medical equipment (Ahmed et al. 2021; Oxford Business Group 2022). The nation has a pattern where its poor citizens spend a greater part of their hard-earned income on healthcare than the richer population (Ahmed et al. 2021).

According to Elkalamawi et al. (2021), there is a shortage of health workers in Egypt. Some scholars have argued that the minimal salary that is paid to doctors and nurses in Egypt, as well as the lack of social respect for healthcare workers has led to a high rate of turnover (Ahmed et al. 2021; Oxford Business Group 2022; Salama 2022). It has also been reported that there have been elevated levels of violence against doctors in emergency rooms in Egypt. Because of lack of safety for doctors as well as underpayment, and overload of work has compelled physicians in the country to feel that society does to appreciate their services (Allianz Care 2022). Some junior doctors in Egypt tend to shuttle between two and three hospitals or clinics every day to make decent living conditions (Ahmed et al. 2021; Allianz Care 2021; USAID 2020). The aftermath of these poor conditions of services for physicians is that they cannot pay enough attention to each patient, as well as prepare to study for career development (Ahmed et al. 2021; Elkalamawi et al. 2021). These challenges that doctors in Egypt face have made the majority of younger physicians migrate to other Gulf Arab states that pay higher wages and provide better working conditions, safety, and modern medical equipment. Although the Arab Republic of Egypt's government made efforts to increase physician salaries, there are many more benefits and conditions of services that need to be provided to enhance the retention of doctors and nurses as well as the number of healthcare providers in the country.

Types of Health Policies

The Arab Republic of Egypt government continues to explore health policies that propel the nation to accomplish its sustainable development goals. One of the most important visions of the government is to achieve universal health coverage. There is no doubt that quality healthcare is a major mechanism for the Government of Egypt's economic development and prosperity for all its citizens. Over the past few decades, the nation has collaborated with the World Health Organization (WHO), and the United States International Development Agency to modernize child health, and maternal health and dismantle HIV/AIDS and COVID-19 pandemics, and healthcare services. Below are some of the major health policies that have been enacted by the Arab Republic of Egypt.

Egyptian Health Insurance Policy enacted in 1964: This policy was extended to cover students' healthcare expenses in the country in 1993. The name of the student version is called Student Health Insurance.

Quality Control Authority Health Policy 2015: The goal of this policy is to regulate and rank Egypt's hospitals and clinics based on a range of metrics, including staff training, and pay, infrastructure, efficiency, and equipment quality (Arab Republic of Egypt Ministry of Health and Population 2015).

The Egypt National Sustainable Strategy Vision 2030 enacted in 2016: The goal of this policy is to effectively address the major challenges facing Egypt's sustainable development process. Egypt Vision 2030 also represents a foothold on the way toward economic and social justice and reviving the role of Egypt in regional leadership. It is also anticipated that by 2030, the nation will achieve a competitive, balanced, diversified, and knowledge-based economy, characterized by justice, social integration, and participation (Arab Republic of Egypt 2016; International Energy Association 2022; United Nations 2022).

The Health Insurance System Policy of 2018: The law covers all citizens, whether they are public or private employees, seasonal or permanent workers, men or women, children, or adults. It also covers workers' spouses, parents, and children as well as work injuries. It applies mandatorily to all citizens existing in Egypt and optionally to Egyptians working or living abroad. It can be also extended to foreigners who are earning their income or living in Egypt subject to reciprocity. The government shall guarantee free healthcare services to people who are unable to pay the contribution fees.

The Arab Republic of Egypt Action Plan 2023–2027 enacted in 2018: The goal of this policy is to develop and invest in human capital; protect natural resources with a view of improved security and sustainability; increase productivity and employment; and improve the efficiency of government performance (Arab Republic of Egypt 2017; Latif et al. 2018).

Universal Healthcare Insurance Policy that will be in place by 2027: The new universal health insurance was formulated, and the full implementation was supposed to be in 2032. However, because of major successes in the initial planning and implementation strategies the Arab Republic of Egypt's Ministry of Health and Population has changed the full implementation date to 2027. According to the Ministry of Health and Population of Egypt (2023), the new universal health insurance will cover medical examination, all health tests, X-rays and scans, surgery, and health treatments. In addition to the new universal healthcare system policy, a General Authority of Healthcare will ensure high-quality oversee services. It is also mandated that citizens could still seek private insurance if they are not eligible for the new universal health insurance (Arab Republic of Egypt Ministry of Health and Population 2023).

The Arab Republic of Egypt has formulated and implemented many vibrant health-related policies over the past three decades. However, despite these policies, the volatile political environment is partially the reason most of the health policies have not been successfully accomplished. Another dilemma facing the country is the numerous changes of presidents due to military coups (Fesseeh et al. 2022; Oxford Business Group 2016). As usual, every nation needs political stability for policies to be effectively implemented. In addition, the rapid growth of the population of the country tends to galvanize tensions in the economy, social, and environmental sectors as well as negatively threaten the health delivery system and capacity-building capability of the majority of the citizens.

Nature of Health Administration

The Arab Republic of Egypt's health system is administered by the Ministry of Health and Population of the country. The nation's health system is divided into five sectors of administration, for example (1) central administration for the minister's office, (2) curative health services, (3) population and family planning, (4) preventative health services, and (5) administration and finance (Columbia University Public Health report 2022; Fesseeh et al. 2022). The administration of the health system by the Ministry of Health and Population is pluralistic because it consists of two functional structures: (a) the administrative structure and (b) the service delivery structure. The Ministry of Health and Population is divided into five administrative sectors (Ministry of Health and Population Egypt 2023). The sectors are: (1) Central administration for the minister's office; (2) Curative health services; (3) Population and family planning; (4) Preventative health services; and (5) Administration and Finance (Ministry of Health and Population Egypt 2023).

The public sector is the largest health sector in the country. It comprises health insurance organizations. The citizens of Egypt that receive services from the health insurance organizations include mostly government ministry and agency employees, private sector employees, pensioners, and the widows of the above staff groups that have passed on (User 2021). Furthermore, all functions of the central headquarters are divided into five broad sector divisions: (1) central administration for the minister's office, (2) curative health services, (3) population and family planning, (4) basic and preventive health services, and (5) administration and finance. There are 13 headquarter undersecretaries in charge of various functions reporting to the minister. Furthermore, the responsibilities of these undersecretaries include preventive care, laboratories, primary health care, endemic diseases, curative care, research and development, pharmaceuticals, dentistry, family planning, and nursing (Ministry of Gericke et al. 2018; Health and Population 2023; Wikipedia 2023).

The public/parastatal sector consists of quasi-governmental organizations such as the Health Insurance Organization and the Curative Care Organization. Citizens can obtain insurance coverage via private insurers who have government support. However, many consider services that public healthcare facilities to be low in quality due to years of underfunding. The lack of medical equipment and qualified personnel in combination with low sanitation and compromised safety measures, especially in facilities located in rural areas, compel citizens to turn to private facilities (Allianz Care 2022; Hammed 2020). It should be noted however that the Ministry of Health and Population is the largest healthcare level that provides inpatient services in the country. In addition, Egypt has four levels of public health hospitals: *First,* the integrated hospitals have 20–60 b0 beds facilities that provide primary healthcare and specialized medical treatment in the rural regions. *Second,* the district hospitals have 100–200 facilities that could provide specialized medical services in every district in the nation. *Third,* is the General hospitals that are equipped with 200 or more beds. The general hospitals are built in every capital of governance in the country. The general hospitals also provide specialist medical treatments. *Fourth,* is the Specialist hospitals. The specialist hospitals are in urban areas in Egypt, and they provide medical treatments in health areas such as (a) gynecology and obstetrics, (b) psychiatric, (c) eye, (d) tumor, (e) heart ophthalmology, (f) cancer, (g) orthopedic, and many other areas (Allianz 2022; Ministry of Health and Populations 2023). This type of hospital is in all governorates in Egypt.

According to Gericke et al. (2018) and User (2021), the private sector is made up of private hospitals, clinics doctors, and pharmacies. Furthermore, the private sector has been rated to provide higher-quality healthcare treatments than the public sector (Gericke et al. 2018; World Health Organization report 2022). The only challenge associated with access to private sector health services is that they can be too expensive for the low-income population of Egypt. This is because many private healthcare treatments are paid for out-of-pocket, and private health insurance may not be acceptable. In most cases, out-of-pocket healthcare payments consist of over 60%, while pharmaceutical drug payments cost over 25% (Gericke et al. 2018; Thelwell 2020). Private healthcare facilities consist of nonprofit organizations and for-profit hospitals, clinics, and pharmacies. In the past two decades, the Arab Republic of Egypt Government has proverbialized more healthcare organizations including clinics with the intention of increasing high-quality healthcare in the country (Allianz Care 2022; Salama 2022; Wikipedia 2023).

The private sector also includes religious hospitals such as Christian and Muslim hospitals, nonprofit and for-profit organizations as well as traditional midwives, private pharmacies, private doctors, and private hospitals that provide health services and treatments to citizens and residents of Egypt (Arab Republic of Egypt Ministry of Health 2023). In addition, there are also several nongovernmental organizations that also provide healthcare services. The nongovernmental organizations include charitable organizations, religious hospitals, and clinics that are in both the urban and rural regions of the country. It is important to note that all the private sector health organizations must be registered with the Ministry of Social Affairs of Egypt in Cairo, the capital city of the country (Gericke et al. 2018; User 2021).

Data Analysis and Discussion

The objective of this chapter is to investigate the nature and impacts of health policies and healthcare services equitably to all the citizens and residents of Egypt. The data used for the analysis of healthcare policy effectiveness were derived from secondary research methods. The secondary research methods adopted include content analysis of the Government of Egypt Ministry of Health reports, World Bank indicators, Development Initiatives report, the World Health Organization reports, United Nations Human Development Index annual report, Center for Disease Control, Country Report, and United States Agency for International Development, academic as well as professional journals articles.

Table 1 analyzes the state of the health system in the Arab Republic of Egypt. The country is experiencing similar health challenges to several other nations in the African continent. The population also has been incrementally increasing in the past decade. The current population in 2023 is 107.5 million people. As discussed in this paper, the healthcare system in Egypt is yet to be effectively consolidated in its health facilities and equipment to align with the population growth rate. Currently, the nation spends an average of 4.4% of its GDP on health annually, this is still below 5.6%–7.6%, which is recommended by the World Health Organization. It should however be noted that the amount that a nation spends on its healthcare system every year does not translate to its ability to accomplish high-quality health system for its citizens. There are many other additional factors that must be in place for a country to have a high-quality healthcare system and practices.

The current rate of medical physicians per 1,000 people in Egypt was 0.75 in 2019. Further, the number of nurses and wives per 1,000 people is 1.9, while the number of hospital beds per 1,000 people was 1.4 in 2017, and 13.5 beds to 10,000 patients in 2019. Further, access to safe and clean water was 99.7% in urban areas and 99.7% of the rural population in 2020. The World Health Organization Indicator (2020) reported that 0.3% of the population in both urban and rural districts in the country do not have access to safe and clean water. In addition, residents of the country that have access to basic sanitation is 98.2% in 2020. While people with no access to basic toilet facilities constitute just 1.8% of the Egypt population. Over the past two decades, the sanitation challenges have been reduced. It has been reported that people with basic sanitation in Egypt constitute 98.2% of the population. In addition, 1.8% of the residents of the country must access basic sanitation facilities or toilets and maybe practicing open defecation mostly in the rural districts (United Nations Human Development Index 2021).

Cardiovascular diseases cancer, diabetes, cancer, stroke, kidney diseases, ischemic heart diseases, and hypertensive heart diseases continue to be the major causes of mortality in Egypt (World Health Organization 2022). Life expectancy has improved in the country. While life at birth is currently 71.8 years. Life expectancy in 2023 for females has increased to 74.7 years. On the other hand, life expectancy for males at birth for male has also increased to 73.5 years in 2023 (World Bank Indicators 2022).

There is also a continued trend of improvement in the mortality rate in the country. On one hand, the mortality rate for female adults per 1,000 people was 16.3% in 2023. Other the other hand, the mortality rate for males at birth for adult males per 1,000 people is 18.2% in the same year. Infant mortality rate per 1,000 people has also reduced

Table 1 Economics and Health Indicators in Egypt

No.	Major Indicators in Zimbabwe	Explanation
1	Population	107.5 million
2	Gross domestic product (GDP)	US$378.11 billion
3	Current health expenditure (% of GDP)	4.4 (2020)
4	Nurses and midwives per 1,000 people	1.9
5	Physicians/doctors per 1,000 people	0.75 (2019)
6	Access to safe and clean water	99.7% Urban; 99.7% rural (2020)
7	Population in rural regions without access to safe drinking water service	0.3% Urban; 0.3 rural (2020)
8	People with basic sanitation	98.2% (2020)
9	Population with no access to sanitation or basic toilet	1.8% (2020)
10	Common diseases	Cancer, diabetes, cardiovascular diseases, stroke, kidney diseases, ischemic heart diseases, hypertensive heart diseases
11	Life expectancy at birth	71.8 years
12	Life expectancy in 2020 at birth for females	74.7 years (2023)
13	Life expectancy in 2020 at birth for males	73.5 years
14	Mortality rate for female adults (per 1,000 people)	16.3%
15	Mortality rate for infants (per 1,000 people)	3.9% (2023)
16	Mortality rate for male adults (per 1,000 people)	18.2%
17	Tuberculosis incidence (per 100,000 people)	11.6
18	Population living below income poverty line PPP $1.90 a day	3.2%
19	Population in multidimensional head count poverty (%)	4.1%
20	Contribution deprivation in health to multidimensional poverty index	6.9 (2014)
21	Number of maternal deaths (per 100,000)	420 (2020)
22	Malaria incidence (per 1,000 people at risk)	0.0%
23	HIV/AIDS prevalence adults' rate (% ages 15–49)	0.07% (2022)
24	COVID-19 vaccination rate (per 1,000 people)	100% (2022)

Sources: World Bank Indicators (2020); World Health Organization. (2022); United Nations Human Development Programme (2021); Global Sustainable Development Indicators Database (2022); World Factbook (2022).

to 3.9% in 2023 (World Factbook 2023; World Health Organization 2023). Further, tuberculosis incidence per 1,000 people has also dropped to 11.6% in 2022. Moreover, the HIV/AIDS prevalence among adults' rate for 15–49 years is 0.07%. Similarly, despite the challenges posed by the COVID-19 pandemic between 2019 and 2022, the vaccination rate per 1,000 people in Egypt has increased to 100%. Thus, it could be argued that the Ministry of Health and Population of the Arab Republic of Egypt and its foreign health patterner have done well in controlling the spread of COVID-19 as well as encouraging the residents of the country to receive free vaccination.

The Arab Republic of Egypt has constantly experienced the spread of noncommunicable diseases. The common noncommunicable diseases that are prevalent in the country including cancer, diabetes, cardiovascular diseases, and chronic respiratory diseases are still recurring in the country. However, the Government of the Arab Republic of Egypt has been engaging in running multiple campaigns to promote increased awareness of the various noncommunicable diseases that have negatively inflicted the Egyptian population in the past decade. Although there are some excellent hospitals and highly trained and specialist physicians in the Arab Republic of Egypt, some of the health facilities in rural districts such as Aswan and Luxor (to mention a few) are inadequate, and of exceptionally low standard because of low funding and understaffing by the government. In addition, despite an ambulance service hotline is 123, the nation's Egyptian ambulance service is not dependable and in some rural regions the emergency services are non-existent (Allianz Care 2022).

Conclusion

This chapter has examined the nature and impacts of health policies and healthcare delivery services equitably to all the citizens and residents of Egypt. It argues that the extent to which health policies in Egypt could reduce the direct pathological effects of various chemicals, physical, and biological agents of disease challenges depends on adequate funding of the sector. This is because the majority of the challenges currently facing the nation's healthcare delivery system are because of a lack of enough budget appropriation.

In addition, the introduction of the universal health insurance scheme in Egypt also set of facilitates another set of challenges for the low-income citizens in the country with respect to high out-of-pocket payments. Therefore, it could be argued that since medicine is not properly covered by universal health insurance in public hospitals and clinics, the poor population is often faced with financial hardship and impoverishment. Further, the lack of a well-managed healthcare delivery and financing system has led to most citizens bearing the majority of expenses. This critical challenge calls for the Government of Egypt to formulate new comprehensive health financing policies that could enhance access to safe, affordable, and quality medicine and health treatment for all citizens of the country soon. Thus, investing more in the socio-economic future of the citizens of the Arab Republic of Egypt could be overly critical to galvanizing equity and social justice as well as the well-being of everyone.

Furthermore, consistent with the public policy-making process future deliberations about amendments to current Egypt's health policy must include citizens and patient representatives in the country. This new initiative in formulating public policy in the health sector could enhance the input and views of various citizens of the country. It is especially important that the Arab Republic of Egypt increase transparency and inclusiveness in all its public policy-making processes. It is not right for just a few administrators in the Ministry of Health and Population and well as their foreign partners to be making health policies that will affect the lives of over 107 million people in Egypt without input to a policy that would affect the lives of the population.

Therefore, it is paramount to distinguish the democratic policy-making process from authoritarian methods of making decrees in the Arab Republic of Egypt.

The analysis in this chapter reveals that there is a shortage of health workers in Egypt. The current 0.7 physician to 1,000 people is a major challenge. The shortage of doctors and nurses is because of brain drain, low salaries, poor facilities, and bad working conditions. Thus, without adequate and qualified healthcare professionals in the country even the best medical hospitals that also have modern and advanced medical equipment will not be able to reinvigorate the health system in the country. Although the Arab Republic of Egypt government had increased the salary of doctors, more needs to be provided to retain enough doctors in the country. The recommended best practice for retention of good doctors and nurses includes good protection policies, sponsoring career development to attain high medical skills, higher salaries that are comparable to those in medium-income countries, good working conditions, and provision of modern medical equipment and facilities. There is an urgent need for the government of Egypt to enact new policies to adequately fund a sustainable health workforce in the country.

Another especially important mechanism that the Arab Republic of Egypt could adopt to pop up its healthcare delivery system soon is new medical technologies. It is, therefore, paramount for the health education system to start incorporating artificial intelligence, data analytics, robotic medical sciences, and genome sequencing in the training of future doctors, nurses, midwives, pharmacies, and other health professionals in the country. Further, our analysis also reveals that Egypt does not have modern national health information systems, as well as a database for its health workforce. These information technology challenges, buttress the need for the nation to strengthen its medical digital technology and telemedicine system to better serve the citizens in both the urban and rural spheres of Egypt.

Finally, the accomplishments of the Arab Republic of Egypt's healthcare policies and initiatives over the past two decades are numerous. There is no doubt that the nation has positively contributed to the economic, health, and social development of many of its citizens. The country has also done a better job in revitalizing the promotion and campaign to increase awareness of communicable and noncommunicable diseases that negatively impact the citizens of the country. The future of health delivery in the future will require more collaboration with new market participants in the global health industry. The collaboration initiative for the effective implementation of universal health insurance could help to change the old pattern of citizens visiting hospitals and health clinics in Egypt.

References

Ahmed M. (2021). Insight into Egypt's Healthcare sector. https://insights.omnia-health.com/management/insight-egypts-healthcare sector. Accessed July 30, 2023.
Ahmed Y., Ramadan R., Sakr M. F. (2021). Equity of healthcare financing: A progressivity analysis for Egypt. *Journal of Humanities and Applied Social Sciences*, 3(1): 3–24.
Allianz Care (2021). Healthcare in Egypt. https://www.allianzcare.com/en/support/health-and-wellness/national-healthcare-systems/healthcare-in-egypt.html. Accessed July 29, 2023.
Arab Republic of Egypt Ministry of Health and Population report (2023). Universal Health Insurance. Ministry of Health and Population Publication.
Arab Republic of Egypt (2017). Egypt STEPS noncommunicable disease risk factors survey. https://ghdx.healthdata.org/record/egypt-steps-noncommunicable-disease-risk-factors-survey-2017. Accessed August 30, 2024.

Arab Republic of Egypt (2016). National strategy for sustainable development: Egypt vision 2030. https://mped.gov.eg/DynamicPage?id=115&lang=en&Egypt-Vision-2030. Accessed September 3, 2024.

Arab Republic of Egypt (2021). Article IV Consultation, Second Review Under the Stand-By Arrangement-Press Release; Staff Report; and Statement by the Executive Director for the Arab Republic of Egypt. https://www.imf.org/en/Publications/CR/Issues/2021/07/22/Arab-Republic-of-Egypt-2021-Article-IV-Consultation-Second-Review-Under-the-Stand-By-462545. Accessed November 8, 2024.

Arab Republic of Egypt Ministry of Health and Population (2015). Egypt health issues survey. https://dhsprogram.com/pubs/pdf/fr313/fr313.pdf. Accessed September 4, 2024.

Bard K. A., Shaw I., (2000). *The Oxford Illustrated History of Ancient Egypt*. Oxford: Oxford University Press.

Botman S. (1991). *Egypt from Independence to Revolution, 1919–1952*. New York: Syracuse University Press.

British Broadcasting Corporation. (2019). Egypt profile—Timeline. https://www.bbc.com/news/world-africa-13315719. Accessed July 25, 2023.

Columbia University Public Health report (2022). Egypt summary. https://www.publichealth.columbia.edu/research/comparative-health-policy-library/egypt. Accessed September 4, 2024.

Daly M. W. (1998). *The Cambridge History of Egypt Volume 2 Modern Egypt, From 1517 to the End of the Twentieth Century*. New York: Cambridge University Press.

Elkalamawi E., Gamal E., Hassan H., Salama N. (2021). Increasing the retention of the health workforce in Egypt: Improving workforce environments, a policy paper. Cairo, Egypt: The Public Policy HUB: The American University in Cairo.

Embassy of the Arab Republic of Egypt (2021). Egypt today. https://egyptembassy.net/egypt-today/egypts-government/.

Fesseeh A., ElEzbawy B., Adly W., ElShahawy R., Georgge M., Abaza S., ElShalakani A., Kalo Z. (2022). Healthcare financing in Egypt: A systematic literature review. *Journal of the Egyptian Public Health Association*, 97(1): 1–11.

Gericke C., Britain K., Elmahdawy M., & Elsisi G. (2018). Health System in Egypt. https://link.springer.com/referenceworkentry/10.1007/978-1-4614-6419-8_7-1(link is external and opens in a new window).

Ghaffar N., Javad S., Farrukh M. A., Shah A. A., Gatasheh M. K., Al-Munqedhi B. M. A., et al. (2022) Metal nanoparticles assisted revival of Streptomycin against MDRS *Staphylococcus aureus*. *PLoS ONE* 17(3): e0264588. DOI:10.1371/journal.pone.0264588.

Ghaffar A., Zennaro L., Nran N. (2022). The African health initiative's role in advancing the use of embedded implementation research for health systems strengthening. *Global Health: Science and Practice*, 10(Supplement 1): e2200318; DOI: 10.9745/GHSP-D-22-00318. Accessed August 22, 2023.

Global Sustainable Development Indicators Database (2022). https:unstats.un.org/sdgs/iindicators/database. Accessed August 18, 2022.

Government of the Arab Republic of Egypt (2021). Embassy of Arab Republic of Egypt Washington DC. https://egyptembassy.net/the-embassy/. Accessed August 21, 2023.

Hammed M. (2020). No hospitals for the poor: How 20,000 beds disappeared from Egypt hospitals. Arab Reporters for investigative journalism. https://arj.net/inestigations/corona-host-Egypt-en/. Accessed July 28, 2024.

Hopwood D., Gordon C., Arthur S., Goldschmidt E. (2023). Egypt. https://www.Britannica.com/place/Egypt/Land. Accessed July 25, 2024.

International Energy Association. (2022). Sustainable Development Strategy: Egypt Vision 2030. https://www.iea.org/policies/14823-sustainable-development-strategy-egypt-vision-2030. Accessed August 24, 2024.

Khalifa A. Y., Jabbour J. Y., Mataria A., Bakr M., Farid M., Mathauer I. (2022). Purchasing health services under the Egypt's new universal health insurance law: What are the implications for universal health coverage. *International Journal of Health Planning Management*, 37(1): 619–631.

Lambert T. (2020). A Brief History of Egypt. https://localhistories.org/a-brief-history-of-egypt/. Accessed July 30, 2023.

Latif A. A., Magdy D., El Sharkawy K., William M., Magid M. (2018). Egypt SDS 2030: Between expectations and challenges to implement. https://documents.aucegypt.edu/Docs/GAPP/Public%20Policy%20Hub%20Webpage/7-stainable%20Development. Accessed August 24, 2023.

Mathauer I., Dkhimi F., Townsend M. (2022). Adjustments in health purchasing as part of the COVID-19 health response: results of a short survey and lessons for the future.2020. https://p4h.world/en/blog-covid-19-and-health-purchasing-response. Accessed September 4, 2024.

Mathauer I., Khalifa A. Y., Mataria A. (2019). Implementing the Universal health insurance law of Egypt: What are the key issues on strategies purchasing and its governance arrangement? World Health Organization Publication.

Memphis Tour (2023). Egypt in the modern era. https://www.memphi stours.com/egypt/Egypt-Wikis/Egypt-History/wiki/Egypt-in-the-Modern-era. Accessed August 20, 2023. in the rn.

Midant-Reynes B. (1992). *The Prehistory of Egypt: From the First Egyptians to the First Kings*. Oxford: Blackwell Publishers.

Office of the Historian (2020). A Guide to the United States' History of Recognition, Diplomatic, and Consular Relations, by Country, since 1776: Egypt. https://history.state.gov/countries/Egypt. Accessed August 20, 2023.

Olassa A. (2020). 7 facts about healthcare in Egypt. https://borgenproject.org/healthcare-in-egypt/. Accessed August 22, 2023.

Oxford Business Group. (2022). Egypt Country Profile. https://oxfordbusinessgroup.com/reports/egypt/2022-report#:~:text=Located%20at%20the%20geographic%20 Centre, positive%20GDP%2growth%20in%202020. Accessed September 4, 2024.

Oxford Business Group (2016). New government policy in Egypt to recalibrate healthcare system. https://oxfordbusinessgroup.com/reports/egypt/2016-report/economy/reform-effort-a-comprehensive-new-government-policy-aims-to-recalibrate-the-health-care-system. Accessed June 15, 2023.

Salama N. (2022). Health equity in Egypt: Reflections in 2022. https://aps.aucegypt.edu/en/articles/786/health-equity-in-egypt-relection-in-2022. Accessed July 24, 2023.

United Nations (2022). Country program document for Egypt (2023–2027). https://www.undp.org/sites/g/files/zskgke326/files/2022-09/N2240578%20-%20UNDP%20Egypt%20 CPD%202023-2027.pdf. Accessed September 4, 2024.

United Nations Human Development Index (2021). https://ourworldindata.org/grapher/human-development-index. Accessed August 31, 2024.

United Nations Human Development Programme (2021). Human Development Report. https;//hdr.undp.org/en/2020-report. Accessed July 10, 2022.

USAID (2020). Egypt Country profile. https://www.usaid.gov/egypt/our-work. Accessed August 25, 2023.

User S. (2021). Egypt's Health Care System. https://www.cghd.org/index.php/global-health-partnerships-and-solutions/profiles/43-egypts-health-care-system. Accessed August 22, 2023.

Wikipedia. (2023). History of Egypt. https://en.wikipedia.org/wiki/History_of_Egypt. Accessed August 20, 2023.

World Bank Indicators. (2022). Egypt: World Health Organization's Global Health Workforce Statistics. https://data.worldbank.org/indicator/SII.MED.NUMW.P3?locations=EG. Accessed August 22, 2023.

World Factbook. (2020). The World Factbook. https://www.cia.gov/the-world-factbook/about/cover-gallery/2020-cover/. Accessed September 4, 2024.

World Factbook (2021). Egypt. https://www.cia.gov/the-world-factbook/countries/egypt/. Accessed November 8, 2024.

World Factbook. (2022). Egypt: The World Factbook. https://www.cia.gov/the-world-factbook/about/archives/2022/. Accessed September 4, 2024.

World Bank Indicators (2020). https://databank.worldbank.org/source/world-development-indicators. Accessed October 30, 2024.

World Health Organization. (2023). Egypt Health Indicators. https://data.humdata.org/dataset/who-data-for-egypt? Accessed August 20, 2023.

World Health Organization. (2022). Egypt Health Indicators. https://data.humdata.org/dataset/who-data-for-egypt? Accessed August 20, 2023.

World Health Organization Indicator (2020). Monitoring Health for the Sustainable Development Goals. https://cdn.who.int/media/docs/default-source/gho-documents/world-health-statistic-reports/2020/en_whs_2020_toc.pdf. Accessed November 8, 2024.

Chapter Seven

HEALTH POLICY AND CHALLENGES IN ETHIOPIA

Robert Dibie and Masey Barekew

Introduction

This chapter examines the major health policy initiatives that the Federal Democratic Government of Ethiopia has taken to improve the nation's healthcare system for all citizens in the country. It also explores some of the major health and social challenges that the government is currently dealing with in the country. It argues that while the Government of Ethiopia is trying to meet the United Nations Millennium Development Goals in respect of healthcare in the country, there is a need for the nation to seek more foreign aid to accomplish its benchmark. The chapter uses data derived from primary and secondary sources to analyze the health policy outcomes and challenges in Ethiopia. The findings show that a better health system in the country could galvanize the private and public sectors in addressing education, healthcare, public health programs, welfare, and economic and social development issues in the rural and urban regions of Ethiopia. In addition, the Ethiopian Government's health policies have not been able to effectively galvanize the private sector and nongovernmental organizations (NGOs) to create more health clinics and hospitals in the rural regions. There is widespread recognition that the Government of Ethiopia does not have infinite healthcare workers and financial resources to provide all the necessary equipment and medical resources needed to accomplish the nation's millennium health goals. This is because of its current unsustainable deficits and civil war. The chapter recommends that the government; private sector, foreign partners, and NGOs should collaborate to establish a mechanism for a better and more efficient approach to providing healthcare, public health prevention services, employment, public goods, and services for all Ethiopians. The chapter also suggests that appropriate monetary and fiscal policies that are necessary for Ethiopia to effectively address its sustainable development and capacity-building challenges should be formulated and effectively implemented.

Brief History of Ethiopia

The Federal Democratic Republic of Ethiopia is the second most populous country in Africa. It also has one of the fastest-growing economies in the African continent. The nation is in the Northeastern Horn of Africa. The nation's population is approximately109.2 million (United Nations Human Development Report 2023). About 50% of the population are women, while the rest are men (African Development Bank Report 2020). Furthermore, 44% of the population is under 15 years of age, and about 52% are between 15 and 65 years old (Africa Facts 2020). The remaining 3% of the population is over 65 years old (African Development Bank Report 2020; Nation Facts 2020). The population living in rural regions of Ethiopia is 83%, while those living the urban areas constitute 16.4% (Ministry of Health Ethiopia, Health Sector Development Program IV 2010). According to the International Monetary Funds (2020) report, the GDP of the country is US$272 billion, while the GDP per capita is US$2,772. The nation's environment is made up of 70% of all the mountains in the African continent (Global Economic Prospects 2021; Nation Facts 2020). The country also has spectacular green plains, vegetation, and landscape (African Facts 2020; Nation Facts 2020). According to the Community Health Poverty Circle (2019) report, green hills and several mountains surround Ethiopia's rural and agricultural communities. The Blue Nile River that derives its source from Lake Tara flows across the country. The official language in the country is Amharic, however, Oroma is spoken by many citizens in the nation. Ethiopia has a federal government and 10 states. The states are Afa, Amhara, Tigray, Oromia, Gambella, Somalia, Benishagul-Gumuz, Southern Nations Nationalist, and Peoples region, Harar the two administrative States Addis Ababa City administration and Dire Dawa Council (Dibie 2018; GlobalEdge 2016).

An especially important historical point is that the Federal Democratic Republic of Ethiopia was never colonized despite two Italian invasions and the European Scramble and Partition of Africa that took place between 1870 and 1914. The Ethiopians' defeat of Italy at the Battle of Adwa is recorded as the first victory of an African nation over a European colonial nation (Africa Facts 2020; GlobalEdge 2016). The Federal Democratic Republic of Ethiopia is the oldest independent country in Africa and one of the oldest in the world (Africa Facts 2020). Ethiopia is a landlocked country and most rural states in the nation are engaged in different forms of traditional economic systems in which the allocation of resources is made based on primitive methods. Many citizens in the rural regions of the country are engaged in subsistence agriculture (GlobalEdge 2016; IMF report 2020). In 2020, it was reported that agriculture constituted almost 45% of the GDP and 85% of the total employment. According to the Federal Democratic Government of Ethiopia (2020) and International Monetary Funds Report (2020), exports of flowers, coffee, oil seeds, and manufactured goods were hit hard by falling global demand due to the coronavirus pandemic and declining prices. However, because of the nation's resilience, the government of the country has adopted measures as well as lower remittances and foreign direct investment (Global Economic Prospects 2021; International Monetary Funds Report 2020).

One of the major challenges to the economic and social development in Ethiopia is that over 900,000 asylum seekers and refugees from Eritrea, South Sudan, migrated to the country as a result of wars that have devasted the economy and livelihood of their respective nations (The United Nations Refugee Agency 2020). The non-employment status of these refugees has contributed to the poor economic and health status of the people of Ethiopia. This is because the refugees neither have land to farm nor finance to start their own businesses. In addition to the above social and economic predicaments created by refugees, more than one million Ethiopian citizens are displaced every year due to rapid urban expansion, the ongoing conflict between the government of the nation and its citizens who are members of the Tigray People's Liberation Front (TPLF) (Mergo 2020).

Health Challenges in Ethiopia

The Democratic Republic of Ethiopia has been making substantial process in its economic development, and the citizens are becoming more productive, educated, and healthy (Adamu 2016; Croke 2020; USAID 2020). However, frequent climate change that leads to drought, disease outbreaks, as well as conflict has often prevented Ethiopia's progress toward its strategic and transformation objective to provide high-quality healthcare services to all the citizens of the country (USAID 2020; Federal Democratic Republic of Ethiopia 2016). According to Mergo (2020), the TPLF of Ethiopia and the Federal Democratic Republic of Ethiopia civil war has claimed the lives of almost one million people as well as displaced several thousand members of its population (Demissie & Negeri 2020). In addition, the civil war has resulted in the misallocation of hard-earned foreign capital that could have been appropriated for economic development healthcare delivery, and capacity building in Ethiopia (Mergo,2020; USAID 2020).

According to the Columbia University School of Public Health report (2024) and Ministry of Health Ethiopia (2015), women in Ethiopia continue to face major problems in maternal and child healthcare. In addition, women in the country are often put under duress to become mothers without the proper infrastructure and care to support them through the nine months of their pregnancy (Gidey et al. 2019; Ministry of Health Ethiopia 2015). Moreover, after the birth of their children, and then the upkeeping of the new children's healthcare is not fully supported by their spouse (Columbia University School of Public Health report 2024; Ministry of Health Ethiopia 2015). Because of the forced childbearing predicament, some women in the country tend to rely on their family or community members for help in transporting them to hospitals and clinics that are often understaffed or do not have specialists to provide high-quality maternal healthcare. These healthcare challenges are also one the major reasons why many infants and children that were delivered in the rural communities do not make it beyond the age of five years or younger due to acute respiratory infection, diarrheal, malaria, and lack of vaccination (Columbia University School of Public Health Report 2024; Croke 2020; and Ministry of Health Ethiopia 2015).

Many scholars contend that in the past one decade, the Federal Democratic Government of Ethiopia has worked diligently to incrementally increase healthcare services to its citizens (Demissie & Negeri 2020; Feysia et al. 2012; Tolu et al. 2020; Reda et al. 2020). Despite these improvements, there have been major challenges to citizens' access to sanitation, immunization, family planning, public health services, and malaria treatment in the country. The Democratic Republic of Ethiopia, Ministry of Health has been implementing the first health sector transformation plan (HSTP-I and HSTP-2), which spanned from 2012, 2015/2016 to 2019/2020. The health transformation plan's major goals are health service delivery; quality improvement and assurance; leadership and governance; and health system capacity (Ministry of Health Ethiopia 2012). These factors constitute a new mechanism for improving the health conditions of the citizens of the country. According to the Ministry of Health Ethiopia report, the COVID-19 pandemic significantly challenged the health system in 2019. It is estimated that by the end of September 2020, more than 77,000 cases were evaluated positive for coronavirus, with a positivity rate of 6% (Croke 2020; Demissie & Negeri 2020; Downie 2016). It is paramount to note that although the Ministry of Health did not foresee the outbreak of the coronavirus when they initiated the plan, they had to adjust the HSPT-2 to accommodate the negative impacts of the COVID-19 pandemic on the health system of Ethiopia (Ministry of Health Ethiopia 2020). This drastic change in the plan created another set of challenges with respect to capita and human resources, as well as governance (Zerfu et al. 2023).

Many scholars have also argued that there is a strong correlation between harmful cultural or traditional beliefs and practices, and the low status of women, as well as male domination (Teller & Hailemariam 2011; Downie 2016; Dynes et al. 2014). Furthermore, marriage has become the principal indicator of women's exposure to the risk of pregnancy, which comes exceedingly early in the lives of girls between 15 and 25 years old in the country (Ministry of Health, Health Sector Transformation Plan 2015/2016–2019/2020). According to Teller and Hailemariam (2011) and Community Health Poverty Circle Report (2019), the tradition in the country requires married girls to bear children as soon as they are married. The outcome of this practice is that women and girls in the rural region of the country die each year from pregnancy complications such as hypertensive disorder, hemorrhage or bleeding, abortion, prematurity of pregnancy, birth asphyxia, neonatal sepsis, and obstructed labor. Another serious healthcare predicament that affects women and girls in the rural regions of Ethiopia is the lack of antenatal and postnatal care, family planning service, safe and clean delivery service, and essential obstetric care (Barros et al. 2012; Teller & Hailemariam 2011; World Health Organization 2020). It is mind-boggling to read about how almost 70% of women in some rural regions of Ethiopia do not see anyone for antenatal care during their pregnancy (Feysia et al. 2012; Poverty Circle Report 2019).

In addition, most poor pregnant women and girls in rural regions are likely to die due to a lack of skilled maternity care during pregnancy and childbirth. The traditional practice of female genital mutilation (or cutting), and early marriage has also contributed to low maternal healthcare service utilization in Ethiopia (Teller & Hailemariam 2011; Feysia et al. 2012; Hill & Narayan 2020).

Although the Federal Democratic Government of Ethiopia may have particularly good intentions and strategic plans to resolve the nation's healthcare delivery challenges, it has been confronted with low financing sources. It has been reported for many years that the government and other public enterprises provide 31% of the financing, NGO donors provide 37%, households mostly from the urban regions provide 31%, and the remaining 2% comes from the private sector employers (Ministry of Health Ethiopia 2021; Wamai 2009). During the 2009–2010 fiscal year, the Ethiopian government and development partners appropriated a budget of US$883.06 million for healthcare service provisions (Debie et al. 2022; Lavers 2019; Ministry of Health Sector Development Program 2010). It also proposed an average annual increase of 9% increase from 2011 to 2015 (Ministry of Health Sector Development Program 2010).

The United States government, and its Central for Disease Control (CDC), the World Health Organization, many NGOs, and nonprofit organizations around the world have been helping to finance Ethiopia's efforts to improve its ability to prevent, detect, and respond to infectious disease outbreak (Central for Disease Control Ethiopia Office Report 2018; Demissie & Negeri 2020; Lavers 2019; Ministry of Health Ethiopia Report 2020; World Bank Group 2022; WHO Report 2020). In addition to the financial challenges in Ethiopia, there is still evidence of a sub-optimal pharmaceutical and medical equipment supply management system and inadequate partnership between the private and public sectors in the administration of healthcare delivery systems in the country.

Hygiene and environmental sanitation are still a major health problem in Ethiopia. According to the Ethiopia Ministry of Health (2021), about 31% of the citizens living in rural regions rely on unprotected water from ponds, rivers, lakes, and other sources of forms of surface water. Further, about 22.3% of rural regions drink unsafe water from hand-dug wells and natural springs (Community Health Poverty Circle 2019). With the support of foreign NGOs, many citizens now have access to safe-managed drinking water than what the situation used to be 15 years ago. It has also been reported that this contaminated water has often become the source of waterborne diseases that have affected many families. Unfortunately, the affected families must pay expensive fees to receive treatment in rural hospitals and clinics (Community Health Poverty Circle 2019). The Ministry of Health—Ethiopia and many charity organizations have been making efforts to educate rural community members on how to use and drink water from safe sources and wash their hands as precautionary health measures from diseases and infection. Safe water sources have also been constructed in many urban and rural communities by the government and NGOs (Ministry of Health 2016).

Sanitation is another major health issue that confronts Ethiopia. Most people living in rural regions and even in the suburban areas of the capital city still practice what is called open defecation (Community Health Poverty Circle. 2019; International Rescue Committee 2020). This means the act of using the forests, fields along the road, and countryside for toilets. The government has adopted health transformation strategic plans to increase the number of households with latrines. Its recent reports show that latrines have been built in the following agrarian regions in higher numbers: Amhara 87.1%, Tigray 70%, Oromia 96.1%, SNNPR 96.3% (Ministry of Health Growth and Transformation Plan II 2016. Health Sector Development Program 2010). In addition to what the Federal Ministry of Health in Ethiopia is doing many foreign NGOs including the IRC have been delivering clean water and sanitation, essential supplies, and protection services for women and girls (World Bank 2020; International Rescue Committee 2020).

Furthermore, the high unemployment rate in the country has also propelled low-income people to start using home-based medicine for therapies to heal their sicknesses

(Bodeker 2000; Hanlon et al. 2017; Wikipedia 2023). Some scholars contend that the use of traditional medicine in Ethiopia among other factors could be traced to testimonies of the effectiveness of traditional herbs. Other reasons for using traditional medicine include the affordability of traditional medicine, perceived inefficacy of biomedicine, perceived incurability of some diseases via biomedicine, and feeling of embarrassment to present medical conditions to practitioners of biomedicine (Demeke et al. 2022; Legesse & Babanto 2023). In addition, poor family members are reported to be dispensing herbal medicine that is like an out-of-home pharmacy. There has been a high rate of false traditional healers in the country as well (Bodeker 2000; Hanlon et al. 2017; Tuasha et al. 2023; Zewdie et al. 2020).

Health Administration in Ethiopia

According to the Federal Democratic Republic of Ethiopia Ministry of Health (2019/2020) report, the health system administration in the country is organized on a multiple level. At the *fourth or highest level*, the Ministry of Health provides central direction with the national health policy formulation and implementation. The Ministry of Health also coordinates the healthcare plans which also regulates all health conditions in the country (Federal Ministry of Health, Health Policy Transitional Government of Ethiopia 1993).

The *third level* comprises a specialist hospital that provides healthcare for over three million people. It should be noted that the decentralization of power and health administrative responsibilities to the regional governments has also resulted in a major shift in the decision-making process for public healthcare services from the Ministry of Health to the regions and down to the district level. Thus, health offices at the three major healthcare levels engage in shared governance in the administration of the nation's health system (Ethiopia Ministry of Health 2020).

Further, the Ministry of Health also is decentralized in such a way that the nine regions and major city administrations play a key role in the health system of the country. The *second level* comprises general hospitals that cover a population of between one and two million people (Federal Ministry of Health, Health Policy Transitional Government of Ethiopia 1993). The city administrations are given some authority to autonomously implement the health plan in the health facilities' that are located with their city. Although the city has some autonomous authority, they are mandated to meet the national set targets for healthcare delivery and outcomes within their metropolitan districts (Ethiopia Ministry of Health 2020).

In addition, the *districts or lower level*, also participate in health planning, and the health officers coordinate the health administration within their region. Thus, the district officers are responsible for supplying a range of services geared toward the specific needs of the populations that reside in their districts. For example, the Woreda District health system also comprises a primary hospital that covers over 60 million people, health centers, and a satellite health post that is connected by a referral system (Adane et al. 2021; Ethiopia Ministry of Health 2010) The district officers are also expected to lead in the health planning from the grassroots, through district-led shared governance models of planning in implementing the process.

Types of Health Policies

The Human Rights Watch (2023) report reveals that the health system in Ethiopia has incrementally improved over the past three decades with government leadership playing a key role in appropriating more funding, and mobilizing other human, and capacity-building resources (Human Rights Watch 2023; Wikipedia 2023). Below are selected health policies that the Federal Government of Ethiopia has enacted over the past four decades.

National Healthcare Quality Strategy 2021–2025: The goal of this policy is to consistently improve the clinical care, patient safety, and patient-centered experience of the citizens and residents of Ethiopia whenever they visit any healthcare facilities in the country. A second mandate of the national healthcare quality strategy is also to increase access to healthcare and equitable delivery of healthcare to all citizens (Amhare et al. 2022; Ethiopia Ministry of Health 2021).

Community-based Health Insurance (CBHI) Policy of 2010: The goal of the community-based insurance company is to help the informal population in Ethiopia achieve universal health coverage (Ministry of Health Ethiopia 2010 & 2015). Since 2010, the Federal Government of Ethiopia has been trying to establish Social Health Insurance (SHI) for the formal sector to achieve universal health coverage however it has not been able to do so because the resistance from the public servants (Columbia School of Public Health 2024). It is anticipated that CBHI will cover over 11 million people, which makes it one of the largest health schemes in Africa (Croke 2020; Gidey et al. 2019; Laver 2019). While there is no mandate to have health insurance, the government does promote CBHI expansion (Ethiopia Ministry of Health 2021; Ethiopia's rural-urban transformation process 2019).

Health Extension Program (HEP) enacted in 2003: The goal of the health extension policy is to train health workers to deliver basic care. The HEP policy was implemented in addition to the large-scale construction of hospitals, health centers, and health posts to house the health extension workers. Further, the health extension policy mandated the Ministry of Health—Ethiopia to recruit and retained highly trained health workforce specifically for rural communities in the country. This policy was also known as the flooring policy. Because it enhanced the public sector workforce by flooding the market with clinical doctors, nurses and midwives, and other healthcare professionals (Asefa et al. 2019; Croke 2020; Ministry of Health—Ethiopia 2010).

Ethiopia Health Policy enacted in 1993: The major goal of this policy is linked to the democratization and decentralization of the health system, and intersectoral collaboration (Ministry of Health—Ethiopia 1993). Other goals of the health policy include (1) Development of the preventive and promotive components of healthcare. (2) Development of an equitable and acceptable standard of health service system that will reach all segments of the population within the limits of recourses. (3) Promoting and strengthening of intersectoral activities. (4) Promotion of attitudes and practices conducive to the strengthening of national self-reliance in health development by mobilizing and maximally utilizing internal and external resources. (5) Assurance of accessibility of healthcare for all segments of the population (Ministry of Health

Ethiopia 1993; Health Policy of the Transitional Government of Ethiopia 1993). The health policy of 1993 has been reported to have led to several health-related programs and strategies that galvanized the health system in the country (Croke 2020; Health Policy of the Transition Government of Ethiopia 1993).

According to Rono et al. (2022) and Ethiopia Ministry of Health (2010), the Federal Ministry of Health of Ethiopia has formulated and adopted other healthcare strategic initiatives in the past two decades such as adolescent and youth reproductive health strategy (2006), maternal and neonatal health, making pregnancy safer (2000), reproductive health strategy (2006), and the revised abortion law (Ministry of Health Ethiopia 2010; Rono et al. 2022). In addition, other strategic initiatives adopted include a healthcare financing strategy, free service for key maternal and child health services, training and deployment of the new workforce of female health extension workers for institutionalizing community healthcare with clean and safe delivery at the health post level, and deployment of health officers with a master of science degree training in integrated emergency obstetric and surgery skills (Ethiopia Ministry of Health 2010; Rono et al. 2022).

Data Analysis and Discussion

The objective of this chapter is to analyze the effectiveness of the healthcare policy and delivery system in Ethiopia. The primary research involves the administration of a questionnaire to 3,500 respondents. Three thousand, two hundred and twenty-five or 92.1% of respondents returned their completed questionnaire. The questionnaire respondents constitute 53% men and 47% women. In addition, 45% of the respondents had visited a hospital or clinic to receive treatment at least twice a year. Another 33% had also visited a hospital or clinic between 3 and 4 times recently to receive treatment. While 22% of the respondents visited 5–6 times in the last year.

Table 1 analyzes the effectiveness of healthcare delivery and health policy in the Federal Democratic Republic of Ethiopia. The result of the questionnaire reveals that 98% of the respondents disagree that the government promotes equity in the delivery of healthcare to underserved citizens in the country. In addition, 98% of the respondents disagree that hospitals and health centers in their city have constant electricity. On one hand, 92% of the respondents indicated that there is a lack of effective health policy implementation and access to hospitals in rural regions of the country. On the other hand, 78.2% of the respondents disagree that the government is effectively regulating medical professional licensing and disciplinary boards. Furthermore, 76.4% of respondents also disagree that corruption and unethical behavior of political and administrative leaders in government negatively affect the health system's funding. The interesting to note that 76.4% of the questionnaire respondents indicated that most hospitals in the country do not have modern equipment. About 76.3% of the respondents also disagreed that they could afford their healthcare treatment and medication costs without government subsidies. Table 1 covers a summary of a questionnaire that was administered in Ethiopia to determine patients' experience of the healthcare system in the country.

Table 1 The Nature of Healthcare Delivery and Policy in Ethiopia

	Questions	Strongly Agree	Agree	Neutral	Strongly Disagree	Disagree	Agree %	Disagree %
1	Healthcare provided by doctors in my city is highly commendable	577	800	54	806	988	1794 55.6%	1377 42.7%
2	Most hospitals in my country do not have modern equipment	327	387	48	1,121	1,342	714 22.1%	2,463 76.4%
3	I can afford my healthcare treatment and medication costs without government subsidies	239	427	100	1,196	1263	666 20%	46 76.3%
4	Most rural public hospitals in my country do not have specialist doctors and nurses.	869	1,741	13	273	329	2,610 80.9%	7 18.7%
5	Competency and skills of doctors, nurses, and malpractice are addressed by the government	634	851	0	796	944	1,485 46%	3 54%
6	Lack of effective health policy implementation and access to hospitals in rural regions of the country	37	109	111	892	2076	146 4.5%	2,968 92%
7	Government promotes equity in the delivery of healthcare to underserved citizens in the country.	23	49	0	1,653	1,500	72 2%	3,040 98%
8	Political leaders and rich citizens of my country prefer to seek healthcare services in foreign nations.	1,238	1,388	19	123	457	2,626 81.4%	0 18%
9	The government is effectively regulating medical professional licensing and disciplinary boards	287	354	63	1,089	1,432	641 20%	2,521 78.2%
10	Hospitals and health centers in my city have constant electricity.	0	63	0	2,413	747	63 2%	3,162 98%
11	Lack of appropriate funding for the healthcare system in my country.	575	1,429	0	483	738	2,004 47%	1,221 30%
12	Corruption and unethical behavior of political and administrative leaders in government negatively affect the health system's funding.	327	387	48	1,121	1,342	714 22.1%	2,463 76.4%
	Mean						31.8%	63.2%

Source: Derived from Field research in Ghana between 2020 and 2023.

In respect of healthcare workers, 80.9% agreed that most rural public hospitals in the country do not have specialist doctors and nurses. Another 81.4% also agreed that political leaders and rich citizens of my country prefer to seek healthcare services in foreign nations. While 55.6% of the respondents agree that healthcare provided by doctors in their city is highly commendable. Among the respondents, 42.7% disagree that the healthcare provided in their city should be commendable. In addition, 46% of the respondents agree that the competency and skills of doctors and nurses' malpractice are effectively addressed by the government in the country are effective. Another 54% of the respondents disagree with the performance of government regulation services in Ethiopia. The mean of the agree was 31.8%, while the mean of disagree is 63.2%. Thus, the respondents confirmed that the healthcare system and health policy in Ethiopia have not been effective.

Table 2 shows the summary of the content analysis of secondary research data that was conducted. The Federal Democratic Republic of Ethiopia currently spends an average of between 3.4% and 4% annually of its gross domestic product (GDP) for healthcare in the past two years. The government appropriated US$3.1 billion or 4.7% of its GDP for the health system in 2016/2017. In 2019–2020, it also spent US$3.62 billion or 6.3% of its GDP on the health system. The trend of funding of the health system in Ethiopia shows that in the past fiscal years, the budget increased from 4.7% of its GDP in 2016/2017 to 6.3% of GDP in 2019–2020 (Ministry of Health 2022). Despite these recurring healthcare spending increases, in 2022, the budget as a percentage of GDP dropped from 6.3% in 2019–2020 to 3.4% in 2022 (Ministry of Health—Ethiopia 2020; World Bank Indicator 2022). This pattern of health sector funding by the Federal Democratic Government of Ethiopia Government is below the 15% of GDP that the government of Ethiopia pledged at the 2001 Abuja Declaration. The GDP of the Federal Democratic Republic of Ethiopia in 2022 was US$126.8 billion.

The physician or doctors per 1,000 was 0.1 in 2020, while the ratio of nurses/midwives per 1,000 people was 0.8 in the same year. Furthermore, the number of hospital beds per 1,000 people was 0.3 in 2015 (World Bank Indicators 2022), In addition, access to safe managed drinking water was 32% in Ethiopia in 2022. Further, people using safely managed sanitation services (% of the population) was 7% in 2022. On the other hand., people practicing open defecation (% of the population) constitute 18% in Ethiopia in 2022 (World Bank Indicators 2023). Among the population of Ethiopia, 94.3% of them has access to electricity.

Furthermore, the common diseases in Ethiopia are neonatal disorders; diarrheal diseases; lower respiratory infections; stroke; tuberculosis; ischemic heart disease; HIV/ AIDS; cirrhosis and other; chronic liver diseases; congenital birth defects; and malaria (World Health Organization 2020). Life expectancy has improved in the country. While life at birth is currently 68 years for females in 2021. The life expectancy in 2021 for males has increased to 62 years. On one hand, the mortality rate for females per 1,000 people will be 177 in 2021. On the other hand, the mortality rate for male adults per 1,000 people is 39 in 2021 (World Bank Indicators 2023). Unfortunately, the mortality rate for infants per 1,000 people dropped to 34 in 2021.

Ethiopia is frequently witnessing various plagues of communicable and noncommunicable diseases. In some instances, these diseases spread from one person

Table 2 Economics and Health Indicators in Ethiopia

No.	Major Indicators in Mali	Explanation
1	Population	123.3 million (2022)
2	Gross domestic product (GDP)	US$126.8 million (2022)
3	Current health expenditure (% of GDP)	3.48% (2020)
4	Physicians/doctors per 1,000 people	0.1 (2020)
5	Nurses and midwives per 1,000 people	0.8 (2020)
6	Population using safe-managed drinking water service	13% (2022)
7	People using safely managed sanitation services (% of population)	7% (2022)
8	People practicing open defecation % of the population	18% (2022)
9	Number of hospital beds per 1,000 people	0.3 (2015)
10	Common disease	Neonatal disorders; diarrheal diseases; lower respiratory infections; stroke; tuberculosis; ischemic heart disease; HIV/AIDS; cirrhosis and other; chronic liver diseases; congenital birth defects; malaria
11	Life expectancy at birth for females	68 years (2021)
12	Life expectancy at birth for males	62 years (2021)
13	Mortality rate for female adults (per 1,000 people)	177 (2021)
14	Mortality rate for male adults (per 1,000 people)	39 (2021)
15	Mortality rate for infants (per 1,000 people)	34 (2021)
16	Tuberculosis incidence (per 100,000 people)	126 (2022)
17	Population living below income poverty line PPP $2.15 a day	14% (2015)
18	Population in multidimensional handout poverty (%)	23.5% (2015)
19	Contribution deprivation in health to multidimensional poverty	No data reported
20	Infants lacking immunization for measles (% of one year old)	65 (2022)
21	Malaria incidence (per 1,000 people at risk)	43.3% (2021)
22	HIV/AIDS prevalence of adults (% ages 15–49)	0.8 (2021)
23	Population (%) with access to electricity	94.3%

Source: World Bank Indicators (2023); United Nations Human Development Program Index (2023).

to another. On the other hand, they could also spread from animal to person. Some of the communicable diseases commonly found in Ethiopia are HIV/AIDs, COVID-19, malaria, tuberculosis, influenza, protists, Ebola, hepatitis, measles, rabies, sexually transmitted diseases, flu, West Nile virus (Center for Disease Control (CDC) Ethiopia Office Report 2018; Health Development Program IV Report 2010). It should be noted that coronavirus causes an acute respiratory disease, which was first reported in Ethiopia in March 2020 (Federal Ministry of Health Ethiopia 2021; Federal Ministry of Health Ethiopia 2022; Tolu et al. 2020).

These diseases could spread through the air, by touch, or through bodily fluids. After reporting the case of COVID-19 in the country, the government started screening people arriving in Ethiopia at the airport in Addis Ababa. Subsequently, the government of Ethiopia selected the Eka Kotebe Hospital as a location for testing, treating, and isolating people infected with the coronavirus in Ethiopia (Debie et al. 2022; Tolu et al. 2020). Noncommunicable diseases are serious health conditions that do not result from an infectious process. Some examples of such diseases are arthritis, Alzheimer's, cardiovascular, cancer, chronic respiratory disease, diabetes, dementia, neurologic disorders, and stroke (CDC 2018). According to the Center for Disease Control (2018) centers, noncommunicable diseases might result from tobacco use, excessive drinking of alcohol, inactivity, and unhealthy diet.

It has been argued that the shortage of skilled health workers has prompted a shift in the provision of selected maternal and newborn health services from facility-based skilled providers to lower-skilled, community-based health workers (Gile et al. 2022; Dynes et al. 2014; Levin et al. 2010; Tilahun et al. 2022). Shortage of professional healthcare workers is a major challenge that the various Health Sector Development programs identified but have not been able to completely resolve (Tilahun et al. 2022; Health Sector Development Program 2010). Although the urban hospitals have reasonable number of professional healthcare workforce, some of the rural regions' hospitals and health centers are still not adequately staffed. The health policies members had that were introduced by the government of Ethiopia have also resulted in substantial increase in the number of private clinics in the nation. There is also construction of more hospitals and health centers in both the rural and urban regions of the country (Haque et al. 2020; Federal Democratic Republic of Ethiopia 2016). One other healthcare challenge that arises from these successful reinvigorations of the healthcare system in Ethiopia is the shortage of doctors, nurses, pharmacists, and other medical practitioners. The migration of higher-skilled professionals to the private sector and abroad has enhanced disparities between regions as well as urban and rural areas (Gile et al. 2022; Levin et al. 2010; World Health Organization 2020). Despite the introduction of the Health Development Army and the Health Extension Programs, the Ministry of Health has fallen short of the goal of increasing coverage for maternal and newborn healthcare skilled works in urban and rural healthcare facilities in the country (Dyne et al. 2014; Gile et al. 2022; Ministry of Health Sector Development Program HSDP III 2021). This major gap in skilled healthcare workers continues to galvanize a community preference for birth care experienced by family members and traditional birth attendants (Barros et al. 2012; Dyne et al. 2014; Haddiya et al. 2020).

Conclusion

This chapter has examined the major health policy initiatives that the Federal Democratic Government of Ethiopia has taken to improve the nation's healthcare system for all citizens in the country. It also explores some of the major health and social challenges that the government is currently dealing with in the country. It argues that while the Federal Democratic Government of Ethiopia is trying a lot to meet the United Nations Millennium Development Goals in respect of healthcare in the country, the challenges to Ethiopia's regulatory capacity system have not been effective at the local level. This is due to insufficient attention to the health regulation system in the country. There is a need for the country to allow more flexibility in allowing regulators to monitor the perceived competence of providers in both the public and private sectors to produce the desired outcomes of regulation.

To address the current healthcare workforce shortage in Ethiopia, there is a need for the government of Ethiopia to establish a new health policy that could allow hospitals to have more autonomy in designing their respective human resources strategies. Thus, moving forward will require senior government health system personnel to collaborate with the private sector to design simplified human resources governance structures for both the specialist health facilities and teaching hospitals. In addition, there is a need for the government of Ethiopia to adopt a strong political will to develop the health sector, human resources, and more financing to support the health system in the country.

Finally, while there has been some improvement in the financing of the health system, the government of Ethiopia is still struggling with low healthcare funding and high out-of-pocket (OOP) expenditure despite the implementation of several reforms in the healthcare financing system. A unified health insurance system that provides the same benefit packages for all, is the most efficient way to attain equitable access to healthcare. In addition, reinvigorating the current strategy to attract more domestic and external resources, aligning donor funding into the government system, and evidence-based allocation of available resources is essential to advance the goal of a vibrant health system in Ethiopia. Therefore, it is paramount for the government of Ethiopia to modify its current health workers' benefit packages, ensuring equal access to healthcare, and introducing an accreditation system to maintain a high-quality health delivery system. This new strategic approach could be helpful in managing service disparities in both urban and rural districts in the country. These strategic doing and evidence-based approaches could become an optional mechanism for generating confidence in the health system as well as help to attract more local and foreign investment in the nation's health system. Therefore, a robust healthcare financing system will be required to speed up the path toward universal healthcare in the country in the future.

References

Adamu K. B. (2016). Designing a resilient health system in Ethiopia: The role of leadership. *Health System & Reform*. 2: 182–186.

Adane A., Adege T. M., Mesoud M. et al. (2021). Routine health management information system data in Ethiopia: Consistency, trends, and challenges. *Global Health Action*. 14(1): 1–17. DOI: 10.1080/16549716.2020.1868961.

Amhare A. F., Tao Y., Li R., Zhang L. (2022). Early and subsequent epidemic Characteristics of COVID-19 and Their Impact on the Epidemic Size in Ethiopia. *Front Public Health.* May 11; 10: 834592. doi: 10.3389/fpubh.2022.834592.

African Development Bank (2020). Federal Democratic Republic of Ethiopia. https://www.afdb.org/en/countries/east-africa/Ethiopia. Accessed February 19, 2024.

Africa Facts (2020). Facts about Ethiopia. https://africa-facts.org/facts-about-ethiopia. Accessed January 8, 2024.

Asefa Y., Gelaw Y. A., Hill P. S., Taye B. W., Van Damme W. (2019). Community health Extension Program of Ethiopia, 2003–2018: Success and challenges towards universal coverage for healthcare services. *Globalization and Health.* 15(1): 24–37.

Barros A. J. D, Ronsmans C., Axelson H., et al. (2012). Equity in maternal, newborn and child interventions in countdown to 2015: A retrospective review of survey data from 54 countries. *Lancet.* 379: 1225–1233. DOI: 101016/S0140-6736(12)60113-5.

Central for Disease and Control Ethiopia Office (2018). Global Health Security: Ethiopia Factsheet. https://www.cdc.gov/global-health/countries/ethiopia.html. Accessed September 6, 2024.

Columbia University School of Public Health (2024). https://www.publichealth.columbia.edu/research/global-health/africa/ethiopia. Accessed September 6, 2024.

Community Health Poverty Circle (2019). 8 Ethiopia Facts: Poverty, Progress, and What You Should Know. https://lifewater.org/blog/8-ethiopia-facts-poverty-progress-and-what-you-should-know/. Accessed December 27, 2023.

Croke K. (2020). The origins of Ethiopia's primary health care expansion: The politics of state building and health system strengthening. *Health Policy and Planning.* 35(10): 1318–1327.

Debie A., Khatri R. B., Assefa Y. (2022). Contributions and challenges of healthcare financing towards universal health coverage in Ethiopia: A narrative evidence synthesis. *BMC Health Services Research.* 22(1): 866.

Demeke H., Hasen G., Sosengo T., Siraj J., Tatiparthi R., Suleman S. (2022). Evaluation of policy governing herbal medicines regulation and its implementation in Ethiopia. *Journal Multidisciplinary Healthcare.* 15(1): 1383–1394.

Demissie B, Gutema Negeri K. (2020). Effect of community-based health insurance on utilization of outpatient health care services in Southern Ethiopia: A comparative cross-sectional study. *Risk Manage Healthcare Policy.* February, 25(13):141-153.

Dibie R. (2018). Business and government relations in Ethiopia. In *Business and Government Relations in Africa.* Edited by Dibie R. New York: Routledge Press, pp. 247-272.

Downie R. (2016). *Sustaining Improvements to Public Health in Ethiopia.* Washington DC: Center for Strategic and International Studies Publication, pp. 247-272.

Dynes M. M., Stephenson R., and Hadley C. (2014). Factors shaping interactions among community health workers in rural Ethiopia: Rethinking workplace trust and teamwork. *Journal of Midwifery & Women's Health.* 59(s1): S32-S43.

Federal Democratic Republic of Ethiopia (1915). National Human Rights Action Plan. https://www.ohchr.org/sites/default/files/Documents/Issues/Education/Training/actions-plans/Excerpts/NHRAP_Ethiopia_Draft_213-2015.pdf. Accessed October 25, 2024.

Federal Democratic Republic of Ethiopia (2016). *Ethiopia 2016 Growth and Transformation Plan II.* Addis Ababa, Ethiopia: Government Press

Federal Democratic Republic of Ethiopia (2021). Ethiopia Economic Outlook. https://www.afdb.org/en/countries-east-africa-ethiopia/ethiopia-bank-intervention-strategy. Accessed October 31, 2024.

Federal Democratic Republic of Ethiopia (2016). Growth and Transformation Plan II (GTP II) (2015/16-2019/20). https://ethiopia.un.org/sites/default/files/2019-08/GTPII%20%20English%20Translation%20%20Final%20%20June%2021%202016.pdf. Accessed September 6, 2024.

Federal Democratic Republic of Ethiopia (2015). Social health insurance scheme. Federal Neagrit Gazette, Council of Ministers Regulation 271/2012.

Federal Democratic Republic of Ethiopia (2016). *Ethiopia 2016 Growth and Transformation Plan II.* Addis Ababa, Ethiopia: Government Press.

Federal Democratic Republic of Ethiopia (2021). Ethiopia Economic Outlook. https://www. afdb.org/en/countries-east-africa-ethiopia/ethiopia-bank-intervention-strategy. Accessed October 31, 2024.

Federal Ministry of Health of Ethiopia (FMOH). (2016). *Health and Health Related Indicators of Ethiopia for the Year 2016/2016.* Addis Ababa, Ethiopia: FMOH Publication.

Feysia B., Herbst C. H., Lemma S., and Soucat A. (2012). *The Health Workforce in Ethiopia: Addressing the Remaining Challenges.* Washington DC: The World Bank Publication.

Gidey M. T., Gebretekle G. B., Hogan M.-E., & Fenta T. G. (2019). Willingness to pay for social health insurance and its determinants among public servants in Mekelle City, Northern Ethiopia: A mixed methods study. *Cost Effectiveness and Resource Allocation.* 17(1): 2–11. DOI: 10.1186/s12962-019-0171-x.

Gile P. P., van de Klundert J. & Buljac-Samardzic M. (2022). Human resource management in Ethiopian public hospitals. *BMC Health Service Research.* 22(1): 763–777.

Global Economic Prospects, (2021). Egypt. /https://thedocs.worldbank.org/en/doc/ 600223300a3685fe68016a484ee867fb-0350012021/original/Global-Economic-Prospects-June-2021.pdf. Accessed November 8, 2024.

GlobalEdge (2016). Market Potential Index (MPI). https://globaledge.msu.edu/mpi/2016. Accessed September 2, 2024.

Haddiya I., Janfi T. and Guedira M. (2020). Application of the concepts of social responsibility, sustainability, and ethics to healthcare organizations. *Risk Management and Healthcare Policy.* 13, 1029–1033.

Hanlon C., Eshetu T., Alemayehu D., Fekadu A., Semrau M., Thormicroft G., Kigozi F., Marais D. L., Petersen I., Alem A. (2017). Health system governance to support scale up of mental health care in Ethiopia: A qualitative study. *International Journal of Mental Health Systems.* 11(1): 38–49.

Haque M., Isalm T., Rahman A. A., Mckimm J. Abdullah A. and Dhingra S. (2020). Strengthening primary health care to help prevent and control long-term chronic non-communicable diseases in low and middle-income countries. *Risk Management and Healthcare Policy.* 13: 409–426.

Health Policy of the Transition Government of Ethiopia (1993). https://faolex.fao.org/docs/pdf/ eth174474.pdf. Accessed September 6, 2024.

Hill R. V., and Narayan, A. (2020). *How is COVID-19 Likely to Affect Inequality? A Discussion Note.* Washington DC: Unpublished report, World Bank.

Human Rights Watch (2023). Ethiopia event of 2023. https://www.hrw.org/world-report/2024/ country-chapters/ethiopia. Accessed September 6, 2024.

International Monetary Funds (2020). Federal Democratic Republic of Ethiopia. IMF Country Report No. 20/150: Washington DC.

International Rescue Committee (2020). Ethiopia Crisis Briefing. https://www.rescue.org/ country/ethiopia?gclid? Accessed January 14, 2024.

Kevin Croke K. (2022). The origins of Ethiopia's primary health care expansion: The politics of state building and health system strengthening, *Health Policy and Planning.* 35(10): 1318–1327.

Lavers T. (2019). Towards universal health coverage in Ethiopia's development state: The political driver of health insurance. *Social Science & Medicine.* 228, 60–67.

Legesse F. M., Babanto A. M. (2023). Factors associated with the use of traditional medicine in Wolaita zone, southern Ethiopia. *SAGE Open.* 13(1). 10.1177/21582440231153038.

Levin S., Munabi-Babigumira S., Glenton C., et al. (2010). Lay health workers in primary and community health care for maternal and child health and the management of infectious diseases. *Cochrane Database System Review.* 17(3): CD004015. DOI: 10.1002/14651858. CD004015.pub3.

Mergo T. (2020). The War in Tigray Is a Fight Over Ethiopia's Past—and Future. https:// foreignpolicy.com/2020/12/18/the-war-in-tigray-is-a-fight-over-ethiopias-past-and-future/. Accessed January 10, 2024.

Ministry of Health—Ethiopia (2022). Ethiopia National Heath Accounts Report, 2019/20. Addis Ababa, Ethiopia: Ministry of Health, Partnership and Cooperation Directorate.

Ministry of Health—Ethiopia (2021). Health Sector Development Program HSDP III 2021. Addis Ababa, Ethiopia: Ministry of Health Publication.

Ministry of Health – Ethiopia (2020). Fact Sheet- Ethiopia 2020. https://www.moh.gov.et/index. php/en/fact-sheets?language_content_entity=en. Accessed September 4, 2024.

Ministry of Health Health—Ethiopia. (2012). Annual Performance Report. file:///C:/Users/ PROFRO~1/ AppData/Local/Temp/Annual_Performance_Report_2012(2019_2020).pdf. Accessed January 10, 2024.

Ministry of Health Health—Ethiopia. (2010). Health Sector Development Program IV. file:///C:/ Users/ PROFRO~1/AppData/Local/Temp/HSDP%20IV.pdf. Accessed January 14, 2024.

Ministry of Health Ethiopia (2015). Health Sector Transformation Plan, Ministry of Health, Ethiopia. YouTube. https://www.youtube.com/watch?v=7-N3PRpF-XU. Accessed February 8, 2024.

Ministry of Health—Ethiopia (2012). Annual Performance Report. file:///C:/Users/ PROFRO~1/ AppData/Local/Temp/Annual_Performance_Report_2012(2019_2020). pdf. Accessed January 10, 2024.

Ministry of Health Sector Development Ethiopia (2010). Health Sector Development Program IV. file:///C:/Users/ PROFRO~1/AppData/Local/Temp/HSDP%20IV.pdf. Accessed January 14, 2024.

Ministry of Health Ethiopia (1993). Health Policy of the Transitional Government of Ethiopia. Addis Ababa, Ethiopia: Ministry of Health Publication. https://faolex.fao.org/docs/pdf/ eth174474.pdf. Accessed February 8, 2024.

Nation Facts (2020). 50 fascinating facts about Ethiopia. https://nationfacts.net/ethiopia-facts/. Accessed August 30, 2024.

Organization for Economic Development (2020). Ethiopia's rural-urban transformation process. https://www.oecd-ilibrary.org/urban-rural-and-regional-development/rural-development-strategy-review-of-ethiopia_8f129f69-en. Accessed November 8, 2024.

Reda M. G., Bune G. T., & Shaka M. F. (2020). Epidemiology of high fertility status among women of reproductive age in Wonago district, Gedeo zone, southern Ethiopia: A community-based cross-sectional study. International Journal of Reproductive Medicine. May 21; 2915628. doi: 10.1155/2020/2915628.

Rono J., Kamau L., Mangwana J. et al. (2022). A policy analysis of policies and strategic plans on maternal, newborn and child health in Ethiopia. International Journal Equity Health. 21, 73. DOI: 10.1186/s12939-022-01656-x.

Teller C. and Hailemariam A. (2011). The Demographic Transition and Development in Africa: The Unique Case of Ethiopia. New York: Springer Press.

Tilahun B., Endehabtu B. F., Gashu K. D., Mekonnen Z. A., Animut N., Belay H., Denboba W., Alemu H., Mohammed M., Abate B. (2022). Current and future needs for human resources for Ethiopia's national health information system: Survey and forecasting study. JMIR Medical Education. 8(2). e28965. DOI: 10.2196/28965.

Tolu L. B., Ezeh A. and Feyissa G. T. (2020). How prepared is African for the COVID-19 pandemic response? The case of Ethiopia. Risk Management and Healthcare Policy. 13: 771–776.

Tuasha N., Fekadu S. & Deyno S. (2023). Prevalence of herbal and traditional medicine in Ethiopia: A systematic review and meta-analysis of 20-year studies. System Review. 12: 232–243. DOI: 10.1186/s13643-023-02398-9.

United Nations Human Development report (2023). Ethiopia Multidimensional Poverty Index 2023. https://hdr.undp.org/sites/default/files/Country-Profiles/MPI/ETH.pdf. Accessed February 6, 2024.

United States refugee Agency (2020). Ethiopia Refugee Crisis Explained. https://www.unrefugees.org/news/ethiopia-refugee-crisis-explained/.

United States International Development Agency (USAID) (2020). Ethiopia Country Profile—December 2020. https://www.usaid.gov/ethiopia/document/ethiopia-country-profile-december-2020. Accessed January 25, 2024.

Wamai R. G. (2009). Reviewing Ethiopia's health system development. *Japan Medical Association Journal*. 52: 279–286.

Wikipedia (2023). Health-in-Ethiopia. https://en.wikipedia.org/wiki/health-in-Ethiopia. Accessed February 9, 2024.

World Bank Indicators (2023). Poverty Data for Ethiopia. https://povertydata.worldbank.org/poverty/country/ETH. Accessed February 6, 2024.

World Bank Group (2022). Ethiopia poverty assessment: poverty rate decline, despite challenges. https://www.worldbank.org/en/country/ethiopia/publication/ethiopia-poverty-assessment-poverty-rate-declines-despite-challenges. Accessed February 6, 2024.

World Health Organization (WHO) (2020). Health topics in Ethiopia. https://www.afro.who.int/countries/ethiopia . Accessed February 6, 2024.

Zewdie S., Andargie A., Kassahun H. (2020). Self-medication practices among undergraduate university students in northeast Ethiopia. *Risk Management and Health Policy*. 13: 1375–1381.

Zerfu T. A., Tareke A. A., Biadgilign S. (2023). Challenges and experience of the Ethiopian rural health extension program: Implications for reform and revitalization. *BMC Health Services Research*. 23(1): 1309. DOI: 10.1186/s12913-023-10253-9.

Chapter Eight

GHANA HEALTH POLICY ANALYSIS

Leonard Gadzekpo and Robert Dibie

Introduction

This chapter investigates the nature of healthcare policies and implementation in Ghana. It argues that although the country's healthcare policies are formulated to accomplish the Millennium Development Goal, there are notable challenges that tend to limit the Government of Ghana's ability to accomplish its various health policy goals. The chapter also describes how some of Ghana's health policies imposed 15%–50% for health service fees. These out-of-pocket fees have negatively affected its citizens' healthcare delivery network and accessibility. The chapter also discussed how citizens' reaction to the negative health policies has led to a major movement from modern medicine to traditional medicine as well as a preference for self-medication for treatment rather than going to hospitals to seek healthcare from physicians. The circumstances that led to the establishment of a new health insurance scheme are also discussed in the chapter. The aftermath of the National Health Insurance Scheme and the current outcomes of the policy's impact on the citizens and residents of Ghana are analyzed. Increased health spending by the government of Ghana has led to an increase in life expectancy, reduced infant mortality, and a reduction in maternal mortality rate. Despite major improvements in the health policy and administration in the country, results show that there is a major gap in access to healthcare between the population in the rural and urban regions. There are disparities between rich and poor citizens and residents of Ghana with respect to the affordability of healthcare services. Some new policies that could be formulated to solve the current challenges are recommended.

Brief History of Ghana

The Republic of Ghana is in West Africa. It has boundaries with the Republic of Togo to the east, Côte d'Ivoire to the west, and Burkina Faso to the north. The Atlantic Ocean is to the south of the country. According to the World Bank Indicators (2022) and Worldometer (2022) report Ghana's population was 33.5 million in 2022 (Worldometer 2023). The nation's gross domestic product (GDP) is estimated to be about US$2,175 billion in 2022 (GlobalEdge 2022; World Bank Indicators 2022; Worldometer 2023). Ghana gained its independence from the United Kingdom on May 6, 1957. The Republic of Ghana currently has a unitary constitutional democracy government.

Ghana formerly called Gold Coast has always been endowed with large mineral deposits since the sixteenth century. However, it is only recently that modern technology has made it possible to locate mineral deposits easily. The mineral resources that have been mined in Ghana in the last few decades include bauxite, crude oil, diamond, dolomite, gold, iron, limestone, manganese, natural gas, and salt (Dibie 2023; World Bank Group 2022; World Economics 2023).

The history of ancient Ghana reveals that there were so many empires in the region that was short-lived. Some of the empires include the Ashanti under King Osei Tutu and the Fante kingdom. Some of the kingdoms that existed in the region include the Songhai Empire, the Ghana Empire, and the Mali Empire. The leaders of these empires, for example, Mansa Musa, were incredibly determined warriors who eventually promoted the trans-Saharan routes (GVI 2023; Owusu-Ansah 2014; Wikipedia 2023). In addition, between the fifteenth and seventeenth centuries, Ghana became a major hob for the transatlantic slave trade. According to Gocking (2005), GVI (2023), and Nehemia (1973), the Ashanti Kingdom of the seventeenth century was recognized for its vibrant tradition as well as its vigorous economic and political systems. King Osei Tutu, the leader of the Ashanti Kingdom also expanded his empire by conquering neighboring states such as the Akan, Bono, Banda, Gonia, and Dagomba Kingdoms (Davies et al. 2023). The King (also called Asantehene) of the kingdom was immensely powerful and participated in several conflicts with the British colonial administration in the region (Boahen 1996; British Broadcasting Corporation 2023; GVI 2023; Buah 1998).

Before the Berlin conference that took place between 1884 and 1885 where the European leaders met to discuss how to control the resources of the African continent, the Portuguese explorers had visited Gold Coast (now called Ghana) in 1470. The British explorers visited the Gold Coast for the first time in 1553 (Brent-Turner 2020; British Broadcasting Corporation 2023). Subsequently, other Europeans such as the British, Danes, Dutch, Germans, and Portuguese settled in several parts of the coastal region of present-day Ghana. According to Meyerowitz (1975) and Gocking (2005), the Fanti chiefs in the southern region of Ghana signed an agreement with the British explorers in 1884. As a result of this agreement, the British subsequently colonized the Gold Coast. The British colonial administration called the territory Gold Cost because of the abundant gold reserve in the region (Brent-Turner 2020; Davies et al. 2023). The name of the nation was changed from Gold Coast to Ghana in 1957 by the British since the majority of the residents relocated south from the formal Kingdom of Ghana (Owusu-Ansah 2014; Wikipedia 2023).

On March 6, 1957, Ghana was granted independence by the British Government after giving up its control of the Ashanti region, the British Togoland, and the Northern Territory Protectorates (Brent-Turner 2020; Davies et al. 2023). Kwame Nkrumah who was one of the leading advocates for Ghana's independence was chosen to be the first Prime Minister and later elected as President of the new Republic of Ghana (Buah 1998; Bretton 1966; Harcourt 2014). During the British colonial administration, the government's role was limited to the provision of basic utilities such as water, electricity, railways, roads, and postal services. Furthermore, other sectors such as agriculture, banking, commerce, and industry were entirely in private hands, with European explorers controlling the greater share in all of them except agriculture.

The Republic of Ghana's first post-independence leader was Kwame Nkrumah (GVI 2023; United States Department of State 2019; Wikipedia 2023). Nkrumah was Prime Minister from 1957 to 1960 and then elected president from 1960 to 1966. After independence, President Nkrumah set out to extend Ghana's control over the economy by establishing many state-owned enterprises in the agriculture and industrial sectors (Davidson 1990; Harcourt 2014). Unfortunately, President Nkrumah's term was replaced by a military coup that was organized by Lieutenant General Joseph A. Ankrah in 1966. Three years later Brigadier-General Akwasi Amankwaa Afrifa, a principal leader of a military coup dethrones General Ankrah's regime. There was another change in the nation's leadership of governance in 1969, and Dr. Kofi Busia was elected President, however on January 13, 1972, General Acheampong overthrew the democratically elected government of Dr. Kofi Busia. Next, Lieutenant-General Frederick W. K. Akuffo became the chairperson of the ruling Supreme Military Council in Ghana from 1978 to 1979. Furthermore, in 1979, Flight Lieutenant Jerry Rawlings led a military coup and overthrew General Akufo. During Rawlings' 112 days role as military leader in Ghana, his regime prosecuted General Ignatius Kutu Acheampong and Lieutenant-General Frederick W. K. Akuffo. Both General Acheampong and General Akuffo were found guilty of corruption and sentenced to death by execution (Harcourt 2014; Wikipedia 2023).

After 112 days as the leader of Ghana, Jerry Rawlings stepped down and Hilla Limann was elected the president on September 24, 1979. After two years of a very weak civilian rule administration during which Ghana's economy continued to deteriorate, Rawlings overthrew President Hilla Limann's government on December 31, 1981. During Rawlings second term as the military ruler of Ghana elections were conducted in 1992, and he was elected President of Ghana. Subsequently, President Rawlings was reelected in 1996. In addition, Jerry Rawlings stepped down from the presidency in 2001 after five years. After Rawling's leadership as a democratic leader of Ghana, John Agyekum was elected President to succeed him from January 7, 2001, to January 7, 2009. Further, after President Agyekum's term, Dr. John Evans Atta Mills was elected President in 2008. President Mills was known for his passion for universal health insurance in Ghana. Unfortunately, President John Evans Atta Mills died in office on July 24, 2012, and his Vice President John Damani Mahama was sworn in as interim President of Ghana (Wikipedia 2023). Later, Dankwa Akufo was elected President of Ghana in January 2017. Further, after the presidential election of December 2020. President Dankwa Akufo was reelected for his second term on January 7, 2021 (Wikipedia 2023).

During the colonial administration, a few health centers were established in the southern regions of Gold Coast territory. In addition, equitable access to health, education, and other social services for all citizens of Gold Coast did not take place during the colonial administration (Addae 1996; Agyei-Mensah & de-Graft Aikins 2010). In the past three decades, the network of hospitals and health clinics that provide primary healthcare for the population all over Ghana has tremendously increased and improved from what it used to be two decades ago.

Health Challenges in Ghana

The Government of Ghana was the first nation in the African continent that introduce the National Health Insurance Scheme in 2003. This health policy was a major mechanism for moving toward the formulation of a Universal Health System in the country in the future (Laar et al. 2020; Opoku et al. 2021). It was originally anticipated that enrollment in the new national health insurance scheme could lay the pathway to Universal Health Coverage in Ghana, as well as enhance access to healthcare in the country for all citizens. Unfortunately, after more than two decades of the enactment of the National Health Insurance Scheme in Ghana, there continues to be low enrollment in the health scheme as well as financial instability for effective implementation (Opoku et al. 2021).

The current healthcare challenges in Ghana include a major disparity in gaining access to the health delivery system between urban and rural regions in the country. There is also a significant gap between rich and poor people in the country with respect to access to healthcare facilities and affordability (Asamani et al. 2018; Obu & Aggrey–Buwey 2021). On the other hand, there are major disparities in access to healthcare among women in rural districts and those working in big cities (Abodey et al. 2020; Okoroh et al. 2018).

According to Laar et al. (2020), the population of Ghana is considered to have a higher rate of increased overweight or obesity. In addition, women in their fertility age in the country have experienced a high rate of obesity. This is due to the lack of promotion of a healthy food environment among other things (de-Giaft Alkins 2016; laar et al. 2020). Despite the new exploration of crude oil, expansion of telecommunications, and afforestation development in the country, some residents of Ghana are moving away from modern medicine to traditional medicine or self-medication treatment due to lack of affordability. Another major challenge of healthcare in Ghana is limited support services to facilitate access to healthcare. Apart from the lack of access for the disabled population to enter buildings around the country, there is also the problem of inadequate financing and transportation for people with disability to have access to healthcare (Abodey et al. 2020; Osafo & Yawson 2020).

Most hospitals in urban areas in Ghana have increased their use of information technology equipment in healthcare delivery. Unfortunately, most hospitals and clinics in the country tend to face some challenges such as a shortage of information technology staff, medical and healthcare practitioners, lack of infrastructure, and shortage of funds (Dibie 2018; Suleiman & Muhammad 2021). Although, medical technology has been used in the past three decades in many countries around the world to treat and prevent diseases, such as malaria fever, cancer; child and maternal healthcare, dengue, Ebola, stroke, and recently COVID-19, the Republic of Ghana health system has not been able to fully embrace the use of digital technology or telemedicine to treat its citizens suffering from noncommunicable diseases due to the lack of adequate funding, modern infrastructure and healthcare facilities (Kumi-Kyereme et al. 2017; Longest 2016; Suleiman & Muhammad 2021).

According to Annobil et al. (2021) and Obu & Aggrey–Bluwey (2021), there have always been major challenges in access to healthcare services in rural regions in Ghana due to inadequate health facilities, deficient healthcare service, and poor road networks linking rural communities to the major towns in the country (Obu & Aggrey–Bluwey 2021). As a strategy for solving the rural community access challenges in 1977, Ghana adopted the Community-based service delivery model through a partnership with community health organizations, community clinic attendants, and traditional birth attendants (Atinga et al. 2019). This alternative health delivery strategy was influenced by the Alma Ata Declaration in 1978 with a focus on access to primary healthcare for all populations in both urban and rural districts (Annobil et al. 2021; Ghana Health Service 2016).

Scholars have argued that distance was a major factor impeding the use of maternity health services in Ghana (Bour 2004; Obu & Aggrey–Bluwey 2021). In addition, to distance, the culture in Ghana just like other African countries relegates women, to be in a situation where they become a vulnerable group mostly in all rural communities. Thus, unfavorable social and cultural practices inhibit women's access to medical care in rural regions of Ghana. In most agricultural societies in Ghana because of women's dependency on their husbands and their weak financial capacity, they cannot independently make decisions about access to health facilities like their male partners in the rural districts (Gadzekpo 2018). Women's weak financial situation or status constitutes a major equity and disparity challenge when it comes to access to healthcare (Osafo et al. 2020).

According to Abor et al. (2022) and Seidu et al. (2020), one of the main causes of poor-quality healthcare delivery in the Ghana public health sector is a frustrated and dispirited labor force who encounter daily obstacles such as lack of equipment and essential tools. It has also been argued that healthcare delivery problems in Ghana reflect two major factors: first, the inability to solve the frustrating working conditions and service quality problems (Abor et al. 2022; Agyepong et al. 2004; and Seidu et al. 2020). Other set of healthcare challenges includes delayed promotion; lack of essential equipment, tools, and supplies; inadequate basic and career development that includes in-service training; effect of job placement and the impact of social factors such as health workers' children care support system when they are working long hours every day of the week (Gobah & Zhang 2011; Osafo et al. 2021; Turkson 2009).

There are disparities in the location of specialist hospitals in Ghana. Specialist and teaching hospitals are in Accra in the southern part of the country with a population of over two million people, as well as Kumasi in the middle belt with a population of over one million people. While the rural regions combine to have more population than the above two cities, there are very few hospitals and clinics that are in the districts (Annobil et al. 2021). The disparity in the location of hospitals in the country makes people living in the rural regions travel more than two hundred miles to see a specialist physician when they are referred. Furthermore, most citizens of Ghana in rural regions who are extremely sick sometimes cannot travel with their serious illness to Accra and Kumasi and end up dead before getting to the two big cities. Another major challenge in the healthcare delivery system in Ghana is that the nation does not have enough physicians and hospitals in small towns where the majority of the citizens and residents of the country live. Moreover, there is also the problem of retaining medical doctors in the remote and underdeveloped rural regions of the country (Abor et al. 2022; Blanchet et al 2012; Drislane et al. 2014). There is also a lack of confidence in the skills of some healthcare staff especially in rural health facilities (Seidu et al. 2020). According to Kweku et al. (2020), and Polychronis (2017), after two decades of formulating the Ghana Health Insurance scheme, the poor population in the rural districts is still very concerned about the nature of ineffective diagnostic equipment, unpredicted opening hours of health facilities in their districts, service availability predicaments, frequent drug stock-outs, insufficiently skilled health workers as well as the unprofessional attitudes of some health staff.

Types of Health Policies

Bawontuo et al. (2022), Dibie (2022), and Opoku et al. (2021) contend that taking a new holistic and comprehensive approach to formulating public health policy is considered critical to ensuring the greatest and most equitable population health gains in any country. As a result, understanding the mechanism of data-driven and collaborative mechanics for policy making is an important part of developing strategies to build the capacity to generate and use research going forward. The Republic of Ghana has enacted several health policies in the form of laws, rules or regulations, implementation decisions, and judicial decisions (Republic of Ghana 2020).

National Health Policy (NHP) of 2020: The National Health Policy was enacted to promote, restore, and maintain good health for all people living in Ghana. The mandate of the policy was intended to ensure that the Government of Ghana works toward the achievement of healthy lives for all people living in the country through an enabling policy framework (Government of Ghana 2020). The National Health Policy was also expected to recognize, empower, and bring together, in a coordinated manner, all stakeholders to work toward the accomplishment of the following goals; (1) strengthen the healthcare delivery system to be resilient; (2) encourage the adoption of healthy lifestyles; (3) improve the physical environment; (4) improve the socio-economic status of the population; and (5) ensure sustainable financing for health (Republic of Ghana 2020; Ghana Health Service 2023). Below are selected health policies that have been enacted and implemented in Ghana.

Disability Act of 2006 and 2012: The object of this policy is to promote issues such as access to quality health services, adequate medical rehabilitation, employment, rights, education, transportation, and housing facilities as well as the participation of persons with disabilities in cultural activities (Ghana Ministry of Health 2013). The policy also mandates unrestricted rights of citizens to access public places and buildings, free healthcare, employment, education, and transportation. The policy also allowed for a 10-year moratorium, within which all public buildings were supposed to be made accessible to disabled people (Abaka 2014; Abodey et al. 2020; Ocran 2019; Republic of Ghana 2006).

Ghana's National Health Insurance Scheme (NHIS) Policy of 2003 amended in 2012: The goal of this policy is to ensure universal access to quality basic healthcare for the citizens and permanent residents of Ghana (Republic of Ghana 2012). The National Health Insurance also covers outpatient services, including diagnostic testing and operations such as hernia repair; most in-patient services, including specialist care, and most surgeries. Furthermore, the NHIS policy also provides coverage for hospital accommodation (general ward); oral health treatments; all maternity care services, including caesarean deliveries; emergency care; and all drugs approved by the National Health Agency (Republic of Ghana 2012).

Ghana Child Health Policy of 1999 and 2007: The objective for enacting this policy is to provide a framework for planning and implementing programs. The amended child health policy in 2027 also builds on the previous act that was enacted in 1999. Furthermore, it also complements the Health Sector Program of Work 2007–2015. The goal of the amended policy is to provide healthcare for mother and child—pregnancy, birth, and immediate newborn period, neonatal period, infants, and children (Republic of Ghana 2006). Another goal of the policies is to expand healthcare to essential areas such as health communication, health systems, human resource, monitoring, evaluation, and research that are important for delivering effective programs to children and their mother (Republic of Ghana 2007).

Community-Based Health Planning and Services Initiative in 1999: The major goal of the Community-Based Health Planning and Services (CHPS) policy is to bring health services closer to communities. The CHPS objective is also to move health services to community locations, develop sustainable volunteerism and community health action, empower women and vulnerable groups, improve health provider, household, and community interaction (Ghana Health Services 2018; Kweku et al. 2020; Ministry of Health Ghana 1995). The CHPS initiative is a national strategy geared toward the delivery of crucial community-based health services involving service delivery and health planning with communities. The policy also seeks to improve accessibility, efficiency and quality of health, and family planning care (Binka et al. 1995; Ghana Health Service 2018; Kweku et al. 2020; Polychronics 2017).

Health Administration in Ghana

In Ghana, the Ministry of Health is responsible for healthcare policy making and setting the strategic direction for the health sector. At the national level, the Ministry of Health headquarters at Accra at the *national level* to the regional and districts levels as well as the private sectors play crucial roles in the delivery of primary healthcare services to the citizens of Ghana (Abor et al. 2022; Asewah-Abor & Abekah-Nkrumah 2008; Ministry of Health Ministry 1997). Meanwhile, the Ministry of Health has mandated the semi-autonomous agency, Ghana Health Service, to implement the national health policies through the management and operation of all public health facilities. To effectively manage healthcare facilities in the country, the Ghana Health Service agency is administratively organized at the national, regional, and district levels in the country (Ministry of Health – Ghana 2020; Heerdegen et al. 2020).

Apart from the Ministry of Health coordinating the healthcare system at the *national level*, Ghana's medical system is centered heavily in the two largest cities: Accra, the capital of the nation on the coast with about two million inhabitants, and Kumasi, with about one million citizens in the center of the country. In addition to the two teaching and specialist hospitals in Accra and Kumasi, a new teaching university at Tamale in the North is also attracting more doctors.

At the *regional level,* the Ghana Health Service Agency also oversee its Regional Health Administrations that are in each of the 10 regions all over the country. At the regional level, the District Health Management Team delivers curative services as well as the public health division of the regional hospital (Ministry of Health 1997). The Regional Health Administration provides supervision and management support to the districts and subdistricts within each region (Abor et al. 2022; Heerdegen et al. 2020). The Republic of Ghana's health system is divided into four main levels. The health administrative levels are (1) Government or public sector, (2) private for-profit, (3) private not-for-profit, and (4) traditional system. The district-level administrators report to the regional level while the regional-level managers report to the national-level Ministry of Health in Accra. This chain of command is mandated by the Ghana Health Service and Teaching Hospital Act of 1996, Section 525 (Abor et al. 2022; Asewah-Abor & Abekah-Nkrumah 2008; Ministry of Health 1997).

At the *district level,* hospitals and clinics provide curative services. The majority of the hospitals at the district's levels are mission-based (Abor et al. 2022). The District Health Administration provides supervision and management support to the subdistricts. In addition, the district's Health management teams, and the public health unit of the district hospitals deliver public health services (Ministry of Health 1997). Further, both preventive and curative services are provided by the health facilities at the district levels, as well as outreach services to the communities within their respective districts. Basic preventive and curative services for minor ailments are being addressed at the community and household level with the introduction of CHPS. The role played by the traditional birth attendants (TBAs) and the traditional healers is also receiving national recognition (Abor et al. 2022; Bawontuo et al. 2022).

In addition, the management of health facilities at the district health level is coordinated by health management teams that consist of 12 core members. Some district hospitals serve an average population of 100,000–200,000 people in a clearly defined geographical area (Drislane et al. 2014; Heerdegen et al. 2020). The District Director of Health who is the head of the team is responsible for the operation and management of public health facilities within their district, including health centers and CHPS (Bawontuo et al. 2022; Drislane et al. 2014).

The healthcare sector in Ghana does not only include government-owned health organizations such as hospitals, clinics, medical laboratories, and maternity homes. The private health sector constitutes non-state organizations such as faith-based organizations, nongovernmental organizations, donors' partners, civil society organizations, and traditional medicine facilities (Abor et al. 2022; Dibie 2022). The private sector is also playing a key role in the health system of Ghana. The private sector also covers more than 40% of the total healthcare service delivery in the country (Abor et al. 2022; Ministry of Health Ministry 1997).

Analysis of Data and Discussion

The purpose of this chapter is to analyze the healthcare delivery system in Ghana as well as the effectiveness of health policies in the country of Ghana. The data used for the analysis of healthcare policy effectiveness were derived from both primary and secondary sources. The secondary research methods adopted include the review of the Republic of Ghana Government's Ministry of Health, World Health Organization reports, United Nations Human Development Index annual report, Center for Disease Control, and United States Agency for International Development, academic as well as professional journal articles.

The primary research involves the administration of a questionnaire to 1,600 respondents. One thousand two hundred and ninety-five or 81% of respondents returned their completed questionnaire. The questionnaire respondents constitute 48% men and 52% women. In addition, 62% of the respondents had visited a hospital or clinic to receive treatment at least twice a year. Another 38% had also visited a hospital or clinic between 3 and 4 times recently to receive treatment. While 20% of the respondents visited 5–6 times a year and 4.2% also visited the hospital more than seven times in the same period. Data were analyzed using SPSS to determine the effectiveness and challenges facing the health policy and quality of the healthcare delivery system in Ghana.

Table 1 analyzes the nature of healthcare delivery and health policy in Ghana. The result of the questionnaire reveals that 100% of the respondents agree that political leaders and rich citizens of my country prefer to seek healthcare services in foreign nations due to lack of trust in the Ghana healthcare system. Furthermore, 100% of the respondents also agree that corruption and unethical behavior of political and senior administrative leaders in government negatively affect the health system's funding in the country. Another 94% of the respondents reported that most rural public hospitals in the country do not have specialist doctors and nurses. On one hand, 89.5% of the respondents agree that because government pay low salary to doctors and nurses that is why they are galvanized to migrate to foreign countries to seek better compensation and working condition. On the other hand, 76.4% also agree that lack of appropriate funding of the healthcare system in Ghana is why health delivery system in not amazingly effective in most rural regions. Further, 74.2% of the respondents agree that the healthcare provided by doctors in their cities is highly commendable. It is especially important to note that most of the specialist hospitals in the country are in the urban cities in Ghana.

Furthermore, while 71.5.2% of the respondents agree that lack of effective health policy implementation or regulations has negatively affected the quality of health delivery in the country, 56.2% also agree that government is effectively regulating medical professional licensing and disciplinary boards. Only 44.2% of the respondents agreed that they could afford to pay for their healthcare treatment and medication costs without government subsidies. The mean of the questionnaire respondents that agree is 69.1% while the disagree mean is 18.2%. In addition, 55.8% of the respondents indicated that they cannot afford to pay their healthcare cost without the support of the government.

Table 1 The Nature of Healthcare Delivery and Policy in Ghana

	Questions	Strongly Agree	Agree	Neutral	Strongly Disagree	Disagree	Agree %	Disagree %
1	Healthcare provided by doctors in my city are highly commendable	280	681	262	42	30	961 74.2%	72 5.6%
2	Most hospitals in my country does not have modern equipment	206	295	481	202	111	501 38.7%	313 24.2%
3	I can afford my Healthcare treatment and medication costs without government subsidies.	365	421	207	331	321	572 44.2%	652 50.3%
4	Most rural public hospitals in my country do not have specialist doctors and nurses.	606	609	76	3	1	1,215 94%	4 0.30%
5	Govt. pay of low salary to doctors and nurses has encouraged their migration to foreign countries.	758	401	70	32	34	1,159 89.5%	66 5.1%
6	Lack of effective health policy implementation or regulations	617	309	96	184	89	926 71.5%	273 21.1%
7	Government promotes equity in the delivery of healthcare of underserved citizens in the country.	220	216	207	331	321	436 33.7%	652 50.3%
8	Political leaders and rich citizens of my country prefer to seek healthcare services in foreign nations.	1227	68	0	0	0	1,295 100%	0 0%
9	Government is effectively regulating medical professional licensing and disciplinary boards	352	376	280	120	167	728 56.2%	287 22.2%
10	Hospitals and health center in my city have constant electricity.	354	310	321	108	202	664 51.3%	310 24%
11	Lack of appropriate funding of the healthcare system in my country.	501	488	106	95	105	989 76.4%	200 15.5%
12	Corruption and unethical behavior of political and administrative leaders in government negatively affects the health system's funding.	766	528	1	0	0	1,294 100%	0 0%
	Mean						69.1%	18.2%

Source: Derived from Field research in Ghana between 2020 and 2023

Table 2 Economics and Health Indicators in Ghana

No.	Major Indicators in Ghana	Explanation
1	Population	33.5 million (2022)
2	Gross domestic product (GDP)	US$2,175.9 billion (2022)
3	Current health expenditure (% of GDP)	3.99% (2020)
4	Nurses and midwives per 1,000 people	3.6
5	Physicians/doctors per 1,000 people	0.2
6	Population using safe-managed drinking water service	41% (2020)
7	People using safely managed sanitation services (% of population)	13% (2020)
8	Common disease	Malaria, stroke, lower respiratory infection, neonatal disorders, ischemic heart disease, HIV/AIDS, diarrheal diseases, diabetes
9	Life expectancy at birth for females	66 years (2021)
10	Life expectancy at birth for males	62 years (2021)
11	Mortality rate for female adults (per 1,000 people)	217 (2021)
12	Mortality rate for infants (per 1,000 people)	33 (2021)
13	Mortality rate for male adults (per 1,000 people)	288 (2021)
14	Tuberculosis incidence (per 100,000 people)	136 (2021)
15	Population living below income poverty line PPP US$1.90 a day	13.3%
16	Population in multidimensional handout poverty (%)	47.8% (2018)
17	Contribution deprivation in health to multidimensional poverty	22.3%
18	Infants lacking immunization measles (% of one year old)	8%
19	Malaria incidence (per 1,000 people at risk)	164.4% (2021)
20	HIV/AIDS prevalence of adults (% ages 15–49)	0.9% (2021)

Source: World Bank Indicators (2022); United Nations Human Development Program Index (2022); Human Development Report (2022), and World Health Organization (2023).

Table 2 shows the summary of the content analysis of secondary research that was conducted. The Republic of Ghana currently spends an average of 3.99% of its GDP on healthcare in the past two years. This is below the 15% of GDP that the Republic of Ghana pledge in honor of the Abuja Declaration. The Abuja Declaration refers to the agreement signed by all Presidents who attended the Islam in Africa conference in Abuja, the capital city in Nigeria between November 24 and 28, 1989. Presidential delegates from Ghana were also in attendance at the conference (Adua et al. 2017). The current ratio of physicians/doctors per 1,000 people is 0.2. While the ratio of nurses and midwives per 1,000 people in Ghana is 3.6 (World Bank Indicators 2022). Further, the population using safe-managed drinking water service in Ghana is 41%, while the contribution deprivation in health to multidimensional poverty constitutes 22.3%.

The practice of open defecation such as human feces in fields, forests, bushes, open bodies of water, beaches, or other open spaces. Lack of safe drinking water, sanitation, and open defecation continues to be a major hygiene and public health challenge in rural Ghana. According to Delaire et al. (2022), the population in rural Ghana that practiced open defecation in 2020 was between 18% and 32% of the nation's population. Open defecation often could lead to serious communicable disease and other public health predicaments. This is because open defecation could contaminate flowing body of water or rivers. Further, the number of people practicing open defecation in Ghana was reported to be 18.75% in 2015 (Osumanu et al. 2019). There is some positive relationship between educational background of respondents and ownership of toilet facilities as 65%. The practice of open defecation in Ghana is associated with lack of good education, diseases, undernutrition, and poverty (Gart et al. 2023) in Ghana are malaria, stroke, lower, respiratory infection, neonatal disorders, ischemic heart disease, HIV/AIDS, diarrheal diseases, and diabetes (Ghana Ministry of Health 2023). In addition, the life expectancy at birth for females in 2021 was 66 years, while that of male citizens of the country was 62 years in 2021 (World Bank Indicators 2022). The mortality rate for female adults per 1,000 people was 217 in 2021, while those for male adults in the same year were 288 per 1,000 people. It was also reported that the mortality rate for infants per 1,000 people in Ghana in 2021 was 33. During the same period, the tuberculosis incidence per 100,000 people 136 (World Bank indicators 2022; United Nations Human Development Index 2022). The number of infants lacking immunization measles (% of one year old) is 8%, while malaria incidence per 1,000 people at risk was 164.4% in 2021. The HIV/AIDS prevalence of adults % of ages 15–49 in 2021 has dropped to 0.9% compared to what the number was in 2019. Thus, while the healthcare of the citizens of Ghana has improved incrementally, there are still a lot of challenges confronting the health system in the country.

Conclusion

This chapter has examined the healthcare delivery system in Ghana as well as the effectiveness of health policies in the country of Ghana. It argues that although the country's healthcare policies are formulated to accomplish the Millennium Development Goal, there are notable challenges that tend to limit Government Ghana's ability to accomplish its various health policy goals. Although the Government of Ghana has accomplished a lot in the healthcare sector in the past two decades, there are still a lot of work that need to be done. The research conducted for this chapter reveals the health system in Ghana has improved in the past two decades. However, the problems facing Ghana's health system could be effective solved if efforts are made by the government to provide adequate financial budget for the health system, good policies for retainment of doctors, building modern hospitals and clinics, and provide state of the act equipment as well as medical information technology.

To increase the retention and number of physicians, nurses and other health professionals in Ghana, the Government will have to invest more to provide incentives as such as good working conditions to prevent the flight of physicians and nurses to other foreign countries. Other incentives to motivate health workers to stay and work in the county must include affordable housing allowance, vehicle allowances, scholarships for aspiring medical doctors and nurses, reasonable work hours, and modern healthcare facilities.

There is no doubt that the appropriation of adequate funding to the health system in the country could enhance healthcare delivery and modern medical equipment in the country. Further, the National Health Insurance Scheme, inadequate hospitals and clinics, lack of funding for transporting emergency patients to well-equipped health facilities, and effective use of information technology to keep patients' records, practice is still a major problem. Thus, evidence-based healthcare, as well as promoting healthcare and lifestyle modification could enhance healthcare. Increasing the number of hospital beds is also an especially important mechanism that could complement the enhancement of health delivery system in the country. Furthermore, the provision of modern medical equipment, logistics, communication, and transportation systems could also enhance patients' access to health services in Ghana.

It should be noted however that the increase in healthcare funding cannot be the only solution to the challenges facing Ghana. What is also needed is a comprehensive fiscal management system established to accompany health spending. The current system tends to condole inefficiencies and misappropriation of health budget funds. The adoption of an effective fiscal management agency to monitor health spending could prevent the misappropriation of millions of dollars due to corruption. Ghana's citizens in some cases, see aspects of the various health policies enacted in the country negatively because the healthcare system does not benefit the population equitable. Some foreign-owned health facilities, especially those that seize opportunities in the country offered less opportunities for the poor people that live in rural districts in Ghana. The junction where government interests, business interests, and international economic and financial institutional interests and pressures converge is another set of challenges of affordability and access to healthcare for the poor or low-income population of Ghana.

Healthy relationships between public and private sector health providers remain the root of robust growth and sustained healthcare delivery system in Ghana. It is therefore very necessary for the nation to attempt to solve some the challenges such as insufficient funding and poor work attitudes. If these predicaments are not resolved the healthcare system might face stagnation and instability soon. Given an extremely optimistic vision, Ghana could become a developed country between 2030 and 2035, where both the government and business could collaborate to unleash public and private resources to galvanize a vibrant economic development in the country. Furthermore, how can energy, capacity building, and potential strategies help to achieve such a goal? What type of transformation leader can lead Ghana to attain real economic development, just as it did over half-century earlier in leading sub-Saharan Africa in overcoming colonization and gaining political independence? Yes, this goal can be accomplished. However, the Government of the Republic of Ghana must be mindful that it will take ethical leadership and the citizens of Ghana to develop their nation's healthcare system.

References

Abodey E., Vanderpuye I., Mensah I., Badu E. (2020). In search of universal health coverage-highlighting the accessibility of healthcare to students with disabilities in Ghana: A qualitative study. *BMC Health Services Research*, 20(1): 270–282.

Abor P. A., Abekah-Nkrumah G., Abor J. (2022). An examination of hospital governance in Ghana. https://www.academia.edu/25767118/An_examination_of_hospital_governance_inGhana. Accessed September 3, 2023.

Addae S. (1996). *History of Western Medicine in Ghana, 1880–1960.* Durham, England: Durham Academic Press.

Adua E., Frimpong K., Li X., Wang W. (2017). Emerging issues in public health: A perspective on Ghana's healthcare expenditure, policies, and outcomes. *EPMA Journal*, 8(1): 197–206.

Agyei-Mensah S., de-Graft Aikin A. (2010). Epidemiological transition and the double burden of disease in Accra, Ghana. *Journal of Urban Health*, 87(1): 879–897.

Annobil I., Dakyaga F., Sillim M. L. (2021). From experts to locals' hands" healthcare service planning in sub-Saharan Africa: An insight from the integrated community case management of Ghana. *BMC Health Services Research*, 21(1): 403–412.

Asewah Abor P., Abekah-Nkrumah G. (2008). An examination of hospital governance. *Leadership in Health Services*, 21(1): 47–60.

Asamani J. A, Chebere M.M, Barton P. M, D'Almeida S. A, Odame E. A, Oppong R. (2018). Forecast of healthcare facilities and health workforce requirements for the public sector in Ghana, 2016–2026. *International Journal of Health Policy Management*, 7(11): 1040–1052.

Atinga R. A, Agyepong I. A, Esena R. K. (2019). Willing but unable? Extending theory to investigate community capacity to participate in Ghana's community-based health planning and service implementation. *Evaluation of Program Plan*, 72(1): 170–188.

Atinga R. A, Agyepong I. A, Esena R. K. (2019). Willing but unable? Extending theory to investigate community capacity to participate in Ghana's community-based health planning and service implementation. *Evaluation of Program Plan*, 72(1): 170–188.

Agyepong I.A., Anafi P., Asiamah E., Ansah E.K., Ashon D.A., Narh-Dometey C. (2004). Health worker (internal customer) satisfaction and motivation in the public sector in Ghana. *International Journal of Health Planning Management.* 19(4):319–36.

Binka F., Nazzar A., Phillips J. (1995). The Navrongo community health and family planning project. *Studies in Family Planning*, 26: 121–139.

Blanchet N. J., Fink G., Osei-Akoto I. (2012). The effect of Ghana's national health insurance scheme on health care utilization. *Ghana Medical Journal*, 46(2): 76–84.

Boahen A. B. (1996). A new look at the history of Ghana. *African Affairs: The Journal of the Royal African Society.* 65(260): 212–222.

Bour D. (2004). Determinants of utilization of health services by women in rural and urban areas in Ghana. *Geo-Journal*, 61(1): 89–102.

Brent-Turner B. (2020). Brief History of Ghana. https://www.african-adventures.co.uk/a-brief-history-of-ghana/#:~:text=The%20Empire%20of%20Ghana%20formed,the%20 region%20as%20'Ghana. Accessed September 8, 2023.

Bretton H. L. (1966). *The Rise and Fall of Kwame Nkrumah: A Study of Personal Rule in Africa*, London: Pall Mall Press.

Buah F. K. (1998). *A History of Ghana.* London: Macmillan Press.

Davidson B. (1990). *Black Star: A View of the Life and Times of Kwame Nkrumah.* London: Allen Lane. Milne, J. Press.

Davies O., Meier D., Boateng A. E. (2023). Ghana. https://www.britannica.com/place/Ghana. Accessed August 27, 2023.

Delaire C., Kisiangani J., Stuart K., Antwi-Agyei P., Khush R., Peletz R. (2022). Can open-defecation free (ODF) communities be sustained? A cross-sectional study in rural Ghana. *PLoS One*, 17(1): e0261674. DOI: 10.1371/journal.pone.0261674.

Dibie R. (2018). *Business and Government Relations in Africa*. New York: Routledge/Taylor and Francis Press.

Dibie R. (2022). Healthcare policy and administration in Nigeria: A critical analysis. *The Journal of African Policy Studies*, 28(1): 101–139.

Drislane F. W., Akpalu A., Wegdam H. H. J. (2014). The medical system in Ghana. *Yale Journal of Biology Medicine*, 87(3): 321–326.

Gadzekpo, L. (2018). Women and Capacity Building in Ghana. In Women's Empowerment for Sustainability in Africa edited Robert Dibie. Newcastle upon Tyne, UK: Cambridge Scholars Publishing, pp. 248-274.

Gart, H., Wemakor, A., Badu, A., and Bukari, M. (2023). Magnitude of undernutrition and its associated factors in children attending Child Welfare clinics in Techiman Municipal Ghana. *Nutrition & Food Science*, 53(7): 1096-1109.

Ghana Health Service (2016). *Community-Based Health Planning and Services: Implementation Guidelines*. Accra Ghana: Ministry of Health Publication.

Ghana Health Service (GHS) (2016). Community-Based Health Planning and Services (CHPS); About CHPS. https://ghs.gov.gh/wp-content/uploads/2022/10/National-CHPS-Implementation-Guidelines-Final-Version-ZNS-13022017.pdf. Accessed November 9, 2024.

Ghana Health Service (2023). Health Administration and support services department. https://ghs.gov.gh/health-administration-and-support-services-department/. Accessed September 3, 2023.

Ghana Ministry of Health (2013). *National Community-Based Health Planning and Services Policy*. Ministry of Health Publication.

Ghana Ministry of Health (2023). *Ghana's Health Sector Annual Summit 2023*. Accra, Ghana: Ministry of Health Publication.

GlobalEdge (2022). Ghana. globalEdge.msu.edu and Export.Gov. Accessed July 10, 2023.

Gobah F. K., Zhang L. (2011). The National Health Insurance Scheme in Ghana: Prospects and challenges: Cross-sectional evidence. *Global Journal of Health Science*, 3(2): 90–101. DOI: 10.5539/gjhs.v3n2p90.

Gocking R. (2005). The History of Ghana. Westport CT: Greenwood Publishing Group, Inc.

Government of Ghana (2020). *National Health Policy: Ensuring Healthy Lives for All*. (Revised Edition). Accra, Ghana: Ministry of Health Publication.

GVI (2023). A Brief History of Ghana. https://www.gviusa.com/contact-us/. Accessed August 30.

Harcourt F. (2014). *Building the Ghanaian Nation-State: Kwame Nkrumah's Symbolic Nationalism*. New York: Palgrave Macmillan.

Heerdegen A. C. S., Gerold J., Amon S., Agyemang S. A., Aikins M., Wyss K. (2020). How does district management emerge within a complex health system? *Insights for capacity strengthening in Ghana*. Frontier in Public Health, 8(1): 1–11.

Human Development Report. (2022). Ethiopia. https://www.google.com/search?q=Human+Development+Report+2022+Ethiopia&sca_esv=6880e701cc3a3908&rlz=1C1GCEA_enUS1031US1031&biw=1707&bih=781&sxsrf=ADLYW. Accessed November 9, 2024.

Kumi-Kyereme A., Amu H., Darteh E. K. M. (2017). Barriers and motivations for health insurance subscription in Cape Coast, Ghana: A qualitative study. *Arch Public Health*, 75(1): 24–37.

Kweku M., Amu H., Awolu A., Adjuik M., Ayanore M. A., Manu E., et al. (2020). Community-Based Health Planning and Services Plus programme in Ghana: A qualitative study with stakeholders in two Systems Learning Districts on improving the implementation of primary health care. *PLoS One*, 15(1): e0226808. DOI: 10.1371/journal.pone.0226808.

Longest Jr. B. (2016). *Health Policy Making in the United States*. Chicago: Health Administration Press.

Meyerowitz E. L. R. (1975). *The Early History of the Akan States of Ghana*. Bucks, UK: Red Candle Press.

Ministry of Health – Ghana. (2020). National Health Policy: Ensuring healthy lives for all. /https://www.moh.gov.gh/wp-content/uploads/2021/08/NHP_January-2020.pdf. Accessed September 6, 2024.

Ministry of Health Ministry (1997). Medium Term Health Strategy. Policy Document. Ministry of Health of Health. Accra, Ghana.

Nehemia L. (1973). *Ancient Ghana and Mali*. New York: Methuen & Co Ltd. p. 3.

Obu N. R., Aggrey–Bluwey L. (2021). A case study of complementary alternative medicines in primary healthcare in Ghana. *Journal of Complementary and Alternative Medical Research*, 15(1): 23–33.

Ocran J. (2019). Exposing the protected: Ghana's disability laws and the rights of disabled people. *Disability & Society*, 34(4): 663–668, DOI: 10.1080/09687599.2018.1556491.

Okoroh J., Essoun S., Seddoh A., Harris H., Weissman J., Dsane-Selby, R. R. (2018). Evaluating the impact of the national health insurance scheme of Ghana on out-of-pocket expenditures: A systematic review. *BMC Health Services Research*, 18(1): 1–15.

Opoku D., Edusei A. K., Agyei-Baffour P., Teddy G., Polin K., Quentin W. (2021). Ghana: Health system review 2021. *European Journal of Public Health*, 31(3): 1–13.

Osafo, J. (2021). Conducting qualitative research on suicide in Ghana using Interpretative Phenomenological Analysis (IPA): A reflection after a decade. New Ideas in Psychology, 60, January https://www.sciencedirect.com/science/article/abs/pii/S0732118X20302117? via% 3Dihub. Accessed September 6, 2024.

Osumanu I. K., Kosoe E. A., Tegeeng F. (2019). Determinants of open defecation in the Wa municipality of Ghana: Empirical findings highlighting sociocultural and economic dynamics among households. *Journal of Environmental and Public Health*, 2019(1): 1–10.

Owusu-Ansah D. (2014). *Historical Dictionary of Ghana*. Rowman & Littlefield.

Polychronis M. (2017). The limitations of Ghana's rural health care access: Case study: Ga East, Greater Accra. https://polisci.rutgers.edu/news-publications/occasional-paper-series/273-occasional-paper-4-maria-polychronis/file. Accessed July 8, 2023.

Republic of Ghana (2006). *Persons with Disability Act (Act 715)*. Accra: Republic of Ghana.

Republic of Ghana (2007). *Under Five's Child Health Policy: 2007–2015*. Accra, Ghana: Republic of Ghana.

Republic of Ghana (2012). *National Health Insurance Act (Act 852)*. Accra, Ghana: Republic of Ghana.

Republic of Ghana (2020). *National Health Policy: Ensuring Healthy Lives for All*. (Revised Edition). Accra, Ghana: Ministry of Health Publication.

Republic of Ghana Ministry of Health (2022). National Food Safety Policy. https://www.moh. gov.gh/wp-content/uploads/2022/07/NFSP-Document-signed-and-launched.pdf. Accessed November 9, 2024.

Seidu A., Darteh E. K. M, Agbaglo E., Louis Kobina Dadzie L. K., Ahinkorah B. O., Ameyaw E. K., Tetteh J. K, Baatiema L., Yaya S. (2020). Barriers to accessing healthcare among women in Ghana: A multilevel modelling. *BMC Public Health*, 20(1): 1916. 10.1186/s12889-020-10017-8.

Suleiman A. B., Muhammad F. (2021). The modern information technology in Healthcare: An African perspective. *International Journal of Health and Life Sciences*. 10.5812/ijhls.107301.

Turkson P. K. (2009). Perceived quality of healthcare delivery in a rural district of Ghana. *Ghana Medical Journal*, 43(2): 65–70.

United States Department of State (2019). Ghana human right report. https://www.state. gov/wp-content/uploads/2020/02/GHANA-2019-HUMAN-RIGHTS-REPORT.pdf. Accessed September 6, 2024.

United States Department of State (2019). Country Reports of Human Right Practice in Ethiopia. https://www.state.gov/reports/2019-country-reports-on-human-rights-practices/ethiopia/. Accessed October 31, 2024.

Wikipedia (2023). History of Ghana. https://en.wikipedia.org/wiki/History_of_Ghana. Accessed August 30, 2023.

World Bank Group (2023). Ghana. http://www.worldbank.org/en/country/ghana. Accessed August 11, 2023.

World Bank Indicators (2022). Ghana. https://data.worldbank.org/indicator/NY.GDP.MKTP. CD.Locations=CM. Accessed August 16, 2023.

World Economics (2023). Ghana's gross domestic product. https://www.worldeconomics.com/Country-Size/Ghana.aspx. Accessed August 30, 2023.

World Health Organization (2023). https://www.who.int/data/gho/data/countries/country-details/GHO/cameroon?countryProfileId=79e4cda0-11b1-4806-9c63-d40904289ced. Accessed August 16, 2023.

Worldometer (2022). Countries where COVID-19 has spread. https://www.worldometers.info/coronavirus/countries-where-coronavirus-has-spread/. Accessed September 6, 2024.

Worldometer (2022). Ethiopia. https://www.worldometers.info/gdp/ethiopia-gdp/#:~:text=GDP%20Growth%20Rate%20in%202022,2.6%25%20in%20GDP%20per%20capita. Accessed November 5, 2024.

Worldometer (2023). Ghana population (2023). https://www.worldometers.info/world-population/ghana-population/. Accessed August 30, 2023.

Chapter Nine

HEALTH POLICY AND CHALLENGES IN KENYA

Robert Dibie and Fredah Mainah

Introduction

This chapter examines how the Government of Kenya has made substantial process in addressing the various health challenges that the nation has been facing. The chapter covers how communicable diseases such as lower respiratory infection, diarrhea, and vaccine-preventable diseases have been controlled to a positive level. It presents an argument that healthcare policy formulation alone cannot postulate positive health outcomes, increase the socioeconomic status of citizens as well as improve sanitation, water quality, and effective regulations to propel better air quality. An additional mechanism is needed in the country to accomplish the positive health needs of both urban and rural citizens of Kenya. Health policies that advocated the expansion of services for immunization to children and the outcomes are also discussed. Analysis of citizens' healthcare needs and their desire to have access to healthcare services show that there are major disparities across regions of the nation. The chapter also provides a clear basis for the assessment of the nation's healthcare system. It is anticipated that the policy analyses and recommendations could help guide the adoption of appropriate healthcare policies to prevent the lives of citizens from danger and the spread of noncommunicable and communicable diseases in Kenya in the future.

Brief History of Kenya

The Republic of Kenya is a country in East Africa. It has a boundary with the Indian Ocean to the east, the Republic of Ethiopia to the north, Somalia to the northeast, and Tanzania to the south. Other countries having boundaries with Kenya are South Sudan to the northwest and Uganda to the west. Lake Victoria is located southwest of the country. According to the World Bank (2022), Kenya has a population of about 44.86 million people. The gross domestic product (GDP) of Kenya was US$132.4 billion in 2022 (World Bank 2022; GlobalEdge 2022).

The East African territory now called the Republic of Kenya was inhabited by Cushitic-speaking people around 2000 AD. The Bantu ethnic extraction who were hunters migrated from West Africa and settled in the region in the first millennium (Askwith 1995). Other groups such as the Nilo-Saharan and Afro-Asiatic ethno-linguistic people also migrated to settle in the Kenya region (Askwith 1995; Embassy of the Republic of Kenya Japan 2023; Frontera-Rial & Ogot 1978). In addition, Arab traders started visiting the region to trade due to the short distance between the Arabian Peninsula and Kenya's region in East Africa (British Broadcasting Corporation 2022; Frontera-Rial & Ogot 1978; Lonsdale 1979). During the first millennium AD, more Nilotic and Bantu hunters also migrated to settle in the eastern African region that is now called the Republic of Kenya (Embassy of the Republic of Kenya Japan 2023; Wikipedia 2024). By the end of the first century AD, the Kenya region had become a multi-ethnic state (Frontera-Rial & Ogot 1978; Wikipedia 2024). As the population of people in the region began to grow there became a desire to establish the Wanga Kingdom toward the end of the seventeenth century. The creation of the Wanga Kingdom galvanized some of the multi-ethnic groups in the region such as Bantu, Cushitic, Kikuyu, Luhya, Nilotic, and other small ethnic groups (Britannia 2024; Wikipedia 2024). The leader of the Wanga Kingdom was called Nabongo (Frontera-Rial & Ogot 1978).

According to McCormack (1984), the foundation of the British colonial history of Africa, and subsequently the Kenya territory can be linked to the Berlin Conference in 1885. The Berlin Conference organized by only European leaders with no African representation produced a resolution to divide the African continent among Western European countries. This was the reason East Africa was first divided into territories by the European leaders who attended the Berlin conference. The United Kingdom explorer established the East African Protectorate in 1895 and soon after, opened the doors for more fertile highlands to white settlers from Europe (Askwith 1995; Lonsdale 1979; McCormack 1984). The United Kingdom also established the East Africa Protectorate in 1895. However, the British colonial administration changed the name of the East Africa Protectorate to Kenya Colony in 1920 (McCormack 1984; Wikipedia 2024).

The Republic of Kenya gained its independence from Britain on December 12, 1963. Between 1963 and 1964 Queen Elizabeth was the first head of state, while Jomo Kenyatta was the first prime minister (British Broadcasting Corporation 2022; Government of Kenya 2022). The nation became a republic in 1964 and Jomo Kenyatta was elected the first President of the new country, while Oginga Odinga was appointed vice-president in the same year. President Jomo Kenyatta was also the leader of the Kenya African National Union and served in both positions between 1964 and 1978 (Government of Kenya 2022). However, after his term as president was over, Daniel Arap Moi succeeded Kenyatta as the next president of the Republic of Kenya. President Daniel Arap Moi served as president of Kenya between 1978 and 2002. During President Moi's presidency, his administration was accused of human rights abuses and corruption. Mwai Kibaki was elected the next president in 2002 and ruled till 2013. Further, Uhuru Kenyatta was elected president of Kenya in 2013 and was also reelected for a second term in 2017 (Embassy of the Republic of Kenya Japan 2023). Uhuru Kenyatta is the son of Kenya's founding President Jomo Kenyatta. Uhuru Kenyatta was elected President in April 2013 and served till September 2022 (British Broadcasting Corporation 2022; Government of Kenya 2022). The current president is William Ruto, he was elected and sworn in on September 13, 2022.

The nation is famous for its glaciers, abundant wildlife, lake, and safari parks. The administrative capital of the country is Nairobi. Nairobi is also the largest city in the country. The country's economy has experienced considerable growth in the past decades due to political stability, and the export of mineral resources and agricultural products. Kenya is endowed with Copper, Gold, Limestone, Soda Ash, Salt, Rubies, ilmenite, tantalum, niobium, fluorspar and fossil fuels, Fluorspar, Garnets, Wildlife, Hydropower, Water, and Arable land (Africa Mining 2023, Embassy of the Republic of Kenya Japan 2023). The discovery of oil in Turkana (northern part of the country) has the potential to further strengthen the nation's economic growth.

Health Challenges in Kenya

The Republic of Kenya's government discarded its national insurance scheme and introduced the National Hospital Insurance Fund cover in 2004. This new insurance scheme constitutes a new mechanism for facilitating access to cheaper health in the country in line with the World Health Organization's Universal health coverage goals (Ajwang 2022; Oraro-Lawrence 2020). However, since the introduction of the National Hospital Insurance Fund, Kenya has struggled to cater to its growing population and the increasing healthcare needs of all its citizens. According to the Ministry of Health of Kenya (2024) and Oraro-Lawrence (2020), only 11% of the population of Kenya is covered by the National Hospital Insurance Fund leaving the majority of the population (89%) without the government-subsidized health plan. Because over 70% of the Kenyan workforce works in the informal sector, most of them are either not eligible or cannot be able to afford the out-of-pocket premiums set by the government to maintain health insurance provision (Blumenthal et al. 2021; Ouma et al. 2020). This constitutes a financial burden on the majority of the low-income population in the country. Many the citizens of the country lack access to health insurance. Those who do not have insurance coverage remain vulnerable to the impact of a possible high prevalence of COVID-19, HIV/AIDS, malaria, and tuberculosis incidence (Ajwang 2022).

The poor network of roads in Kenya makes access to health facilities very difficult for the huge population of the country that is living in rural communities. Thus, another area that needs substantial improvement in Kenya is its roads. Although the country has few good roads. The decapitated conditions of some of its rural roads are terrible, especially during the rainy season (Oyugi et al. 2023). The nation's capital city Nairobi is the commercial center and transportation hub of Eastern and Central Africa and the largest metropolitan town between Cairo and Johannesburg (Dibie 2018). On the nation's eastern coast is the Port of Mombasa. The city of Mombasa is the most important seaport in the region, supplying the shipping needs of more than a dozen countries despite equipment deficiencies, inefficiency, and corruption (GlobalEdge 2022). It has been reported that the Government of Kenya has been unable to provide a secure environment for businesses and families, particularly in urban settings (Dibie 2018). Frequent property crime and violence are major concerns and have become unavoidable in Kenya.

There has been considerable improvement in the health system in Kenya in the past two decades however the country is still faced with a magnitude of challenges. There continues to be limited access to hospitals and clinics in the country, especially for the population living in the rural regions. In addition, there has been a major shortage of healthcare workers to respond to the medical needs of the low-income population of the country (Kenya Health Federation 2021; Masaba et al. 2020). According to the World Bank report (2018), the ratio of physicians to 1,000 people is 022. While the ratio of nurses and midwives per 1,000 people was 1.2 in 2018. Further, the ratio of registered medical officers per 100,000 population in 2021 was 27.1. It is, however, reported that the ratio slightly increased in comparison to those of 2018–2020. Kenya counted 13,376 registered medical doctors in 2021. This number constitutes 26 physicians per 100,000 population (Cowling 2023). This healthcare workers ratio is below the WHO-recommended average of 21.7 doctors and 228 nurses per 100,000 people, which is the required standard for optimal delivery of services (Ashigbie et al. 2020; Kenya Health Federation 2021). Therefore, the inadequate number of healthcare workers in government hospitals and clinics has been recognized as a major predicament to a resilient and responsive health system in Kenya (Ashigbie et al. 2020; Kenya Medical Association 2023). In as much as the nation tends to have highly skilled workers in other sectors, it does not have enough doctors and nurses to provide healthcare services to the larger low-income population. The people who mostly need these services, still have challenges accessing the services of specialized health workers to assist them (Masaba et al. 2020).

According to the Kenya Medical Association (2023) and Oyugi et al. (2023), traditionally Universal Health Coverage is governed by the following three factors: (1) appropriate financing; (2) health service delivery; and (3), superior health management and governance. Unfortunately, over the past two decades, Kenya's total government health system budget in the country has been between 4% and 6% of its GDP each year (Oyugi et al. 2023). If this rate of funding the healthcare system in Kenya is compared with the 12% recommended in the Kenya Health Sector Strategic Plan and the 15% in the Abuja Declaration which Kenya is a party to. It could be argued that the health system is poorly funded (Oyugi et al. 2023). In addition to this inadequate financing are weak accountability systems, and structures, and terrible corruption at both the National and 47 County Governments levels in the country (Center for Disease Control and Prevention 2024). The current health delivery predicaments will make it very difficult for Kenya to accomplish its desire to accomplish universal health coverage, an equitable health system, a good health status, an acceptable health system, efficiency, and sustainable health system that is free from disparities (Kenya Medical Association 2023; Masaba et al. 2020; Oyando et al. 2022).

There are also other challenges due to expensive private sector hospitals and clinics despite the fact that the government of Kenya has adopted a policy to subsidize user fees (Ilinca et al. 2019; Masaba et al. 2020). Furthermore, although over 80% of the nation's population tends to depend on government funding for their healthcare, the other 20% of the inhabitants who are rich could afford to seek the expensive healthcare provided by the private sector. This practice constitutes the nature of disparity in the health system in Kenya (Ashigbie et al. 2020; Oyugi et al. 2023).

According to the Kenya Health Federation (2021) and Ngigi et al. (2017), poor medical infrastructure has often prevented most government hospitals and clinics from managing the medical challenges facing patients (Makoni 2023; Mauti et al. 2019). The public hospitals that are highly equipped with specialized equipment do not have effective processes and specialist physicians and professional nurses in place to implement the tasks, as well as provide access to medical records and healthcare financing (Masaba et al. 2020; Ngigi et al. 2017). Other precarious health challenges in the health system in Kenya are the supply chain of medicine and poor financing and medical technology innovations (Ashigbie et al. 2020. Kenya Health Federation 2021; Oyando et al. 2022). In addition, there has been a limited increase in financing and investment in the health system in Kenya. In addition, limited progress has been made toward achieving the commitments of the Abuja Declaration, in which countries committed to spending at least 15% of their public expenditures on health (Ashigbie et al. 2020; Ministry of Health of Kenya 2014b; Oyando et al. 2022).

Furthermore, the free maternal health policy implementation in Kenya has been confronted with many challenges due to shortage of drugs, and supplies, insufficient funding, shortage of skilled healthcare workers, noninvolvement of stakeholders in maternal health, late reimbursement of the costs incurred in providing free maternal healthcare services, heavy workloads, and demotivation of health workers (Ashigbie et al. 2020; Buitendyk et al. 2023; Gitobu et al. 2018; Oyugi et al. 2023). In addition, the poor investment in healthcare has recently propelled several health workers to strike. Since 2013, it has become common practice for health workers to go on strike nearly every week because of low salaries and poor working conditions (Buitendyk et al. 2023; Kenya Medical Association 2023).

Health Administration in Kenya

Before the Health Policy of 2014–2030 was enacted by the Republic of Kenya's government in 2024, the healthcare system was structured in a hierarchical manner that begins with primary healthcare, with the lowest unit being the community, and then complicated cases being referred to higher levels of healthcare at the national level. One of the major goals of the Republic of Kenya Health Policy 2024 was recognizing the right of communities to manage their own health affairs and to further their development of a decentralized system (Ministry of Health Kenya 2014a). The policy acknowledges the need for new governance and management arrangements at both levels of government and outlines governance objectives.

The *primary care level* consists of dispensaries and health centers. The current structure consists of the following six levels: (1) Level 1: Community, (2) Level 2: Dispensaries; (3) Level 3: Health centers; (4) Level 4: Primary referral facilities; (5) Level 5: Secondary referral facilities; and (6) Level 6: Tertiary referral facilities (Ministry of Health, Kenya 2014a). Under the old structure of health administration, the National referral hospitals are at the apex of the healthcare system, providing sophisticated diagnostic, therapeutic, and rehabilitative services (Ministry of Health of Kenya 2014a). The major two national referral hospitals are Kenyatta National Hospital in Nairobi and Moi Referral and

Teaching Hospital in Eldoret (Masaba et al. 2020; Wikipedia 2023). In addition, the private sector referral health facilities are the Nairobi Hospital, and Aga Khan Hospital in the same city.

At the *provincial level*, the general hospitals function as referral hospitals to their districts. The private health facilities at the provincial level also provided specialized care as well for the regional population. The only shortcoming is that the cost of healthcare treatment at private hospitals is very high when compared with that of public health facilities. The structure also makes it possible for the provincial-level health facilities to act as an intermediary between the national central level and the districts (Masaba et al. 2020; Ministry of Health Kenya 2014).

According to Masaba et al. (2020) and Tama et al. (2018), the transition into the devolution of health services began in 2013. The old six-level health administration structure of the Kenya system was devolved into two levels: (1) the national government and (2) 47 semiautonomous county governments (Masaba et al. 2020; Tama et al. 2018).

On one hand, the national government was mandated to continue to manage health policy formulation and regulatory functions in Kenya. The national government is also responsible for planning, management, and budgeting (Ilinca et al. 2019; Masaba et al. 2020; McCollum et al. 2018). The new function of the national government or the Ministry of Health of Kenya includes not only health policy formulation and regulation but also national referral to public health facilities as well as capacity building and technical assistance to 47 counties' healthcare departments (Ministry of Health of Kenya; 2014). In addition, the national referral services also include all tertiary hospitals, national reference laboratories, and services; blood transfusion services as well as research and training health institutions that train specialist health professionals workers. The Ministry of Health of Kenya was also mandated to oversee the discipline specialization and the geographical specialization (Masaba et al. 2020; Tama et al. 2018). The Ministry of Health of Kenya was also required to be in charge of training and research services on issues of cross-county importance (Masaba et al. 2020; McCollum 2018; Ngigi et al. 2019).

On the other hand, the 47 counties in Kenya were assigned to administer health service delivery in all the hospitals and clinics in their respective county (Ba-Diop et al. 2014; Ministry of Health 2014). It should be noted that the decentralization policy also mandated county governments to make decisions on priorities by drafting county integrated development plan; annual planning and budgeting; service delivery for public health, disease surveillance, community health services, primary health services, ambulance, county hospital services; recruitment, and human resource management (includes facility and community health workers) and partner coordination (McCollum et al. 2019; Ministry of Health of Kenya 2014). The 2014–2023 health policy also requires the county government to form the county health system together with those managed by nonpublic sector stakeholders such as for-profit and non-profit partners in the nation's health industry. The county health facilities are also responsible for comprehensive patient diagnostics medical, surgical, habilitative, and rehabilitative care such as specialized outpatient services and reproductive services (Ministry of Health of Kenya 2014). The sub-county health facilities also operate ambulatory and emergency services as well basic out-patient diagnostic services (Masaba et al. 2020; Ouma et al. 2020; Ministry of Health of Kenya 2024; Ngigi et al. 2017; Wikipedia 2024).

The Kenya health decentralized system succeeded in consolidating service areas into four main categories for ease of governance and responsibility. The policy was originally designed to share the Republic of Kenya's healthcare responsibility between the national and county governments (English et al. 2020; Oyando et al. 2022). Despite the set goals, some scholars contend that the devolution of the system in Kenya has been confronted with many challenges. For instance, since the formulation of the decentralization policy in 2014, there have been recurrent health workers' strikes in different counties, and more migration of doctors and nurses from many counties to foreign countries to seek better salaries, and good working conditions (Ilinca et al. 2019; Masaba et al. 2020; Ngigi et al. 2019).

Types of Health Policies

Healthcare is considered to be human right in Kenya and many other countries around the world. To accomplish this goal, the Republic of Kenya has been enacting various health policies to promote the well-being of its citizens since it became an independent country in 1963. There have been two categories of policies formulated in Kenya over the past 60 years. The first type of health policy focused on curative health treatment for the population in the country. The second type of health policy focused on the prevention of communicable and noncommunicable diseases in the country. The crucial role played by the government and health workers also requires policymakers to enact performance management strategies or plans that could galvanize effective administration of the health system in the country. Below are selected health policies that have been enacted and implemented in Kenya to ensure its citizen's rights to good health.

Kenya Universal Health Coverage Policy 2020–2030 enacted in 2020: Kenya is investing in UHC to ensure its people remain healthy. Besides health financing, UHC implies putting in place efficient health service delivery systems, adequate health facilities and human resources, information systems, good governance, and enabling legislation. This policy embraces the principles of equity, people centeredness, efficiency, social solidarity, and a multi-sectoral approach (Ministry of Health of Kenya 2020a). It focuses on four objectives and their related strategies to support the attainment of the government's goal in health. The policy is cognizant of the functional responsibilities between the National and County levels of government with their respective accountability mechanisms and frameworks (Ministry of Health of Kenya 2020a). It is envisaged that the national and county governments will benefit from this policy as a guide for planning and budgeting for healthcare services at all levels of care. The detailed strategies and program packages will be elaborated in specific strategic and investment implementation plans (Ministry of Health of Kenya 2020a).

National Community Health Digitization Strategy 2020–2025 enacted in 2020: The major objective of the National Community Digitization strategy is to enhance access to healthcare, thereby improving productivity, reducing poverty, and combating hunger and preventable death and disease (Ministry of Health of Kenya 2020b). The National Community Digitization strategy envisages the development of a national electronic Community Health Information System to respond to the gaps identified in community health service delivery and data management through the Landscape Assessment and intensive stakeholder engagement (Ministry of Health of Kenya 2020b). The policy also has a fundamental principle that demands statistical data and health information be made liberal and readily accessible as a "Public good" and in a timely manner. It also promotes use of existing data (Ministry of Health of Kenya 2020b).

Kenya Health Policy 2014–2030 enacted in 2014: The goal of this policy is to work toward achieving the highest standard of health in a manner responsive to the needs of the Kenyan population (Ministry of Health, Kenya 2014a). The health policy was formulated to enhance the accomplishment of fundamental human rights in the nation, including the right to health as enshrined in the Constitution of Kenya 2010. Other major objectives of the 2014–2030 health policy include (1) The promotion of democracy and accountability in delivery of healthcare; (2) Fostering of seamless service delivery during and after the transition period; (3) Facilitating powers of self-governance to the people and enhancing their participation in making decisions on matters of health affecting them; and (4) Recognizing the right of communities to manage their own health affairs and to further their development (Ministry of Health, Kenya 2014b).

Free Maternal Healthcare Policy enacted in 2013: The goal of this policy is to promote the professional delivery of children and reduce pregnancy-related mortality in Kenya. The policy also mandates that pregnant mothers are required to delivery their new baby or babies free of charge at any government hospitals or clinics in the country (Gitobu et al. 2018; Ministry of Health of Kenya 2013). The government also promised to pay between US$25 and US$175 for each child that is delivered to public health facilities in the country. The government reimbursement covers all types of delivery process such as caesarian sections or through spontaneous vaginal process (Gitobu et al. 2018; Ministry of Health of Kenya 2013). Further, the amount of money that reimbursed to hospitals and clinics for the delivery of children is contingent on the facility's status, as well as the nation's health system capacity to effectively manage complications during the delivery of children (Gitobu et al. 2018).

Data Analysis and Discussion

The purpose of this chapter is to analyze the healthcare delivery system in Kenya as well as the effectiveness of health policies in the country. The data used for the analysis of healthcare policy effectiveness were derived from both primary and secondary sources. The secondary research methods adopted include the review of the Republic of Kenya Government's Ministry of Health policies, National Strategic Plans, World Health

Organization reports, United Nations Human Development Index annual report, Center for Disease Control, and United States Agency for International Development, Work Bank reports, and academic and professional journals articles.

The primary research involves the administration of a questionnaire to 105 respondents. Sixty-eight or 65% of respondents returned their completed questionnaire. The questionnaire respondents constitute 31.4% men and 33.3% women. In addition, 55% of the respondents had visited a hospital or clinic to receive treatment at least twice a year. Another 31% had also visited a hospital or clinic between 3 and 4 times recently to receive treatment. While 10% of the respondents visited 5–6 times a year and 4% also visited the hospital more than 7 times the same period. Data were analyzed using SPSS to determine the effectiveness and challenges facing the health policy and quality of healthcare delivery system in Kenya.

Table 1 analyzes the nature of healthcare delivery and health policy in Kenya. The result of the questionnaire reveals that 81.6% of the respondents agree that corruption and unethical behavior of political and administrative leaders in government negatively affect the health system's funding. In addition, 88.2% of the respondents also agree that political leaders and rich citizens of my country prefer to seek healthcare services in foreign nations due to a lack of trust in the Kenya healthcare system. Furthermore, 78.1% of the respondents agree that the lack of appropriate funding for the healthcare system in the country constitutes why hospitals and clinics are not well-equipped and poorly staffed. Another 71.2% of the respondents acknowledge that most rural public hospitals in the country do not have specialist doctors and nurses. On one hand, 64.2% of the respondents agree that because the government pays low salaries to doctors and nurses that is why they are compelled to migrate to foreign countries to seek better compensation and working conditions. On the other hand, 69.7% also agree that the lack of effective health policy implementation or regulations is one of the reasons there are several cases of mortality due to errors during surgery conducted by some physicians in Kenya. Further, 63.2% of the respondents confirm that hospitals and health centers in the rural regions of their county do not have constant electricity. While 65.1% of the respondents acknowledge that they cannot afford to pay for their healthcare treatment and medication costs without government subsidies, only 16.7%. agree that they could pay for healthcare treatments. In addition, 50% of the respondents disagree that the Government of Kenya promotes equity in the delivery of healthcare to underserved citizens in the country. Similarly, 46.1% also disagree that the government in Kenya effectively regulates medical professional licensing and disciplinary boards in both the public and private hospitals and clinics in the country. It is especially important to note that most of the specialist hospitals in the country are in urban cities.

Furthermore, while 42.4% of the respondents agree that most hospitals in my country do not have modern equipment, 45.5% also contend that healthcare provided by doctors in their respective counties and urban cities is highly commendable. The mean of the questionnaire respondents that agree the nature of health delivery in Kenya is not good is 55.5% while those that contend that the health system in the country is doing well is 30%.

Table 1 The Nature of Healthcare Delivery and Policy in Kenya

	Questions	Strongly Agree	Agree	Neutral	Strongly Disagree	Disagree	Agree %	Disagree %
1	Healthcare provided by doctors in my city is highly commendable	7.6%	37.9%	30.3%	10.6%	13.6%	45.5%	24.2%
2	Most hospitals in my country do not have modern equipment	3.0%	25.8%	28.8%	10.6%	31.8%	28.8%	42.4%
3	I can afford my healthcare treatment and medication costs without government subsidies.	0	16.7%	18.2%	22.7%	42.4%	16.6%	65.1%
4	Most rural public hospitals in my country do not have specialist doctors and nurses.	28.8%	42.4%	13.6%	10.6%	4.6%	71.2%	15.2%
5	Government pays of low salaries to doctors and nurses has encouraged their migration to foreign countries.	35.8%	28.4%	19.4%	7.5%	9%	64.2%	16.5%
6	Lack of effective health policy implementation or regulations	28.8%	40.9%	13.6%	7.6%	9.1%	69.7%	16.7%
7	Government promotes equity in the delivery of healthcare to underserved citizens in the country.	0	23.5%	25%	25%	26.5%	23.5%	50%
8	Political leaders and rich citizens of my country prefer to seek healthcare services in foreign nations.	57.4%	30.8%	5.9%	2.9%	2.9%	88.2%	5.8%
9	Government is effectively regulating medical professional licensing and disciplinary boards	6.2%	29.3%	18.5%	13.8%	32.3%	38.2%	46.1%
10	Hospitals and health centers in my city have constant electricity.	10.3%	26.5%	11.8%	11.8%	51.4%	36.8%	63.2%
11	Lack of appropriate funding for the healthcare system in my country.	48.4%	29.7%	6.3%	7.8%	7.8%	78.1%	15.6%
12	Corruption and unethical behavior of political and administrative leaders in government negatively affect the health system's funding.	55.4%	26.2%	7.7%	3.1%	7.1%	81.6%	10.2%
	Mean						53.5%	30%

Table 2 Economics and Health Indicators in Kenya

No.	Major Indicators in Kenya	Explanation
1	Population	54.03 million (2022)
2	Gross domestic product (GDP)	US$113.4 billion (2022)
3	Current health expenditure (% of GDP)	4.2% (2022)
4	Physicians/doctors per 1,000 people	0.2 (2018)
5	Nurses and midwives per 1,000 people	1.2 (2018)
6	Population using safely managed drinking water service	63% (2022)
7	People using safely managed sanitation services (% of population)	Urban areas 28%; Rural regions 33% (2022)
8	People practicing open defecation % of the population	6% Urban areas; rural 9% (2022)
9	Common disease	HIV/AIDS, lower respiratory infections, diarrheal diseases, neonatal disorders, stroke, tuberculosis, ischemic heart disease, cirrhosis, malaria, and diabetes.
10	Life expectancy at birth for females	64 years (2021)
11	Life expectancy at birth for males	59 years (2021)
12	Mortality rate for female adults (per 1,000 people)	311 (2021)
13	Mortality rate for male adults (per 1,000 people)	28 (2021)
14	Mortality rate for infants (per 1,000 people)	419 (2021)
15	Tuberculosis incidence (per 100,000 people)	57 people (2021)
16	Population living below income poverty line PPP $2.15 a day	29.4% (2015)
17	Poverty head count ratio at national poverty lines (% of population)	36.1% (2015)
18	Contribution deprivation in health to multidimensional poverty	None
19	Infants lacking immunization for measles (% of one year old)	89% (2021)
20	Malaria incidence (per 1,000 people at risk)	64.5 (2021)
21	HIV/AIDS prevalence of adults (% ages 15–49)	1% (2021)

Source: World Bank Indicators (2022); United Nations Human Development Program Index (2022); World Health Organization (2023).

Table 2 shows the summary of the content analysis of secondary research that was conducted. The Republic of Kenya currently spends an average of 4.29% of its GDP on healthcare in the past two years. This is below 15% of GDP that the Republic of Kenya pledged in the Abuja Declaration.

According to the World Bank Indicators (2022) and the Global Health (2023), the common diseases in Kenya include HIV/AIDS, lower respiratory infections, diarrheal diseases, neonatal disorders, stroke, tuberculosis, ischemic heart disease, cirrhosis, malaria, and diabetes. According to the Centers for Disease Control and Prevention (2023) report, in Kenya, malaria is the leading cause of outpatient morbidity. Prevalence accounts for one-third of all new cases reported in the country. After malaria, the most common illnesses seen in outpatient clinics are diseases of the respiratory system, skin diseases, diarrhea, and intestinal parasites. Other frequent health problems include accidental injuries, urinary tract infections, eye infections, rheumatism, and other infections (World Health Organization 2023).

Furthermore, while the number of physicians per 1,000 people was 0.2 in 2018, and nurses and midwives per 1,000 people in the same, respectively, the ratio has not improved over the past few years. To buttress the challenges of shortage of health workers in the country in the increase in doctors and nurses' migration to foreign countries. Life expectancy at birth for females in Kenya was 64 years in 2021, and that of men was 59 years in the same year. In addition, the mortality rate for female adults per 1,000 people was 311 in 2021, while that for male adults per 1,000 people was 419 in 2021. The good news however is that the mortality rate per 1,000 infants has declined to 28 children in 2021. On one hand, the population living below income poverty line PPP of $2.15 a day in 2015 was 29.4%, while the poverty head count ratio at national poverty lines per percentage of the population was 36.1%. The Government of Kenya should however be mindful that there is a positive correlation between a high rate of poverty and a high mortality rate.

Conclusion

This chapter has examined how the Government of Kenya has made substantial process in addressing the various health challenges that the nation has been facing. It also explored how several health challenges especially the disparities in the access to healthcare have not been effectively resolved in Kenya. It presents an argument that healthcare policy formulation alone cannot postulate positive health outcomes, increase the socioeconomic status of citizens as well, and improve sanitation, and water quality, and effective regulations to propel better air quality are also required. It argued that there is an urgent need for policymakers in Kenya to acknowledge the complexity and dynamics of the health system factors that may affect the fabric of their respective societies and culture of good healthcare delivery professional and ethical management.

The research conducted by the author of this chapter reveals that shortage of doctors and nurses, a lack of appropriate funding of the health system in the effective supply chain of medicine and medical equipment, as well as corruption and poor management of the health system in Kenya has drastically impeded access to professional healthcare by over 75% of the population of the country. Because of the shortage of physicians and nurses the low-income citizens of Kenya who mostly need healthcare services, continue to be frustrated due to their inability to receive quality treatment from specialized health workers within the country.

Moving forward will require the Republic of Kenya's government to reinvigorate measures that could be effectively utilized to reduce health inequalities and to reverse the downward trend in the dissatisfaction of over 75% of the nation's population about the health system. It should be noted that health inequalities in the country exist mostly in the rural regions of Kenya. It is mind-boggling to notice that while the low-income people in the country do not have access to professional healthcare, the government of Kenya is engaged in sponsoring its minister and members of the national assembly to seek health treatment in foreign. Future health policies to enhance the system in the country should involve collaboration and partnership with all stakeholders in the country. This approach could positively impact new healthcare outcomes in Kenya. In addition, there is an urgent need to change unethical and immoral practices in the current governance structure and management of public resources to achieve social justice where every citizen in the country is treated equally before the law as well as equitably has access to health treatment.

Furthermore, to promote efficiency in the health system in Kenya, there is a need for the government to galvanize efficiency. The fact that there are medicine supply chain challenges in the country, requires a strategy to do so that stuck of drugs are ordered several months before the government hospital runs out of supply. Information and technology could be effectively utilized to monitor the usage of the current stock of drugs available to ensure that there is no gap in the supply chain process of the healthcare system in Kenya. The nation needs to upgrade its medical information systems as soon as possible so telemedicine can be practiced enhancing communication and the sharing of medical records between urban specialist hospitals and rural medical facilities. It is also very important to enhance health workers' density with the use of medical information technology by providing training to doctors and nurses to become technically more efficient.

Finally, current health policies in Kenya need to be enforced effectively. Further, a vibrant regulation system that promotes ethical and professional etiquette needs to be practiced in the health system including the Ministry of Health of Kenya. In addition, the corruption challenges in the health sector need to be taken seriously given the precarious experiences in other African countries. The Republic of Kenya's government must be mindful that precautionary public health mechanism needs to be adopted to prevent the loss of lives that resulted from the previous pandemics in Kenya. The need to address the coordination of the supply chain of medicine and health equipment in Kenya cannot be emphasized enough. It should be noted that "once beaten twice shy."

References

Africa Mining (2023). Mining in Kenya. https://projectsiq.co.za/mining-in-kenya.htm#:~:text=Mining%20in%20Kenya%20yields%20high,niobium%2C%20fluorspar%20and%20fossil%20fuels. Accessed December 8, 2023.

Ajwang N. W. O. (2022). Rethinking public health insurance coverage in Kenya in the wake of a global pandemic. *Open Access Library*, 9: e9603.

Ashigbie P. G., Rockers P. C., Laing R. O., Cabral H. J., Onyango M. A., Buleti J. P. L, et al. (2020). Availability and prices of medicines for non-communicable diseases at health facilities and retail drug outlets in Kenya: A cross-sectional survey in eight counties. *BMJ Open*. 10: e035132. DOI: 10.1136/bmjopen-2019-035132.

Askwith T. (1995). Lewis, J (ed.). *From Mau Mau to Harambee: Memoirs and Memoranda of Colonial Kenya*. Vol. 17. Cambridge, UK: Cambridge University Press.

Ba-Diop A., Marin B., Druet-Cabanac M., Ngoungou E., Newton C. R., Preux P. (2014) Epidemiology, causes, and treatment of epilepsy in sub-Saharan Africa. *The Lancet Neurology*, 13(10): 1029–1044.

Blumenthal J. A, Hinderliter A. L, Smith P. J, Mabe S, Watkins L. L, Craighead L, Ingle K, Tyson C, Lin PH, Kraus WE, Liao L, Sherwood A. (2021). Effects of lifestyle modification on patients with resistant hypertension: results of the ruimph randomized clinical trial. Circulation, 12;144(15): 1212–1226.

Britannia (2024). Kenya. Encyclopedia Britannica. https://www.britannica.com/place/Kenya Accessed September 10, 2024.

British Broadcasting Corporation (2022). Kenya profile. https://www.bbc.com/news/world-africa-13682176. Accessed December 7, 2023.

Buitendyk M., Kosgei W., Thorne J., Millar H, Alera J. M., Kibet V, Bernard C. O., Bernard C., Christoffersen-Deb A. (2023). Impact of free maternity services on outcomes related to hypertensive disorders of pregnancy at Moi Teaching and Referral Hospital in Kenya: A retrospective analysis. *BMC Pregnancy Childbirth*. 23(1): 98. DOI: 10.1186/s12884-023-05381-3.

Center for Disease Control and Prevention. (2023). Kenya: https://wwwnc.cdc.gov/travel/destinations/traveler/none/kenya. Accessed October 31, 2024.

Center for Disease Control and Prevention. (2024). CDC in Kenya. https://www.cdc.gov/global-health/countries/kenya.html. Accessed September 8, 2024.

Cowling N. (2023). Number of registered medical officers in Kenya from 2016 to 2021 per 100,000 people. https://www.statista.com/statistics/1240311/ratio-of-medical-doctors-to-100-000-population-in-kenya/. Accessed December 8, 2023.

Dibie R. (2018). *Business Government Relations in Africa*. New York: Routledge Press, pp. 340–370.

Embassy of the Republic of Kenya Japan (2023). Brief history on Kenya. http://www.kenyarep-jp.com/en/kenya/history/. Accessed December 6, 2023.

English D., Lambert S. F., Tynes B. M., Bowleg L., Zea M. C., Howard L. C. (2020). Daily multidimensional racial discrimination among Black U.S. American adolescents. *Journal of Applied Developmental Psychology*. 66:101068. doi: 10.1016/j.appdev.2019.101068.

English M., Irimu G., Akech S., Aluvaala J., Ogero M., Isaaka L., Malla L., Tuti T., Gathara D., Oliwa J., Agweyu A. (2021). Employing learning health system principles to advance research on severe neonatal and paediatric illness in Kenya. *BM Journal of Global Health*, 6(3): e005300.

English, M.C.W., Gignac, G. E., Visser, T.A.W. *et al.* (2021). The Comprehensive Autistic Trait Inventory (CATI): development and validation of a new measure of autistic traits in the general population. *Molecular Autism* 12, 37 DOI: 10.1186/s13229-021-00445-7.

Frontera-Rial B. A., Ogot. (1978). Kenya before 1900: Eight regional studies. *The American Historical Review*, 83(5): 1314–1331.

Gitobu C. M., Gichangi P. B., Mwanda W. O. (2018). Satisfaction with delivery services offered under the free maternal healthcare policy in Kenyan health facilities. *Journal of Environmental and Public Health*. 4902864, DOI: 10.1155/2018/4902864. Accessed December 6, 2023.

GlobalEdge (2022). Kenya: introduction. https://globaledge.msu.edu/countries/kenya. Accessed September 8, 2024.

Global Health (2023). Kenya: Country health profile. https://www.afro.who.int/health-topics/kenya-country-health-profile. Accessed November 10, 2024.

Government of Kenya. (2022). Vision (2030). https://vision2030.go.ke/about-vision-2030/. Accessed November 9, 2024.

Ilinca S., Di Giorgio L., Salari P., Chuma J. (2019). Socio-economic iInequality, and inequity in use of health care services in Kenya: Evidence from the fourth Kenya household health expenditure and utilization survey. *International Journal Equity Health.* 18(1): 196. DOI: 10.1186/s12939-019-1106-z.

Kenya Health Federation. (2021). Challenges of Kenya's healthcare systems. https://khf.co.ke/blog/2021/01/08/challenges-in-kenyas-healthcare-systems/. Accessed December 8, 2023.

Kenya Medical Association. (2023). Moving together to build a healthier world. https://kma.co.ke/component/content/article/79-blog/125-challenges-facing-the-attainment-of-universal-health-coverage-in-kenya?Itemid=437. Accessed December 8, 2023.

Lonsdale J. B. B. (1979). Coping with the contradictions: The development of the colonial state in Kenya, 1895–1914. *Journal of African History Cambridge University Press.* 20(4): 487–505.

Makoni M. (2023). New laws bring major reform to Kenyan health care. *Lancet.* 402(10413): 1613. DOI: 10.1016/S0140-6736(23)02451-0.

Masaba B. B., Moturi J. K., Taiswa J., Mmusi-Phetoe R. M. (2020). Devolution of healthcare system in Kenya: progress and challenges. *Public Health.* 189: 135140.

Mauti J., Gautier L., De Neve J. W., Beiersmann C., Tosum J., Jahn A. (2019). Kenya's health in all policies strategy: A policy analysis using Kingdon's multiple streams. *Health Research Policy System.* 17(15): 1–12.

McCollum, D., Zhou, W., Bertram, C., de Boer, H.-S., Bosetti, V., Busch, S., Despres, J., Drouet, L., Emmerling, J., Fay, M., Fricko, O., Fujimori, S., Gidden, M., Harmsen, M., Huppmann, D., Iyer, G., Krey, V., Kriegler, E., Nicolas, C., Pachauri, S., et al. (2018). Energy investment needs for fulfilling the Paris Agreement and achieving the Sustainable Development Goals. Nature Energy 3(7): 589–599.

McCollum D. L., Echeverri L. G., Busch S., Pachauri S., Parkinson S., Rogelj J., Krey V., Minx J., Nilsson M., Stevance A., Riahi K. (2018). Connecting the sustainable development goals by their energy inter-linkages. *Environmental Research Letters,* 13(3): 1–12.

McCollum R., Taegtmeyer M., Otiso, L. et al. (2019). Healthcare equity analysis: applying the Tanahashi model of health service coverage to community health systems following devolution in Kenya. *International Journal for Equity in Health* 18, article number: 65.

McCormack R. (1984). The Giriama and colonial resistance in Kenya. 1800–1920. by Cynthia Brantley The Giriama and Colonial Resistance in Kenya. 1800–1920. by Cynthia Brantley. Berkeley, University of California Press, 1981. xiii. 196 pp. $30.00. *Canadian Journal of History,* 19(1): 147–148.

Ministry of Health – Kenya. (2024). Government of Kenya launches PHC assessment report to boost universal health coverage efforts. https://www.health.go.ke/ministry-health-launches-phc-assessment-report-boost-universal-health-coverage-efforts. Accessed September 8, 2024.

Ministry of Health of Kenya (2020a). *Universal Health Coverage Policy 2020–2030.* Nairobi, Kenya: Ministry of Health Publication.

Ministry of Health of Kenya (2020b). *National Community Health Digitization Strategy 2020–2025.* Ministry of Health of Kenya. Nairobi, Kenya: Ministry of Health Publication.

Ministry of Health of Kenya (2014a). *Health Information System Policy 2014/2030.* Ministry of Health of Kenya. Nairobi, Kenya: Ministry of Health Publication.

Ministry of Health Kenya (2014b). *Kenya Health Policy 2014–2030.* Nairobi, Kenya: Ministry of Health Publication. https://publications.universalhealth2030.org/uploads/kenya_health_policy_2014_to_2030.pdf. Accessed November 9, 2024.

Ministry of Health of Kenya (2013). *Free Maternal Healthcare Policy Enacted 2013.* Kenya: Ministry of Health Publication.

Ministry of Health of Kenya. (2024). National Guidelines for Safe Management of Healthcare Waste. http://guidelines.health.go.ke:8000/media/HCWM_Guidelines_final_print_version___Final_FiRzql0.pdf. Accessed November 9, 2024.

Ngigi M. W, Mueller U, Birner R. (2017). Gender differences in climate change adaptation strategies and participation in group-based approaches: an intra-household analysis from rural Kenya. *Ecological Economics*, 138(1): 99–108.

Oraro-Lawrence T. W. K. (2020). Policy levers and priority-setting in universal health coverage: A qualitative analysis of healthcare financing agenda setting in Kenya. *BMC Health Services Research*. 20: 182. DOI: 10.1186/s12913020-5041-x.

Ouma P. N., Masai A. N., Nyadera I. N. (2020). Health Coverage and what Kenya can Learn from the COVID-19 Pandemic. *Journal of Global Health*. 10(2): 020362. DOI: 10.7189/jogh.10.020362. Accessed December 6, 2023.

Oyando R., Barasa E., Ataguba J. E. (2022). Socioeconomic inequity in the screening and treatment of hypertension in Kenya: Evidence from a national survey. *Front Health Services*. 2: 786098.

Oyugi B., Kendall S., Peckham S., Orangi S., Barasa E. (2023). Exploring the adaptations of the free maternity policy implementation by health workers and county officials in Kenya. *Global Health Science Practice*, 11(5): e2300083. DOI: 10.9745/GHSP-D-23-00083.

Smith W. M., Opare-Addo P. M. A. (2023). Creative approach to central venous access in a Kenyan intensive care unit. *Journal of Global Health Reports*, 7: e2023019.

Tama E, Molyneux S, Waweru E, Tsofa B, Chuma J, Barasa E. (2018). Examining the implementation of the free maternity services policy in Kenya: A mixed methods process evaluation. *International Journal of Health Policy Management*. 1;7(7):603–613.

United Nations Human Development Program Index (2022). Human development report. https: hdr.undo.org/en/2022-report. Accessed December 10, 2023.

World Bank. (2022). World Development Indicators. https://databank.worldbank.org/source/world-development-indicators. Accessed November 9, 2024.

World Bank Report (2018). Kenya economic update, No. 17: policy options to advance the big 4. https://openknowledge.worldbank.org/entities/publication/58d5deda-d54d-5de4-a577-eafeb6298a91. Accessed September 10, 2024.

Wikipedia. (2023). History of Kenya. https://en.wikipedia.org/wiki/History_of_Kenya. Accessed November 9, 2024.

Wikipedia (2024). History of Kenya. https://en.wikipedia.org/wiki/History_of_Kenya. Accessed September 10, 2024.

Chapter Ten

MALI HEALTH ANALYSIS

Robert Dibie, Mariam Konaté, and Hassimi Traore

Introduction

The purpose of this chapter is to assess the healthcare policy's impact on the citizens and residents of Mali. It will also explore whether the formulation and implementation of health policy were delivered as intended both at the facility level or training sector level or the individual or provider delivery level. It argues that the perception of healthcare providers in Mali has not effectively strengthened and sustained the positive intervention of health policies in the country. The quality of the resources used to deliver healthcare services including qualified staff, training, implantation, monitoring costs, and infrastructure will be used to determine the effectiveness of health policy in Mali. The main goal of the chapter is to describe the effects of the current health policy and services as well as identify challenges associated with community-based health schemes in Mali. The research methods adopted for collecting data involve qualitative and quantitative analysis. The research findings show that rural regions of the country do not have equal access to community-based health schemes as their urban counterparts in Mali. The research findings also reveal the challenges of poor healthcare quality of service delivery, weak policy strategies, unequal gender bias lifestyle, and poverty. The chapter provided some health policy recommendations that could enhance healthcare delivery in Mali in the future.

Brief History of Mali

The Republic of Mali is a country in West Africa. It has a boundary with the Republic of Algeria to the northwest, the Republic of Niger to the northwest, and the Republic of Mauritania to the east. The Republic of Mali has a boundary with many countries in the south. The countries include the Republic of Senegal, The Republic of Gambia, The Republic of Guinea Bissau, The Republic of Guinea, and the Republic of Cote d'Ivoire. It also has a boundary with the Republic of Burkina Faso to the southeast. Although the Republic of Mali is regarded as a landlocked country due to no direct boundary with the Atlantic Ocean, the River Niger flows through its interior, functioning as the main trading and transport artery in the country. The river Niger also provides the much-needed fertile agricultural land along its banks in Mali to enhance agriculture and rearing of livestock (Hill 2023; South African History Online 2023). According to

World Bank (2022), Mali has a population of about 22.6 million people in 2022. The gross domestic product (GDP) of Mali was US$18.8 billion in 2022 (World Bank 2022; GlobalEdge 2022). The capital city of the Republic of Mali is Bamako. The abundant gold deposits in the west and southwest of Mali and other commodities have served as a major resource in the economic life of early businesses and the constant succession of the political system for several decades (Britannia 2023; GlobalEdge 2022).

The Mande, Malinke, and Soninke ethnic tribal people were reported to have resided in the region now called the Republic of Mali as far back as 600 BC (Mcintosh & Mcintosh 1979). These inhabitants of the land also created a series of early cities and towns along the middle Niger River (in Mali) including at Dia which began around 900 BC and reached its peak around 600 BC (McIntosh & McIntosh 1979, 2003). As far back as the first millennium AD, the Mande and Soninke people were known for using the cylindrical brick technology architecture to build their city wall (Mcintosh & Mcintosh 1980; Shaw 1993; Wikipedia 2024). The Bambara, Mandinka, and French are some of the major languages spoken in Mali by millions of people in the country (Britannica 2024).

According to many history scholars, the Mali region has had many empires (Levtzion & Hopkins 2011; Boddy-Evans 2020; Hill 2023; Martin 2023). Some of the empires in the region include Ghana 100 C–1200, Mali 1230–1600, Songhai 1591–1712, Bambara 1753–1854, Messina 1818–1862, Toucouleur 1864–1890, and Wassoulou 1878–1998. Other kingdoms that existed in the region include Kaarta 1753–1854, and Kenedougou 1887-1892. Martin (2023) and Boddy-Evans (2020) contend that the Mali Empire was a powerful West African Kingdom that existed from the 13th to the 17th century. The Mali empire spread from present-day Mauritania to Mali, Gambia, Senegal, and Guinea, as well as Burkina Faso and the Niger Republic. The Mali empire was founded by Sundiata Keita in 1230 (Hill 2023, South African History Online 2023). Other major rulers of the Mali empire include Sundiata Keita and Mansa Musa I (Middleton 1997; South African History Online).

According to Hill (2023) and Martin (2023), in 1324, Mansa Musa embarks on a pilgrimage to Mecca, bringing with him a large entourage and vast amounts of gold. Mansa Musa's pilgrimage to Mecca earns him fame throughout the Islamic world and establishes Mali as a major center of trade and scholarship (Hill 2023; McIntosh & McIntosh 1979; Wikipedia 2023). In addition, many scholars argued that the Mali Empire had a vibrant culture and scholarship. For example, the city of Timbuktu became a major center of Islamic scholarship and learning and was home to many universities and madrasas. Timbuktu City was also known for its libraries, which contained thousands of manuscripts on a wide range of subjects, including science, mathematics, medicine, and literature (Middleton 1997; Hill 2023; Shaw 1993; Wikipedia 2023). In addition, the thriving trade network of the Mali Empire enables traders to exchange gold, salt, ivory, and slaves for goods such as textiles, spices, and luxury items like silk and ceramics. Traders who visited the empire spread from North Africa across the Sahara Desert and into the Middle East (Boddy-Evans 2020; Hill 2023; Martin 2023).

France explorers invaded and captured the Mali region during the scramble and partition of Africa in the late nineteenth century. During the late nineteenth century,

French colonial explorers expanded their control from Senegal in the west toward the Mali empire territory (Martin 2023; Middleton 1997; Wikipedia 2023). Some historians also contend that during the latter part of the nineteenth century, Islamic religious wars had led to the establishment of theocratic states in some regions in West Africa (Al-Bakri 1981; Hill 2023; Shaw 1993). In 1855, French colonial explorers established a military fort at Médine in western Mali. During the same period, the French colonial explorers viewed the Ségou Tukulor empire as the principal obstacle to their acquisition of the Niger River valley (Middleton 1997). Most of the nineteenth century was characterized by French colonial expansion from Senegal in the west and by Islamic jihads or religious wars that led to the establishment of theocratic states (Britannica 2024). In 1898, France's military conquered the Mali Empire. Subsequently, France's colonial administration changes the name of the Mali Empire to French Sudan (British Broadcasting Corporation 2020; Britannica 2024; Wing 2023).

The African inhabitants of the former Mali Empire were now deplored to supply human labor to France's colonies on the coast of West Africa (Wing 2023). The French colonial administration granted the French Sudanese Republic autonomy to join the French community in 1958. After many negotiations between political leaders and the French Sudan colonial administration, the Sudanese Republic and Senegal formed the Federation of Mali in 1959 (World Factbook 2023). In addition, on March 31, 1960, the French colonial administration formally approved Mali to become a fully independent nation. Subsequently, on June 20, 1960, the Republic of Mali formally became an independent nation (World Factbook 2023; Wing 2023). Since granted independence by France in 1960, there have been a lot of military coups and counter-coups, and political instability in the Republic of Mali.

In 1960, Modibo Keita was appointed the first president of the new Republic of Mali. President Keita was noted for practicing a socialist approach to economic development. His term in office as president was cut short after eight years by 1968 General Moussa Traoré in 1968, who planned a coup to overthrow Modibo Keita (Hill 2023; Wing 2023). The Republic of Mali experienced 31 years of dictatorship until 1991, when a military coup led by Amadou Toumani Touri ousted the government, established a new constitution, and instituted a multi-party democracy (Wikipedia 2023; World Factbook 2023). President Alpha Oumar Konare won Mali's first two democratic presidential elections in 1992 and 1997, respectively. In keeping with Mali's two-term constitutional limit, Alpha Oumar Konare stepped down in 2002 and was succeeded by Amadou Toumani Toure, who won a second term in 2007 (Hill 2023; Wikipedia 2023). Subsequently, Amadou Toumani Toure's administration was toppled by another military coup in March 2012.

Further, Ibrahim Boubacar Keita won the presidential elections of the Republic of Mali in 2013 and 2018. Some scholars argued that despite security and logistic challenges, the international election observers confirmed that the 2013 elections in Mali were credible (Boddy-Evans 2020; Britannica 2023; Wing 2023). The characteristics of political instability propel banditry, activities, ethnic-based violence, terrorism, and extra-judicial military killings that plagued the country during President Keita's second term (World Factbook 2023). Because of these catastrophes in the Republic of Mali, the military junta in the country arrested President Keita in August 2020 (Hill 2023; Wing 2023; Wikipedia 2023). In addition, his prime minister, and other senior members of the government civil service were arrested. After this debacle, the military junta that toppled the government established a transition regime in September 2020. Subsequently, a retired army officer by the name of Bah N'daw was appointed interim president, while Colonel Assimi Goita who happened to lead the coup appointed himself interim vice president of the Republic of Mali (Britannica 2024; World Factbook 2023). Thus, the political instability in the Republic of Mali has negatively affected the health delivery system in the country for many years.

Health Challenges Mali

The multiple military coups that have occurred in the Republic of Mali in the past two decades tend to have disrupted the health delivery system in the country. This is because violence and insecurity associated with the military operation often escalated the destabilization of health workers as well as the inability of the sick population to trade and seek healthcare for hospitals and clinics around the country. In some cases, it has also been reported that innocent people were kidnapped by bandits on their way to the hospitals. These precarious situations made the health system in Mali to be very fragile. Furthermore, the lack of access to healthcare also escalated the nutritional conditions in some of the regions of the country.

The number of government hospitals and clinics in Mali is very limited. Most of the specialist hospitals are located in Bamako the capital city. In addition, there are very few health facilities outside the urban city of Bamako. Because of the shortage of public hospitals, the citizens and residents of the nation have to depend on international development organizations, traditional medicine, and foreign missionary groups for much of their healthcare services (Grosse-Frie et al. 2019; Wikipedia 2023; Williams 2020).

In the Republic of Mali, the status of women is lower than that of their men because of religious and cultural values. In addition, women tend to seek more medical health-related treatment than men who try to fight through illnesses themselves (Bove et al. 2012; Debarre 2019; Witter et al. 2016). There is a disparity in access to healthcare in both the urban and rural regions of the country. Apart from these major health challenges, there are inadequate numbers of physicians in rural regions (Sangare et al. 2021). While the women living in urban regions of the nation have access to specialist hospitals, those in rural regions tend to depend more on their family members or others around them for their health needs. Further, women are also influenced by their community and the number of people with at least secondary education (Sangare et al. 2021; Witter et al. 2016). Those in rural regions depend on traditional medicinal healing than their counterpart in the Urban region. Further, because of the prohibitive cost of modern medicine in rural regions, poor people succumb to traditional medicine (International Peace Institute 2019; Sangare et al. 2021; Williams 2020).

In addition, because of the frequent military coups, security challenges, and violence associated with the political instability in Mali, women and girls have increasingly been exposed to sexual violence (Williams 2020). Mali, like many other African countries, engages in female genital-cutting practices, which negatively impact women's health (Jones et al. 1999; Wikipedia 2024). According to the World Health Organization (2023a), the practice of female genital mutilation has no health benefits for girls and women. In addition, women in the country have especially high rates of pregnancy at a young age (younger than 18 years of age), even compared to other African countries (Mahe et al. 1995; Wikipedia 2024). Another set of challenges that are associated with a high rate of child morbidity and mortality for women and children is the lack of access to specialist health facilities. As a result, many of the population of Mali including women face major threats from infectious diseases including diarrhea, and malaria (HP+ Health policy plus 2022; World Health Organization 2023a).

As a result of over two decades of lack of a functional government in Mali health policies that were previously enacted or those that were partially promulgated by the military juntas were never effectively implemented. In most cases, there was a major gap in both the government structure and strategies for implementation (International Peace Institute 2019; Toure 2015; Williams 2020). These challenges made the health system to remain poor. Some of the best hospitals in Bamako also continue to suffer from overcrowding, and lack of modern medical equipment as well as insufficient supply of medicine. These shortages of healthcare resources also spill over to the regional hospitals. While some progress has been made in the last few years, the situation at the regional hospitals has not changed (International Peace Institute 2019; World Health Organization 2020). Another implication of a failed state of governance in Mali is the lack of enough health workforce in both the urban and poor regions of the country. In the northern and central parts of the country, more than 15% of hospital buildings have been destroyed and are no longer functioning according to occupational and health safety standards (HP+ Health Policy Plus 2022; Williams 2020; World Health Organization 2023).

According to the United Nations OCHA Services Report 2022, Mali is continuing to be confronted with limited access to basic health and social services. These predicaments in the country are propelling severe humanitarian needs, especially in the poor rural regions of the country. In addition, the Economic Community of West African States (ECOWAS) sanction imposed on Mali in 2022 has made the living conditions of people terrible (United Nations OCHA Services 2022). The current authoritarian regime has also reduced government investment in healthcare delivery and other social services in conflict-affected areas. Food insecurity affects 1.8 million people or 10% of the population, and more than 1,950 schools are closed, affecting more than 587,000 children. Insecurity has triggered the displacement of more than 440,000 people (United Nations OCHA Services 2022). Further, the Republic of Mali continues to be home to 57,444 refugees from neighboring countries, and 182,107 Mali citizens are also refugees in neighboring countries such as Burkina Faso, Ivory Coast, and Senegal (United Nations OCHA Services 2023).

Another major health challenge is the low national expenditure on health (World Health Organization 2020b). Mali has one of the lowest health spending rates in the world ($35.45 per capita with 44% of spending coming from households). In addition, the pattern of underfunding nature of the health system in the past decade is propelling frustration and a brake for the possibility of accomplishing the goals of the universal health coverage reform policy that was enacted by the government of Mali (Touré et al. 2023). The lack of financial incentives was a source of frustration for many doctors and nurses. Furthermore, late payment of salary to health workers, and access to modern health equipment posed a series of problems that limited the motivational effects of incentives. The allocation of the budget is 4.3% of the nation's Gross Domestic Product (GDP) in 2022 (World Bank Indicators 2022). This amount is far below the 15% that African leaders agreed to in the Abuja Declaration. Further, the Republic of Mali's health system is dependent so much on foreign funding for its health system. Because of the dependency trap the nation's health delivery system may collapse whenever the foreign funding stops (International Peace Institute 2019; World Health Organization 2023b).

The Republic of Mali also faces with lowest densities of health workers (Williams 2020; World Health Organization 2023b; Zitti et al. 2021). In addition, Mali just like any other developing country does not have enough medical doctors and nurses that could play a very important role in the healthcare of the population in the country. The shortage of health workers is considered a negative factor that increases the mortality rate in Mali (Zitti et al. 2021). Among other factors that often propel the sub-standard performance of health workers in the country is the lower rate of salary that physicians and nurses are paid. There has been a migration of several physicians and nurses to foreign countries to seek better pay and working conditions. Thus, financial, and non-financial incentives, career development, continuing education, the state of infrastructure, the availability of human and material resources, the management and leadership skills of managers, and job satisfaction are crucial mechanisms that could help to retain the healthcare workforce (Willis-Shattuck et al. 2019; Zitti et al. 2021).

Some scholars have also argued that the nation's hospitals and clinics do not have high-quality and modern health equipment. Most of the hospitals operating in Bamako, the nation's capital city, still use suboptimal laboratory systems in the delivery of healthcare services to patients (Sangare et al. 2021; Willis-Shattuck et al. 2019; World Health Organization 2020; Zitti et al. 2021).

Moreover, the mortality rate of children has incrementality escalated in Mali due to the lack of availability of appropriate medicines and medical equipment. Therefore, it has been argued that appropriate and timely access to quality-assured medical products is critical to reversing these trends and saving lives in Mali. According to USAID (2022), the health system in Mali has been experiencing a shortage in medicine supply. In Mali, poor-quality medical products threaten the public's health and undermine national health programs. Pharmaceutical supply chains are vulnerable to substandard and falsified medical products. Continuous monitoring across all levels of the supply chain is critical to ensure the safety and efficacy of medical products available to the public (Touré et al. 2023; USAID 2022; World Health Organization 2020).

Health Administration in Mali

Mali's health system is pyramidal at three levels (peripheral, intermediate, and central). The Ministry of Health is responsible for the formulation of health policies, as well as the development of national health priorities at the central level. There are national hospitals and university hospitals (Ministry of Health Mali 2020). Health policies that are formulated by the Ministry of Health of Mali are normally implemented by the National Health Directorate. At the intermediate level are reference health centers and district hospitals (Ministry of Health Mali 2020; Severe Malaria Observatory 2020).

At the *peripheral level*, community health centers provide primary-level care (International Peace Institute 2019; Ministry of Health Mali 2020). One other responsibility of the Ministry of Health in Mali is to ensure the security of physicians and nurses in the central regions of Mali (International Peace Institute 2019). Typically, because of the insecurity in the country, the Ministry of Health often collaborates with the Ministry of Defense and the Ministry of Security to ensure the safety of doctors, nurses, and midwives so that they are able to perform their responsibilities in a secure environment. In addition, the administration of the public health system is decentralized in the following format (1) Seven tertiary-level referral public hospitals/ university hospitals at the central level; (2) Eight secondary referral public hospitals at the intermediate level; and (3) Sixty-five referral health centers and 1,404 community health centers at the operational level (Ministry of Health Mali 2020; Severe Malaria Observatory 2020).

Furthermore, The Republic of Mali has three national hospitals that are located in the national capital city Bamako. These three national hospitals are also referred to as specialist health facilities. Patients are typically referred to the national hospitals from the regional health facilities. The National Health Directorate is also responsible for coordinating or supervising the regional health programs all over the Republic of Mali (Ministry of Health Mali 2020). There are also seven regional hospitals in the Republic of Mali that implement health programs that are developed by the Regional Health Directorates (Severe Malaria Observatory 2020).

The next level of health facilities is the *referral centers*. It should be noted that each of the referral centers supervises a few community health centers in the country. In addition, the community health centers provide primary healthcare with a primary goal on maternity and pediatric or children's healthcare services in the country (Devlin et al. 2023; International Peace Institute 2019). In some bigger and commercial villages, a reasonable number of community health practitioners such as nurses and midwives are posted to health centers to respond to critical health cases as the need arises (Devlin et al. 2023; International Peace Institute 2019).

In addition to the five levels of government health administration units in the Republic of Mali, there are also a considerable number of private health providers, that are nonprofit, a for-profit providers in the country. The for-profit private health facilities are very expensive and the low-income people in the rural regions of the country cannot afford to seek healthcare from such expensive hospitals and clinics. There are also a number of foreign humanitarian healthcare providers in Mali. Humanitarian healthcare providers not only provide their services free, but they also support emergency services as well as support government hospitals with several modern medical services.

Types of Health Policies

Since the Republic became an independent country in 1960, it has enacted several health policies to primarily try to solve its citizens' healthcare problems. According to some scholars, the main purpose of public policy is to the enlightenment of the political system, the fuller development of individuals in a country, and the development of consensus (Chakrabarty & Kandpal 2020; Denhardt et al. 2014; Dibie 2014). In addition, public policy involves improving the democratic and political capacities of the people of a nation, and not simply the efficiency and effectiveness of the delivery of the health system in Mali (Chakrabarty & Kandpal 2020). In the Republic of Mali and many other countries, public and private health providers are two sides of the same solution mechanism. The partnership of the two sides cannot be separated. Below are selected health policies that have been enacted by the Republic of Mali.

Mali Action Plan (MAP), Policy of 2019: The health reform framework of the Government, known as the Mali Action Plan (MAP), expresses Mali's vision "to become the first country to nationalize and implement the Global Action Plan for Healthy Lives and Wellbeing for All." To coordinate financing for the MAP and to strengthen national capacity to implement it, the Government has established a management unit in the Ministry of Health and Social Affairs and is exploring opportunities to establish a MAP "basket fund" (Ministry of Health and Social Affairs of Mali 2019).

Universal Health Insurance Scheme Policy enacted in 2018: The goal of the universal health scheme is to promote and extend mutual health insurance in rural areas of Mali. This new health insurance system is composed of a compulsory health insurance plan for employees in the formal economy, a medical assistance plan (5% of the indigent population), and Voluntary health insurance covering 78% of the population (rural world and informal sector) (Ministry of Health and Social Services Mali 2018; USAID 2023). It has been argued that a major barrier for the Republic of Mali to accomplish universal health coverage is its current fragmented national health insurance scheme with very limited coverage, high out-of-pocket health expenditure, and geographical barriers to accessing services (World Health Organization 2020).

Artemisinin-Based Combination Therapy ACT Policy of 2005 and 2007: The goal of this policy is to exempt children aged below 5 years from paying healthcare treatment fees in Mali. The policy started in a district in the southern part of Mali in 2005. However, the Government of Mali expanded the exemption fee for infants all over the country. The Ministry of Health also modified the methods of reimbursement mechanism for parents who previously paid out of pocket for the treatment of their children all over Mali (Heinmuller et al. 2013; Ministry of Health Mali 2007).

The Policy of Free Healthcare for Malaria enacted in 2007: The goal of this policy was the exemption from the payment of healthcare fees for the treatment of malaria disease for children under five years old and pregnant women in Mali. The free healthcare treatment for malaria as well as preventive treatment. For the citizens of Mali to be qualified for free malaria healthcare service, the malaria diagnosis must be confirmed by rapid diagnostic testing or thick blood smear (Ministry of Health Mali 2007; Toure 2015; Witter et al. 2016).

The Free Healthcare Policy for Cesareans enacted in 2005: The major objective of the policy is to improve technical facilities and human resources for maternal health in Mali. The cesareans policy was also a measure introduced by the Republic of Mali Government to reaffirm its sovereignty in decisions about national healthcare policies with its technical and foreign donors (El-Khoury et al. 2011; Ministry of Health Mali 2007; Toure 2015).

Data Analysis and Discussion

The objective of this chapter is to assess the healthcare policy impact on the citizens and residents of Mali. It will also explore whether the formulation and implementation of health policy were delivered as intended both at the facility level or training sector or the individual or provider delivery levels. The data used for the analysis of healthcare policy effectiveness were derived from both primary and secondary sources. The secondary research methods adopted include the review of the Republic of Ghana Government's Ministry of Health, World Health Organization reports, United Nations Human Development Index annual report, Center for Disease Control, and United States Agency for International Development, academic as well as professional journal articles.

The primary research involves the administration of a questionnaire to 105 respondents. Sixty or 81% of respondents returned their completed questionnaire. The questionnaire respondents constitute 34% men and 26% women. In addition, 43% of the respondents had visited a hospital or clinic to receive treatment at least twice a year. Another 37% had also visited a hospital or clinic between 3 and 4 times recently to receive treatment. While 17% of the respondents visited 5–6 times a year. The limitation of this research is that the insecurity due to political conflict in Mali prevented the administration of the questionnaire in some regions of the country.

Table 1 analyzes the nature of healthcare delivery and health policy in the Republic of Mali. The result of the questionnaire reveals that 80% of the respondents disagree that the Government of the Republic of Mali promotes equity in the delivery of healthcare to underserved citizens in the country. Furthermore, 99.3% of the respondents agree that political leaders and rich citizens of the country prefer to seek healthcare services in foreign nations due to a lack of trust in the Ghana healthcare system. In addition, 82% of the respondents also agreed that corruption and unethical behavior of political and senior administrative leaders in government negatively affect the health system's funding in the country. Another 53.3% of the respondents reported that most rural public hospitals in the country do not have specialist doctors and nurses. On one hand, 60% of the respondents agree that because the government pays low salaries to doctors and nurses that is why health workers are galvanized to migrate to foreign countries to seek better compensation and working conditions. On the other hand, 47% also agree that the lack of appropriate funding for the healthcare system in Mali is why the health delivery system is not effective in most rural regions.

Table 1 The Nature of Healthcare Delivery and Policy in Mali

	Questions	Strongly Agree	Agree	Neutral	Strongly Disagree	Disagree	Agree	Agree %	Disagree	Disagree %
1	Healthcare provided by doctors in my city is highly commendable	0	28	8	0	17	28	47%	17	32%
2	Most hospitals in my country do not have modern equipment	0	16	4	0	30	16	27%	30	50%
3	I can afford my Healthcare treatment and medication costs without government subsidies.	0	12	0	8	38	12	20%	46	77%
4	Most rural public hospitals in my country do not have specialist doctors and nurses.	7	35	7	2	5	32	53.3%	7	12%
5	Government pay of low salaries to doctors and nurses has encouraged their migration to foreign countries.	17	25	11	2	1	36	60%	3	5%
6	Lack of effective health policy implementation or regulations	3	23	19	12	0	26	43.3%	12	20%
7	Government promotes equity in the delivery of healthcare to underserved citizens in the country.	0	1	8	14	34	1	2%	48	80%
8	Political leaders and rich citizens of my country prefer to seek healthcare services in foreign nations.	52	4	0	0	4	56	99.3%	0	0%
9	Government is effectively regulating medical professional licensing and disciplinary boards	11	6	36	0	4	17	28.3%	4	7%
10	Hospitals and health centers in my city have constant electricity.	14	17	22	0	5	31	52%	5	8.3%
11	Lack of appropriate funding for the healthcare system in my country.	3	25	7	0	18	28	47%	18	30%
12	Corruption and unethical behavior of political and administrative leaders in government negatively affect the health system's funding.	26	23	10	0	0	49	82%	0	0%
	Mean							50%		27.6%

Further, 47% of the respondents agree that the healthcare provided by doctors in their cities is highly commendable. It is especially important to note that most of the specialist hospitals in the country are in the urban cities of Bamako, the nation's capital city. In addition, 77% of the respondents confirm that they cannot afford to pay for their healthcare treatment without government subsidies. While 52% of the respondents agreed that hospitals and health centers in their town or city have constant electricity, another 8.3% reported that there was no care in their hometown. Further, 50% of the respondents also confirmed that most rural public hospitals in my country do not have specialist doctors and nurses. It is also important to note that 43.3% of the respondents reported that the lack of effective health policy implementation or regulations is a major challenge to the health delivery system in Mali. They also reported that the lack of appropriate regulation of healthcare delivery in the country has negatively affected the quality of health services or treatment that has been offered to people in Mali. The lack of effective regulation of health policies, as well as accountability for health workers, has resulted in high mortality rates in some regions of the country. On the other hand, only 20% of the respondents disagree that lack of regulation is not a major health problem in the country. This is because doctors and nurses are not held accountable for medical malpractice in Mali. Only 20% reported that the Ministry of Health in Mali is making efforts to effectively regulate the current policies as well as holding physicians accountable in the country.

Moreover, 47% of the questionnaire respondents indicated that healthcare provided by doctors in their city or town is highly commendable. However, 32% disagree that physicians and nurses in their hometowns of the city should be commended for their services. The mean of the agreement that the health system policy in Mali is doing fine is 50%, while the mean of disagreement with the quality of health policy in the country is 27.6%.

Table 2 shows the summary of the content analysis of secondary research that was conducted. The Republic of Mali currently spends an average of 4.3% annually of its GDP on healthcare in the past two years. This is below 15% of GDP that Republic of Mali pledged at the Abuja Declaration. The GDP of the Republic of Mali in 2022 was US$18.8 billion. The physician or doctors per 1,000 was 0.1 in 2018, while the ratio of nurses/midwives per 1,000 people was 0.4 in the same year. According to the World Health Organization (2009) report, on one hand, without sufficient availability and accessibility to health workers healthcare cannot be guaranteed. On the other hand, if physicians and nurses are available but they are not acceptable the health services might not be used, when the quality of the health workforce is inadequate, improvements in health outcomes will not be satisfactory. Therefore, the chronic shortage of doctors and nurses in Mali is well recognized as one of the main obstacles to the delivery of effective health services to those who need them most especially in the rural regions of the country. Shortage of Health workers is also regarded as one of the most fundamental constraints to achieving international health and development goals such as the Millennium Development Goals and universal access to HIV prevention, treatment, care, and support in Mali (Dibie 2022; World Health Organization 2009).

Table 2 Economics and Health Indicators in Mali

No.	Major Indicators in Mali	Explanation
1	Population	22.6 million (2022)
2	Gross domestic product (GDP)	US$18.8 billion (2022)
3	Current health expenditure (% of GDP)	4.3% (2022)
4	Physicians/doctors per 1,000 people	0.1 (2018)
5	Nurses and midwives per 1,000 people	0.4 (2018)
6	Population using safely managed drinking water service	84% (2022)
7	People using safely managed sanitation services (% of population)	16% (2022)
8	People practicing open defecation % of the population	4.5% (2022)
9	Common disease	Neonatal disorders, malaria, diarrheal diseases, lower respiratory infections, stroke, ischemic heart disease, congenital defects, malnutrition, HIV/AIDS, and meningitis
10	Life expectancy at birth for females	60 years (2021)
11	Life expectancy at birth for males	58 years (2021)
12	Mortality rate for female adults (per 1,000 people)	254 (2021)
13	Mortality rate for male adults (per 1,000 people)	311 (2021)
14	Mortality rate for infants (per 1,000 people)	62 (2021)
15	Tuberculosis incidence (per 100,000 people)	50 (2021)
16	Population living below income poverty line PPP $2.15 a day	2% (2021)
17	Population in multidimensional handout poverty (%)	34.7% (2021)
18	Contribution deprivation in health to multidimensional poverty	No data Found
19	Infants lacking immunization for measles (% of one year old)	77% (2021)
20	Malaria incidence (per 1,000 people at risk)	353.6 (2021)
21	HIV/AIDS prevalence of adults (% ages 15–49)	0.4% (2021)

Source: World Bank Indicators (2022); United Nations Human Development Program Index (2022); World Health Organization (2023a).

In addition, 84% of the population of Mali have access to safely managed drinking water services in 2022 (World Bank Indicators 2022). People using safely managed sanitation services as a percentage of the population constitute only 16% in 2022. Further, people practicing open defecation percentage of the population constitute 4.5% in 2022. The common diseases in the Republic of Mali are neonatal disorders, malaria, diarrheal diseases, lower respiratory infections, stroke, ischemic heart disease, congenital defects, malnutrition, HIV/AIDS, and meningitis (World Health Organization 2023). The Republic of Mali is reported to be facing health challenges, such as high maternal and child mortality rates (Williams 2020; World Health Organization 2020).

Further, the life expectancy at birth for females was 60 years old. While the life expectancy at birth for males is 58 years in 2021. The mortality rate for female adults per 1,000 people was 254 in 2021, and the mortality rate for male adults per 1,000 people was 311 in 2021. This means that there are more men dying every year than women in Mali. It should be noted also that the mortality rate for infants per 1,000 people in 2021 was 62. This is a major improvement in the healthcare system in Mali (World Bank Indicator 2022). Another good news is the number of tuberculosis incidence per 100,000 people has dropped to just 50 in 2021 from over 250 a few years ago. Despite the civil war, political instability, and climate change's negative impact in Mali, the population living below the income poverty line PPP of $2.15 a day was only 2% in 2021. However, the percentage of the population in multidimensional handout poverty in Mali was 34.7%.

Conclusion

This chapter has examined the healthcare policy's impact on the citizens and residents of Mali. It will also explore whether the formulation and implementation of health policy were delivered as intended both at the facility level or training sector level or the individual or provider delivery level. The research reveals that health policies in Mali were sometimes incoherent and ineffectively implemented in the country. Because of the security dangers, and sexual violence faced by women and girls in some regions of Mali, there is an urgent for neonatal and obstetric services, mental health, and trauma services, as well as primary healthcare services for female citizens and residents of Mali. Funding the health system in Mali is still a major challenge. Moving forward would require more collaboration between the Government of Mali and nongovernmental organizations is provide funding for the already established free user fees for children below 5 years and pregnant women in the country.

There is also an urgent need for the government of Mali to enhance the promotion of how the populations in both the urban and rural regions of the country could have access to urgent care. This new marketing initiative could reverse the negative impact is a lack of access to essential health services and prevention of diseases. Sharing more healthcare information accessibility, drug distribution, emergencies, clinical care, and life-saving interventions such as childhood immunization, safe pregnancy and delivery services for mothers and access to treatment for AIDS, tuberculosis, and malaria could reverse the current trend of disparities in healthcare delivery in Mali (Dibie 2022; International Peace Institute 2019; World Economic Forum 2019).

There need more efforts to increase the demand for diagnostic services among women with breast-related symptoms nationwide could therefore lead to an excessive demand for the few specialized services at the tertiary hospitals in Bamako. In the twenty-first century, it is time for the Mali culture of de-humanizing body need to stop.

In order to develop a vibrant health system in Mali in the near future, two mechanisms need to be developed and effectively implemented (1) performance management and internal accountability mechanism; (2) political, military, and humanitarian actors in the country need to preserve humanitarian space in the country. Finally, the world leaders need to ask the France government to stop exploiting French-speaking countries in the African continent. It is the right time for the French-speaking African countries to completely be allowed to manage their resources, and funds for the common good of their citizens.

References

Al-Bakri A. (1981). Abd al-'aziz al-Bakri on West Africa. https://jjcweb.jjay.cuny.edu/history/worldspring09/paperdemo/albakri.html. Accessed November 9, 2024.

Boddy-Evans A. (2020). A Brief History of Mali. https://www.thoughtco.com/brief-history-of-mali-44272. Accessed December 19, 2023.

Bove R. M, Vala-Haynes E., Valeggia C. R. (2012). Women's health in urban Mali: Social predictors and health itineraries. *Social Science & Medicine*. 75(8): 1392–1399.

Britannica (2023). History of Mali. https://www.britannica.com/topic/history-of-Mali Accessed November 5, 2024.

Britannica (2024). Mali. *Encyclopedia Britannica*, https://www.britannica.com/place/Mali-historical-empire-Africa. Accessed September 10, 2024.

British Broadcasting Corporation (2020). Mali Profile-timeline. https://www.bbc.com/news/world-africa-13881978. Accessed December 19, 2023.

Chakrabaryty B., Kandpal P. C. (2020). *Public Administration in a Global World: Theories and Practices*. Thousand Oaks, CA: Sage Press.

Debarre A. (2019). Providing Healthcare in Armed Conflict: The Case of Mali. https://www.ipinst.org/2019/01/providing-healthcare-in-armed-conflict-mali. Accessed September 10, 2024.

Denhardt R., Denhard J. V., Blanc T. A. (2014). *Public Administration: An Action Orientation*. Boston, MA: Wadsworth, Cengage Learning.

Devlin K., Egan K. F., Rajani T. P. (2023). Community Health System in Mali. https://www.theglobalfund.org/media/13439/crg_community-systems-responses-gc7-grants_presentation_en.pdf. Accessed December 27, 2023.

Dibie R. (2014). *Public Administration: Theory Analysis and Application*. Ilishan-Remo, Ogun State, Nigeria: Babcock University Press.

Dibie R. (2022). Healthcare policy and administration in Nigeria. *The Journal of African Policy Studies*. 28(1): 101–139.

El-Khoury M., Gandaho T., Arur A., Keita B., Nichols L. (2011). Improving access to life saving maternal health services: The effects of removing user fees for caesareans in Mali. *Health System*. 20(1): 20–29.

GlobalEdge (2022). Mali: Economy. https://globaledge.msu.edu/countries/mali/economy. Accessed September 10, 2024.

Grosse-Frie K., Kamaté B., Traoré C. B., Mallé B., Kantelhardt E. J. (2019). Health system organization and patient pathways: Breast care patients' trajectories and medical doctors' practice in Mali. *BMC Public Health*. 19, 204–211. DOI: 10.1186/s12 889-019-6532-8.

Heinmuller R., Dembele Y. A., Jouquet G., Haddad S., Ridde V. (2013). Free healthcare provision with an NGO or by the Milian government. *The Journal of Field Action*. 8.

Hill R. (2023). The Mali Empire. https://www.blackhistorymonth.org.uk/article/section/african-history/the-mali-empire/#:~:text=The%20Mali%20Empire%20was%20a,legendary%20warrior. Accessed December 19, 2023.

HP+ Health Policy Pus (2022). Legacy Impact: Mali. http://www.healthpolicyplus.com/pubs.cfm?get=18561. Accessed September 10, 2024.

International Peace Institute (2019). *Providing Healthcare in Armed Conflict: The Case of Mali*. Vienna, Austria: International Peace Institute Publication.

Jones H. D., Nafissatou A. I., Kabore I. (1999). Female genital cutting practices in Burkina Faso and Mali and their negative health outcomes. *Studies in Family Planning*. 30(3): 219–230.

Levtzion N., J. F. Hopkins. (2011). (eds.) *Corpus of early Arabic Sources for West African History*. Princeton, NJ: Markus Wiener Publishers.

Mahe A., Prual A., Konate M., Bobin P. (1995). Skin diseases of children in Mali: A public health problem. *Tropical Medicine & Hygiene*. 89(5): 467–470.

Martin J. M. (2023). *The Mali Empire: The Complete History of the Mali Empire*. New York: Trafford Publishing.

McIntosh R. J., McIntosh S. K. (1980). Jenne-Jeno: An ancient african city. *Archaeology*. 33(1): 8–14.

McIntosh R. J., McIntosh S. K. (2003). Early urban configurations on the middle Niger: Clustered cities and landscapes of power. In Smith, Monica L. (ed.). *The Social Construction of Ancient Cities*. Washington, DC: Smithsonian Books. pp. 103–120. ISBN 9781588340986.

McIntosh S. K., McIntosh R. J. (1979). Initial perspectives on prehistoric subsistence in the Inland Niger Delta (Mail). *World Archaeology*. 11(2 Food and Nutrition): 227–243. DOI: 10.1080/00438243.1979.9979762.

Middleton J. (1997). Mali. Encyclopedia of Africa South of the Sahara. Vol. 3. Charles Scribner's Sons.

Ministry of Health Mali (2007). *Artemisinin-Based Combination Therapy ACT Policy of 2005 and 2007*. Bamako, Mali: Ministry of Health Publication.

Ministry of Health Mali (2020). Mali's Action Plan 2020–2030 – towards better health for all. Accessed September 10, 2024.

Ministry of Health and Social Services Mali (2018). Mali health thematic country report. Accessed September 10, 2024.

Ministry of Health and Social Affairs of Mali (2019). National Action Plan. . peacewomen.org/wp-content/uploads/2021/08/Mali-2019-2023.pdf. September 10, 2024.

Sangare M., Coulibaly Y. I., Coulibaly S. Y., Dolo H., Diabate A. F., Atsou K. M., Souleymane A. A., Rissa Y. A., Moussa D. W., Abdallah F. W., Dembele M., Traore M., Diarra T., Brieger W. R., Traore S. F., Doumbia S., Diop S. (2021). Factors hindering health care delivery in nomadic communities: A cross-sectional study in Timbuktu, Mali. *BMC Public Health*. 28;21(1): 421. DOI: 10.1186/s12889-021-10481-w.

Severe Malaria Observatory (2020). Mali Health System. https://www.severemalaria.org/countries/mali/mali-health-system. Accessed December 27, 2023.

Shaw T. (1993). *The Archaeology of Africa: Food, Metals and Towns.* New York: Routledge, Press. p. 632.

South African History Online (2023). Mali History. https://www.sahistory.org.za/place/mali. Accessed December 19, 2023.

Toure L. (2015). User fees exemption policies in Mali: Sustainability jeopardized by the malfunctioning of health system. *BMC Health Service Research.* 15(3): 58–70.

Touré L., Boivin P., Diarra Y., Diabaté S., Ridde V. (2023). Innovations in mutuality: Challenges and learnings for the universal health insurance plan in Mali. *BMJ Glob Health.* 7(Suppl 9): e011055. DOI: 10.1136/bmjgh-2022-011055.

United Nations Human Development Program Index (2022). Human Development Report. https://hdr.undo.org/en/2022-report. Accessed December 20, 2023.

United Nations OCHA Services (2022). Overview of the humanitarians response in Mali https://www.unocha.org/mali#:~:text=The%202023%20Humanitarian%20Response%20Plan,protecting%20the%20most%20vulnerable%20people. Accessed December 23, 2023.

United Nations OCHA Services (2023). Mali: humanitarian response lan 2023. https://reliefweb.int/report/mali/mali-humanitarian-response-plan-2023. Accessed December 23, 2023.

USAID (2022). Ensuring quality medical products in Mali. https://www.usaid.gov/mali/news/ensuring-quality-medical-products-mali. Accessed December 23, 2023.

USAID (2023). The U.S. Government supports universal health coverage in Mali. https://www.usaid.gov/mali/press-release/dec-12-2023-us-government-supports-universal-health-coverage-mali. Accessed December 23, 2023.

Wikipedia (2023). History of Mali. https://en.wikipedia.org/wiki/History_of_Mali. Accessed November 9, 2024.

Wikipedia (2024). History of Mali. https://en.wikipedia.org/wiki/History_of_Mali. Accessed December 19, 2023.

Williams E. (2020). What to know about healthcare in Mali. https://borgenproject.org/healthcare-in-mali/. Accessed December 22, 2023.

Willis-Shattuck M., Bidwell P., Thomas S., Wyness L., Blaauw D., Ditlopo P. (2019). Motivation and retention of health workers in developing countries: systematic review. *BMC Health Services Research.* 2008; 8(1): 247. [cité 16] : 10.1186/1472-6963-8-247.

Wing S. (2023). Mali. https://www.oxfordbibliographies.com/display/document/obo-9780199846733/obo-9780199846733-0104.xml. Accessed December 20, 2023.

Witter S., Boukhalfa C., Cresswell J. A., Daou Z., Filippi V., Ganaba R., et al. (2016). Cost and impact of policies to emove and reduce fees for obstetric care in Benin, Burkina Faso, Mali and Morocco. *International Journal of Equity Health.* 15(1). DOI: 10.1186/s12939-016-0412-y. Accessed December 27, 2023.

World Bank Group (2022). The World Bank in Mali. https://www.worldbank.org/en/country/mali/overview#:~:text=The%20economy%20proved%20resilient%20in,resilience %20of% 20the%20mining%20sector. Accessed September 10, 2024.

World Economic Forum (2019). Mali just took a huge step towards universal healthcare. https://www.weforum.org/agenda/2019/03/mail-just-took-a-huge-step-towards-universal-healthcare/. Accessed September 11, 2024.

World Factbook (2023). Photo of Mali. https://www.cia.gov/the-world-factbook/countries/mali/. Accessed December 20, 2023.

World Health Organization (2009). Health workforce: The health workforce crisis. https://www.who.int/news-room/questions-and-answers/item/q-a-on-the-health-workforce-crisis. Accessed December 27, 2023.

World Health Organization (2020). Leveraging the GAP to Support the Mali Action Plan On Primary Health Care. https://www.who.int/news-room/feature-stories/detail/mali. Accessed December 22, 2023.

World Health Organization (2023a). Female Genital Mutilation. https://www.who.int/en/news-room/fact-sheets/detail/female-genital-mutilation. Accessed December 22, 2023.

World Health Organization (2023b). https://www.who.int/data/gho/data/countries/country-details/GHO/cameroon?countryProfileId=9e4cda0-11b1-4806-9c63-d40904289ced. Accessed December 20, 2023.

Zitti T., Fillol A., Lohmann J. et al. (2021). Does the gap between health workers' expectations and the realities of implementing a performance-based financing project in Mali create frustration? *Global Health Research Policy.* 6(5) DOI: 10.1186/s41256-021-00189-0.

Chapter Eleven

NIGERIA HEALTH POLICY ANALYSIS

Robert Dibie and Josephine Dibie

Introduction

The Federal Republic of Nigeria is a country in West Africa. It has boundaries with the Republic of Niger in the northwest and the Republic of Chad in the northeast. The Republic of Cameroon is located to the east of Nigeria. While the Republic of Benin is located in the west of Nigeria. The Atlantic Ocean is located in the southern part of Nigeria. The population of Nigeria is estimated to be 223.8 million in 2023, while the gross domestic product (GDP) was US$1.115 trillion in the same year (World Bank Indicator 2023; World Economics 2023).

This chapter examines the perception of the healthcare system's effectiveness in Nigeria by citizens and residents of the country. It specifically researched the positive and negative benefits that citizens are deriving from the current healthcare system. It argues that the Nigerian government needs to adopt more pragmatic healthcare policies that could be effectively implemented. The chapter uses quantitative and qualitative data derived from a questionnaire survey administered to 3,202 Nigerian citizens and residents including professional medical staff at federal state and local government levels in the country. Interviews of 600 citizens, officials of public and private sectors as well as foreign NGO stakeholders were conducted. The secondary data consisted of the review of related government reports, government websites, and academic and professional journals. Data were analyzed to determine the impacts of perception and challenges facing the healthcare system administration in Nigeria. The conceptual framework is based on strategic doing, benchmarking, stewardship leadership theory, and an integrated healthcare system model. Recommendations were provided on how to reform and galvanize the healthcare system in Nigeria in the future.

Health Challenges in Nigeria

According to Asakitikpi (2019), Balogun (2022), and Sotunde et al. (2020), the health system in Nigeria health system has been confronted with many challenges over the past decade. The health system has been characterized having deteriorating medical infrastructure, inadequate control of the circulation of fake drugs, massive engagement of the elite medical tourism, lack of enough funding, corruption, poor working condition, poor supply chain of medicine to health facilities, poor compensation of physicians and nurses, and mass emigration of skilled healthcare workers to foreign countries (Aljazeera 2020; Balogun 2022; Oloribe et al. 2018; International Trade Administration 2023). In addition, a major challenge facing the Nigerian healthcare system is the migration of highly qualified health professionals such as doctors with different specialties, pharmacists, nurses, and dentists to developed countries (Adeloye et al. 2017; Balogun 2022; Dibie 2022, 2017). Chukwuma (2024) and Salami et al. (2016) contend that the migration of healthcare professionals has preponderance negative implications on the human resources for the health capacity and outcomes in Nigeria in the past three decades.

Although Nigeria is endowed without standing specialist physicians within the country and foreign nations, the government of the country has continuously failed to appoint honest and charismatic physicians to participate in reinvigorating the nation's health system (Dibie 2022; Oloribe et al. 2018; Onyemelokwe 2023). These laps in the administration of the health delivery system in Nigeria have propelled the underdeveloped and lack of modern medical facilities. The International Trade Administration (2023) reported that the current healthcare indicators are very disappointing for a nation that is endowed with natural and human resources. Although Nigeria is one of the fastest growing populations globally with 5.5 live births per woman and a population growth rate of 3.2% annually, the government of the country does realize the positive correlation between the high population and the healthcare needs of its citizens. The Federal Government of Nigeria appropriated 5% of its budget to health in 2021, compared to the 15% it pledged as part of the 2001 Abuja Declaration. Although the Federal Government of Nigeria has been under obligation of the 2001 Abuja Declaration to allocate not less than 15% of its GDP annually to the nation's health system, that has never happened. Unfortunately, the Federal Government of Nigeria has not been able to even meet the 6% mark since 2001. The Nigerian Government's priority tends to be the few privileged political leaders and senior public administrators and not the general public (Christian Connection for International Health 2021; Chukwuma 2024; Severe Malaria Observatory 2022).

Further, rather than investing in its health system, most elites in the country especially elected politicians and senior public administrators engage in seeking healthcare in foreign countries. It is estimated that Nigeria loses at least $2 billion every year to medical tourism, according to the Nigerian Medical Association (NMA). The United Kingdom, the United States, and India account for more than half of this foreign outflow of funds that could have been invested within Nigeria to revamp its health system (International Trade Administration 2023).

Accessibility to public hospitals all over Nigeria is also a major challenge to citizens who need urgent care healthcare (Sama and Nguyen 2008; World Health Organization 2017). Research reveals that there is an uneven distribution of hospitals in the six geopolitical regions in Nigeria. Other related challenges include a lack of strategic planning for the nation's health system, low technology usages such as telemedicine, mismatch in the allocation of resources, poor condition of health service delivery, and political instability (Balogun 2022; Dibie 2022; International Trade Administration 2023). Thus, Nigeria continues to be one of the African countries that have not effectively developed its healthcare capacity to address the list of communicable diseases and noncommunicable diseases above (Olufemi & Akinwumi 2015; Salami et al. 2016).

Healthcare policies and issues are currently a major problem in Nigeria because there is no consensus on how the federal and state governments, as well as the private sector, should provide optimal healthcare equitably to all the citizens and residents of the country (Adeloye et al. 2017; Abimbola et al. 2016; Alubo et al. 2022; Dibie 2022). While healthcare policy is expected to be influenced by value-driven issues in Nigeria, the current practice falls short of cutting across the entire national landscape of the country (Enabulele et al. 2016; Mclaughlin and Mclaughlin 2008). Unfortunately, the Nigerian model of health governance tends to be ambivalent (Petterson 2018; Reddy 2016).

According to Harrison (2016), the most successful healthcare organizations create a culture that fosters, professional development of medical staff, innovation, creativity, and transformation leadership as well as equipped with state-of-the-art equipment. In the case of Nigeria however, inadequate compensation and unconducive working environment for healthcare workers have often resulted in frequent industrial strikes in the health sector of Nigeria (Akinyemi & Atilola 2013; Omoluabi 2014; Sotunde et al. 2020). Scholars have argued that an estimated 40,000 of the 75,000 registered Nigerian doctors, were practicing abroad while 70% in the country were thinking of picking jobs outside (Salaudeen 2018; Odusote 2017). Between 2005 and 2015, Nigeria educated physicians who migrated and now practicing in the United States constitute about 3,669 (Duvivier et al. 2017). In addition, 50% of the medical doctors out of the 72,000 that are registered with the Medical and Dental Council of Nigeria are also reported to be practicing in foreign countries (Abang 2019). In addition, the World Health Organization (2006) and Lohr et al. (1996) have reiterated the negative consequences of midwives, nurses, and physicians leaving the African continent. They contend that such exodus migration could result in inadequate qualified medical professionals to provide healthcare for the citizens (Chukwuma; 2024).

The healthcare system in Nigeria has not been effectively managed for over two decades (Balogun 2022; Sotunde et al. 2022). The aftermath of these challenges has been needless deaths and an unhappy workforce. Further, most of the state hospitals are in terrible dilapidated conditions and are considered breeding grounds for the spread of harmful diseases (Abang 2019; Awwire & Okumagba 2020; Salaudeen 2018; Odusote 2017). The dilapidated health infrastructure and inadequate administration of the health system have resulted in high-rate wealthy citizens traveling out of the country to seek better or advanced healthcare. At the current time, there are only one or two universities in Nigeria offering a doctorate in Medicine (Ph.D.), a doctorate in Nurse Practice (DNP), or a Master of Science in Medicine. This predicament in made it difficult for prospective medical students to seek clinical specialist training and effective pedagogical training within the country (Agbodia 2012; Dibie 2022; Ezeonnwu 2013). Therefore, the migration of indigene medical doctors to foreign countries has reduced citizens' access to better healthcare in Nigeria.

It is estimated that Nigeria has a population of 226.4 million people and the average and the life expectancy for men is 54 years, while that of women is 56 years (World

Bank Indicators 2023; GlobalEdge 2020). According to the World Health Organization Report (2017–2018), the estimated probability of dying rate is between 15 and 60 years at 341 per 1,000 people. Further, although the government owns 62% of all the healthcare institutions in the country, and the private sector 38%, it has been reported that the private sector contributes 65% of the healthcare services in Nigeria (Adeloye et al. 2017; Omoluabi 2014). It has also been reported that there is only one medical doctor per 5,000 people in Nigeria (Abang 2019; Odusote 2017). While the National Health Act of 2014 has yet to be fully implemented, another new healthcare policy was enacted in 2016. At the same time, the National Health Insurance Scheme that was proposed has only achieved 4% coverage of the citizens of the country after almost 12 years (Adeloye et al. 2017). The citizens and residents in the country co-payment of healthcare is estimated to be about 70% per capita expenditure (Omoluabi 2014).

In the past three decades, there has been increased attention to why the senior leaders political and administrative leaders including the president often travel to the United Kingdom, the United States, United Arab Emirates, Dubai, and India to seek healthcare while there are many hospitals in Nigeria. These political leaders often take the money that should have been invested in the health system in Nigeria to make it a state-of-the-art institution to treat members of their family in foreign countries while the middle class and poor citizens do not have access to good healthcare. Adegboyega and Abdulkareem (2012) and Adeloye et al. (2017) argued, respectively, that the lack of appropriate funding of the health system by corrupt political and administrative myopic leaders is the primary cause of the poor healthcare institutions in the country. It is indeed mind-boggling to imagine the type of stewardship that these Nigerian leaders practice. The Ministry of Health (2016) report shows that 86% of women with children in the urban areas of the country receive antenatal care from skilled professional providers while only 48% of mothers in rural areas receive the same treatment (Adeloye et al. 2017; Chukwuma 2024; Dibie 2022; Ministry of Health 2016).

According to Dibie (2022) and Salami et al. (2016), despite the enactment of National Health Policies in 1988, 2004, the National Health Act of 2014, and the National Healthcare Policy of 2016, the country the negative challenge of corruption and lack of a prudent justice as well as law enforcement system in the country has led to a disparity between the poor and rich in the country. Adegboyega and Abdulkareem (2012), Salami et al. 2016 and Adeloye et al. (2017) contend that corruption in the petroleum industry in Nigeria has drastically and negatively affected the implementation of healthcare policy in the country. On the other hand, Akinyandenu (2013) and Otte et al. (2015) acknowledge that counterfeit drugs have been identified as having serious implications for the health system and the poor people in the country.

There is growing recognition that there is a major healthcare disparity between low and high socio-economic status in Nigeria. Malaria, tuberculosis, lower respiratory tract infections or diarrheal, schistosomiasis, and HIV/AIDS have been reported as the leading communicable diseases in Nigeria (Petterson 2018). On the other hand, accidents, mental illness, substance abuse, dementia, violence against women and children, asthma, and epilepsy constitute major challenges (Chukwuma 2024; Petterson 2018). While death from HIV has declined in Nigeria, malaria, typhoid, diabetes cancer, prevalence of high systolic blood pressure, chronic respiratory and cardiovascular diseases continue to be the cause of death in the country. In addition, the lack of capacity building in the healthcare system in Nigeria, and the low level of influence that medical doctors play in the policy formulation and implementation process in the country is another set of problems (Abimbola et al. 2012; Dibie 2022).

Further, healthcare professionals in the country tend to be less focused on policy compliance because the federal and state governments in the country have not been engaged in prosecuting them for medical malpractice (Adegboyega & Abdulkareem 2012; Dibie 2022). The country also faces a major challenge to health disparities between urban and rural residents in the country. People living in the rural regions of the country tend to have extremely poor healthcare due to a shortage of doctors and nurses and well-equipped hospitals.

Scholars have argued that the lack of foresight to rationalize the health system in Nigeria has resulted in the low quality of the health system (Adeloye et al. 2017; Enabulele & Enabulele 2016) (Chukwuma 2024; Oleribe et al. 2018). All the public and private hospitals visited during the research between 2019 and 2023, respectively, did not have constant electricity and adequate medical resources, modern infrastructure, and equipment. Many of the state hospitals in rural regions were dilapidated and not fit for human beings yet sick people were habituated. Dibie (2022) and Chukwuma (2024) argued that stewards of healthcare in any country ought to be responsible for protecting and ensuring healthcare delivery to all citizens and residents of the nation who need it. This principle is missing in Nigeria.

Types of Health Policies

The Constitution of the Federal Republic of Nigeria postulates that health is a human right. Therefore, one of the social responsibilities of the government is to work diligently to improve the healthcare of all its citizens. Although Nigeria's health system continues to face several challenges, the nation continues to explore mechanisms that could help it accomplish the goal of vibrant universal health coverage for all its citizens soon. Below are selected health policies that the Federal Republic has enacted and continues to strive toward attaining its healthcare goals.

The National Strategic Health Development Plan II, 2018–2022: The goal of this policy is to ensure better healthcare outcomes by 2022 through consolidation of the gains made and by incorporation of the lessons learned from National Strategic Health Development Plan 1. This policy is expected to ensure better cohesion that guarantees greater participation, ownership, sustainability, and full implementation of the plan. It is expected to enable an environment for the attainment of sectoral outcomes that focus on leadership, governance, and community participation in healthcare. The other objective of the policy includes increasing the utilization of essential packages of healthcare services which cover nutrition, communicable and noncommunicable diseases, and mental health, care for elderly people (Federal Ministry of Health 2018).

National Child Health Policy enacted in 2018: The goal of this policy is to provide a long-term direction for protecting and promoting the health of children.

The policy also provides a holistic and integrated vision for bringing together in one document all the key policy elements for promoting the health and development of children. The other major objectives of the policy are: (1) End preventable deaths of new-born and under-five children by 2030; (2) Reduce by one-third, pre-mature mortality from noncommunicable diseases through prevention and treatment and promote mental health and well-being by 2030 (Federal Ministry of Health 2018).

The National Health Policy enacted in 2016: The objective of this policy is to strengthen the nation's health system particularly the public healthcare sub-system to deliver quality, effective, efficient, equitable, accessible, affordable acceptable, and comprehensive healthcare services to all the citizens of Nigeria. The policy also guarantees a minimum service package for all citizens and residents of Nigeria through the establishment of the basic healthcare provision fund (Federal Ministry of Health 2016).

National Quality Assurance Policy for Medicines and Other Health Products enacted in 2015: The goal of this policy is to establish a uniform system that works in conjunction with other applicable guidelines, rules, regulations, and policies to ensure the quality, safety, and efficacy of medicines, and other health products within Nigeria. Other objectives of the policy include: (1) Ensure that medicine and other health products distributed in Nigeria are in accordance with regulatory requirements and fit for intended use, (2) Procurement meets predetermined norms and standards in terms of safety, quality, and effectiveness, and (3) Ensure that consumers receive medicines and other health products appropriate to their health needs (Federal Ministry of Health 2015).

National Policy on Food Safety and Its Implementation Strategy enacted in 2014: The goal of this policy is to build the capacity of both the public and private sectors to strengthen the activities of the Food Safety Control Agencies, considering recent developments at national and international levels. It is anticipated that the policy will help to reduce public health maintenance costs, as well as enhance a sustainable expansion of the food and agro-based industries in Nigeria. The policy will also mandate the engagement of the private sector stakeholders to take greater responsibility for food safety and agricultural health through the development and implementation of programs such as Good Agricultural Practices, Good Manufacturing Practice, and the Hazard Analysis and Critical Control Point System (Federal Ministry of Health 2014).

Traditional Medicine Policy for Nigeria enacted in 2007: The objective of the policy is to address the relevant issues such as legislation and regulation, strategy, system management, management information system, human resources development skills, and culture. The policy also serves and promotes the interest of the various stakeholders in the realm of traditional medicine including traditional medicine practitioners, researchers, regulatory agencies, policymakers, culture practitioners, law enforcement agents, business entrepreneurs, and so on. The policy is also expected to enhance the practice of traditional medicine in Nigeria as well as become a respectable mode of treatment, preserving the nation's cultural heritage with respectable practitioners and providers delivering quality healthcare to all Nigerians (Ayodele et al. 2024; Federal Ministry of Health 2007; Li 2020).

Health Administration in Nigeria

The administration of the health system in Nigeria is decentralized. The Federal Ministry of Health plays a key role in coordinating the health system in the country. The Minister of Health heads the Federal Ministry of Health. The nation has three tiers of health administration. This requires Federal, State, and Local to share responsibilities for providing health services and programs in Nigeria. The three levels of government, that is, federal, state, and local governments share responsibilities for the management of health services in the country by providing health services and programs. They also bear the burden of coordinating health affairs under their purview (Balogun 2022; Onyemelokwe 2023; Welcome 2011). The Federal Ministry of Health is responsible for providing policy guidance, planning, and technical assistance, coordinating the state-level implementation of the National Health Policies, and establishing health management information systems. According to Balogun (2022) Dibie (2022), Christian Connection for International Health (2021), Onyemelokwe (2023), the healthcare system in Nigeria is driven by the public sector. Approximately 66% of the country's 34,000 health facilities are owned by three tiers of government: federal, state, and local (Chukwuma 2024; Federal Ministry of Health 2018).

The Federal Government of Nigeria constitutes *the highest or tertiary level*. Tertiary healthcare refers to the highest level of the health system, in which specialized consultative care is provided usually on referral from State (secondary), and Local Government (primary) medical facilities. In Nigeria, the tertiary care service is provided by medical colleges and advanced medical research institutes (Ministry of Health 2018). The Federal Ministry of Health is reported to be responsible for disease surveillance, drug regulation, vaccine management, and training health professionals. It also oversees the University Teaching Hospitals, and specialist psychiatric and orthopedic hospitals that are established all over the country (Balogun 2022; Federal Ministry of Health 2018; Welcome 2011).

At the *state or secondary level*, the administration of government hospitals and clinics as well as programs are shared by 36 States' Ministries of Health and State Hospital Boards, respectively, in Nigeria. Further, the secondary-level health system in Nigeria is the state hospitals to which patients from local government health facilities are referred. The secondary health facilities are considered state specialist hospitals for treatment (Balogun 2022; Federal Ministry of Health 2018; KPA 2024). Most state hospitals in Nigeria are located in urban areas.

The *local government or primary-level* health facilities are managed in the 774 Local Government Areas in Nigeria. The local governments are also involved in the management of health facilities in their domain (Christian Connection for International Health 2021; Onyemelokwe 2023). The primary level in Nigeria is considered to be the first level of contact between individuals and families with the health system. Primary Health facilities basically take care of mother and child treatments, family planning, immunization, prevention of locally endemic diseases, treatment of common diseases or injuries, provision of essential facilities, health education, provision of food and nutrition, and adequate supply of safe drinking water (Balogun 2022; Federal Ministry of Health 2018; KPA 2024). In addition, most of the primary health facilities are located in rural communities in local governments.

The private health sector in Nigeria comprises not-for-profit, for-profit, and traditional medicine health facilities. The private sector hospitals and clinics also play a key role in the provision of health services in Nigeria (Ministry of Health 2018). Faith-based health facilities typically respond in Nigeria and perform two roles. First, they provide health or medical services of different kinds. Second, private faith-based health organizations serve as an advocate for ethical health behavior, community mobilization, prevention, care, and other humanity support services. In addition, it is estimated that faith-based, and the private sector contribute up to 70% of the total health services provision in the rural areas and the hard-to-reach places in Nigeria (Balogun 2022, Federal Ministry of Health 2018). At this level, the impact of Christian-related organizations has also been significant (Christian Connection for International Health 2021).

Further, the actual number of hospitals and clinics in Nigeria is not well documented by the Federal Ministry of Health. The estimated figure provided by the Federal Ministry of Health reveals the total number of health facilities in Nigeria is about 40,821. This is broken down into 34,675 primary healthcare facilities: 5,780 secondary care facilities; and 166 tertiary care facilities (Federal Ministry of Health 2018). It should be noted that in Nigeria faith-based hospitals and clinics constitute Christian and Islamic health facilities. Other nongovernmental hospitals and clinics are normally lumped together as "private" health facilities Christian Connection for International Health (2021).

Analysis of Data and Discussion

The objective of this chapter is to examine the nature, and effectiveness of healthcare policies in Nigeria. In-depth one-to-one interviews of six hundred people were randomly conducted. Four thousand and fifty questionnaires were administered in Nigeria. Four thousand and five hundred 4,500 questionnaires were administered in Nigeria. A total of 3,225 (71.7%) questionnaire was completed and returned by the respondents. The secondary data consisted of the review of related government reports in Nigeria, government websites, and academic and professional journals. The research was conducted between 2019 and 2023 in Nigeria.

The demography of the respondents for this research includes 3,225 (questionnaires) and 600 (interviewed) citizens and residents of Nigeria. The respondents are employed in both the public and private sectors in the country. A few also the respondents worked for non-governmental organizations (NGOs), and a few foreign companies in the petroleum industry. Further, 1,367 (42%) of the respondents were women and the remaining 1,867 were men. Sixteen percent of the questionnaire respondents hold doctoral degrees, while 21% have master's degrees and hold professional jobs in the country. In addition, 28% of the respondents hold a Bachelor's degree or Higher National Diploma (HND). It was interesting to note that 13% of this group of respondents with first degree were not employed. A total of 35% of the questionnaire respondents only graduated from high school and partially worked in the retail sector. Among the 600 interviews, 48%

were women, while 52% were women from various private and public sectors. Data collected were also analyzed with the SPSS statistical tool and presented in correlations, frequency tables, and percentile.

The central research questions are: (1) What are your perceptions and experiences of the healthcare system in Nigeria? (2) What do you consider to be the barriers to high-quality hospitals and healthcare systems in Nigeria? The limitation of the study is that as a result of the Boko Haram insurgency and kidnapping in some northern states in Nigeria, respondents were selected only from residents in the southern and middle belt states of Nigeria. Tables 1 and 2 are utilized to analyze the respondents' responses to the four research questions.

Table 1 shows provide a summary of patients' perceptions of their healthcare experiences in Nigeria. Questionnaire items 8–18 provide an overview of respondents' experiences based on their visits to every hospital in the country. The table reveals that 98% out of the 3,225 respondents stated that hospitals and health centers that they had visited do not have constant electricity. Thus, it was exceedingly difficult for medical doctors and nurses to perform their duties diligently. In addition, 76.7% of the questionnaire respondents indicated that hospitals and health centers where they received treatment were not particularly good.

Another serious observation made by 76.4% of the respondents is that most hospitals that they had visited around Nigeria do not have modern state-of-the-art equipment. While 72% of the respondents stated that they were not satisfied with the type of healthcare services that were provided to them in the hospitals, 27% of the group reported that they very satisfied with the treatment that they had received. On the other hand, 55.6% of the respondents indicated the healthcare provided by doctors in the hospitals that they had visited is highly commendable.

Research Question 1: What are your perceptions and experiences of the healthcare system in Nigeria?

In addition, 64.9% of the questionnaire respondents indicated that they could not afford to pay for all the healthcare services that they had received from the hospitals. An interesting observation made is that 71.2% of the respondents contend that the hospitals that they had visited to seek healthcare in Nigeria were kept exceptionally clean. Another 62.1% reported however that all the hospitals in the country do not provide emergency services. On one hand, 46% of the respondents indicated that the doctors and nurses, and other medical practitioners were very skillful. On the other hand, 56% of the respondents stated that most of the medical practitioners in the hospitals that they had visited seemed not to know what they were doing. While only 27.8% of the questionnaire respondents indicated that they would prefer to receive their healthcare services from government hospitals in the country, only 23.3% of the respondents agree that the hospitals and health centers in the country are particularly good. Further, while the average agreed positive citizens' perception of healthcare experiences is 38.5%, the average disagree factor good healthcare delivery system is 61%. Table 1 confirms that the citizens of Nigeria believe that the government of Nigeria does not have a good Healthcare policy and has not been effective in the administration of good affordable healthcare to all the residents in the country.

Table 1 Patients' Perception of Their Healthcare Experience in Nigeria

Questions	Strongly Agree	Agree	Neutral	Strongly Disagree	Disagree	Agree %	Disagree %	Total 3225
1 Hospitals and health centers in my city are particularly good.	206	417	130	1,293	1,180	752 23.3%	2,473 76.7%	3,225
2 Healthcare provided by doctors in my city is highly commendable.	577	800	54	806	988	1,794 55.6%	1,377 42.7%	3,225
3 I prefer to receive my healthcare in the government hospitals in my country.	219	679	0	1439	888	898 27.8%	2,327 72.2%	3,225
4 Competences and skills of medical practitioners in my city hospital are particularly good.	634	851	0	796	944	1,485 46%	1,740 54%	3,225
5 Most hospitals in my country do not have modern equipment	327	387	48	1,121	1,342	714 22.1%	2,463 76.4%	3,225
6 Hospitals in my country do not provide emergency services.	575	1,429	0	483	738	2,004 62.1%	1,221 37.9%	3,225
7 Hospitals and health centers in my city have constant electricity.	0	63	0	2,413	747	63 2%	3,162 98%	3,225
8 Doctors and nurses in my city hospitals are professional and friendly.	249	1,427	0	687	862	1,676 52%	1,549 48%	3,225
9 Government hospitals in my country are kept exceptionally clean.	984	1,312	34	134	761	2,296 71.2%	895 27.8%	3,225
10 I can afford to pay for all my healthcare services	391	742	0	688	1404	1,133 35.1%	2,092 64.9%	3,225
11 I am satisfied with the type of healthcare services provided in my country.	286	586	37	1,198	1,118	872 27%	2,316 72%	3,225
Average						38.5%	61%	

Source: Derived from Field research in Nigeria in 2019 and 2023.

In addition, among the 600 interview respondents (79%) indicated that they would prefer to travel to the United States, Canada, England, India, or Dubai to seek medical treatment if they could afford it just like the president and other political leaders as well as their family members do in Nigeria. It was also mind-boggling to note that 83% of the respondents who hold a bachelor, or higher degree were furious that doctors in Nigeria are not held accountable or reprimanded for medical malpractice. Almost, 97.8% of the interview respondents stated that they feel that the Government in Nigeria is not serious about providing good healthcare services to all the citizens in the country. To buttress this point, 64% of the respondents indicated that there were occasions when they could afford their medical bills and the hospital, they visited refused to provide treatment. In such situations, they had to go and borrow money from friends and relatives before they could receive treatment. Among the respondents living in rural regions in the country, 43% indicated that they did not bother to go to the hospital since they were not nearby, all they did was go to the local pharmacy and buy drugs with a prescription from a doctor hoping that such medications would help to cure their illnesses. Those that cannot afford to buy drugs, resort to traditional medicine. Below are some comments made by interview respondents:

The Nigerian Healthcare policy is just printed in the book or website of the government does not make appropriate efforts to implement what it proclaims to do.

Instead of funding the hospitals in the country to buy modern equipment that would benefit all the citizens, the president, governors, and other political leaders keep the money and use it to travel to foreign and developed countries to receive the best healthcare while the citizens die in Nigeria.

I worked for the Nigeria army for 37 years before I retired. Since I retired, I have no way to receive a good healthcare service from the government, I must pay the healthcare bills even though we are not paid our retirement benefits regularly.

As far as I am concern, we do not have a government that cares for the citizens in Nigeria. Thank God that I have good friend who provide for me to get healthcare if not I would have been dead since I retired as a civil servant almost 18 years ago.

Research Question 2: What do you consider to be the barriers to high-quality hospitals and healthcare systems in Nigeria.?

Table 2 data explain the major barriers to an effective healthcare system in Nigeria. The table shows that 91% of the questionnaire respondents reported that a major barrier to a good healthcare system in Nigeria is corruption. In addition, 93% of the respondents indicated that there is no mandatory health insurance for all the citizens in the country. Another 80% agree that political leaders and rich citizens prefer to seek healthcare services in foreign countries, as a result, they are less concerned about enacting or appropriating enough funding to enhance the healthcare system in the country.

Closely related to the above is that 73.4% of the respondents indicated that lack of appropriate funding for the healthcare system in Nigeria is another major barrier why most hospitals are not up to date, and the public does not have access to a good healthcare system in the country. While 70.4% of the respondents indicated that lack

Table 2 Barriers to High-Quality Healthcare Systems in Nigeria

No	Barriers	Strongly Agree	Agree	Neutral	Strongly Disagree	Disagree	Agree %	Disagree %	Total 2025
1	Lack of appropriate funding for the healthcare system in my country.	1,358	1,009	0	277	581	2,367 73.4%	858 26.6%	3,225
2	Political leaders and rich citizens prefer to seek healthcare services in foreign countries	1,246	1,341	0	194	444	2,587 80.2%	638 19.8%	3,225
3	Lack of trust in the poor healthcare services in the country.	983	1,511	0	346	385	2,494 77.3%	731 22.7%	3,225
4	Low salaries of doctors, nurses, and pharmacists in the country	807	1,105	92	658	593	1,912 59.3%	1,251 38.8%	3,225
5	Lack of modern medical equipment in the country.	853	1,418	0	377	577	2,271 70.4%	954 29.6%	3,225
6	Very few specialist hospitals in the country	624	1,399	48	482	672	2,023 62.7%	1,154 35.8%	3,225
7	Ineffective healthcare policy, and the implementation of the National Health Act of 2014.	927	989	67	514	728	1,916 59.4%	1,242 38.5%	3,225
8	Corruption and unethical behavior of political and administrative leaders	1,401	1,563	0	84	207	2,964 91%	291 9%	3,225
9	Inability to retain qualified doctors and medical experts in the country.	879	1,410	102	387	446	2,289 70.9%	833 25.8%	3,225
10	Public, private, and community partnership, in healthcare provision is not strongly encouraged	392	1,088	59	571	1,115	1,480 46%	1,686 52.3%	3,225
11	No mandatory health insurance in the country	1,342	1,655	18	10	200	2,997 93%	210 6.5%	3,225
12	Lack of strategic doing vision of government in the country.	825	1,579	74	298	449	2,404 74.5%	747 23.2%	3,225
	Average						71.5%	27.38%	

of modern medical equipment constitutes a major barrier to a good healthcare system in the country, another 77.3% reported that lack of trust in the state of the hospitals in Nigeria is reason why efforts are not made by the political and administrative leaders in the country are not compelled to seriously make efforts to resuscitate the health institutions in Nigeria. On one hand, 74.5% indicated that lack of strategic doing vision and approach are serious impediments to the delivery of a good health system in Nigeria. On the other hand, 70.9% of the questionnaire respondents reported that the inability of the government to retain highly qualified doctors and medical experts in the country is a major barrier to a good healthcare system. Further, 59.4% reported that low salaries of doctors, nurses, and pharmacists in the country, and 59.3% stated that the ineffective healthcare policy, as well as the inability to implement the National Health Act of 2014, were major barriers to a valuable healthcare system in Nigeria. Table 2 analysis shows that the barriers to an effective health system in Nigeria includes; (a) Lack of appropriate funding of healthcare operations; (b) political leaders and rich citizens preferring to seek healthcare services in foreign countries, instead of investing in the nation's hospitals; (c) ineffective healthcare policy; (d) lack of effective implementation of the National Health policies; (e) corruption; and (f) unethical behavior of political and administrative leaders. These predicaments have prevented the government of Nigeria from providing good affordable healthcare to all the citizens in Nigeria.

The respondents who disagreed that these barriers to the healthcare system in Nigeria do not exist in all ramifications varied from an average of 23.2% to 27.3%. These respondents believe that the inability to retain qualified doctors and other medical experts as well as public, private, and community partnerships in healthcare delivery are issues that could be resolved if there is the political will to provide a good healthcare system for all citizens. There is a consensus among all the respondents however that collaboration to expand access to primary healthcare and testing in the country could better benefit all the citizens of the country than the current focus of the public sector approach.

The data analysis of this research seeks to determine the factors that may be necessary to optimize the best strategies to physically deliver good and modern functional healthcare as well as enhance the quality of life to all citizens and residents of Nigeria.

The lack of mandatory health insurance for all citizens was confirmed by 94% of the interview respondents to be the major barriers to affordable healthcare in Nigeria. In addition, 56% of the interview respondents also disagreed that the low salary of doctors, nurses, and pharmacists was a barrier. Below are some statements made by respondents:

Nigeria is a crazy country because the political leaders only care for their family members and themselves. It is shame that both the federal and state governments no-longer represent the citizens. If they do, Nigeria will have modern hospitals, schools, electricity, and good roads.

Why is it that a rich country like Nigeria will increasing degenerate into a society where the citizens are socially excluded, stigmatized, and inhumanly deprived of a good healthcare system. How are we going to rediscover our human and civil rights as well as cooperate ethically in the financial, political, and partnership front to strive for reform in our quest for sustainable development.

Public Policy Recommendations

According to the United States Department of Health and Human Services, Office of Disease Prevention and Health Promotion (ODPHP) Report (2020) and Emerson (2017), prevention and the ability of the government to collaborate in expanding the awareness of nonclinical issues play a vital role in keeping the nation's citizens health condition to improve and get better.

It is recommended that the Federal Government of Nigeria need to effectively solve the following issues that affect their citizens. The nation's federal and state governments should also be mindful that citizens' ability to have access to quality healthcare is paramount to their ability to sustain good health (Healthy People 2020). High drug prices have also made it difficult for poor citizens in Nigeria to buy drugs when they are sick. Therefore, new efforts to reduce drug prices and the adoption of national health insurance could make the healthcare system in Nigeria more affordable.

In addition to funding, and equipping the hospitals in Nigeria with modern medical facilities and specialist doctors, it should be noted that public health concerns are part of every crisis that confronts the citizens of the country. Therefore, providing solutions to the social barriers influencing citizens' healthcare could resonate well as a remedy to their predicament (Domestic Public Health Achievements Team 2010; Rowitz 2009).

The Federal Government of Nigeria should also facilitate the use of technology to foster a patient-centered approach that could promote the encouragement of hospitalization (Dibie & Quadri 2019). Technology kits could be remotely used to send biometric information directly to a command center in a specialist hospital to alert medical experts about issues such as symptoms of heart attack, sudden weight change low blood sugar, and many other issues (Domestic Public Health Achievements Team 2010; United States Department of Health and Human Services Report 2020).

It is also paramount for the effective healthcare leader to work with economic development, nongovernmental organizations, and business leaders to reinforce the connection between health and economic vitality in Nigeria (Dibie 2022; Emerson 2018; Holsinger & Calton 2018). In order to effectively accomplish the new strategic doing healthcare revitalization goals in Nigeria the leaders must be ethical, provide the right funding for the health system, and be willing to do the right ethical thing (Dibie & Dibie 2017) This is because ethical leaders must engage in monitoring and coaching relationships, building trust, maintaining confidentiality, and providing a safe working environment that could foster the attainment of the proposed health system goals for Nigeria. (Dibie & Dibie 2018; Holsinger & Calton 2018).

Conclusion

This chapter has examined the perception of the health system by citizens and residents of Nigeria.

It argues that the Nigerian government needs to adopt a pragmatic healthcare policy that could be effectively implemented. This is because the current health policies in the country are ineffective, and the government seems not to care about the distinct roles health professionals could play in setting and implementing healthcare policy in the country. Therefore, good governance is paramount for achieving a dynamic or superb healthcare system in the country. The innovative approach to healthcare delivery should involve strategic doing, collaborative new public management, network or cluster of health and business brainpower, accountability, transparency, coordination of priorities as well as a partnership with various stakeholders from the private sectors including nongovernmental organizations and foreign agencies across international boundaries.

The key problems associated with the current healthcare system in Nigeria in this study include ineffective healthcare policies in the past three decades, inadequate collaborative health system, dictatorship instead of sustainable health development, corruption among leaders of the public health system, lack of basic healthcare services, poor or dilapidated healthcare infrastructure including hospital buildings, lack of modern equipment, no central health information system, unethical health administrators, lack of constant electricity in hospitals all over Nigeria, and lack of appropriate funding of the healthcare system in the country.

In addition, steward leaders in network clusters or coalition healthcare experts in the business, nongovernmental organizations, and public sectors could provide coherent leadership on how better to achieve set healthcare goals. Instead of dancing around the bush, the Nigeria government should seek a network or clusters of health and business brainpower, as well as partnerships with various stakeholders from the private sectors including nongovernmental organizations and foreign agencies across international boundaries to help the nation rebuild a new healthcare system. According to Cole et al. (2004), a nation seeking superb healthcare needs to adopt or build on the methods that have been successfully utilized in other nations. This is because the adopted models must have been evaluated and refined to maximize their proficiency and acceptance.

The political and administrate leaders of Nigeria should be mindful that a good health system should provide vertical, longitudinal, and horizontal integration of medical treatment to all citizens in a country (Denhardt et al. 2014; Peterson 2006). Therefore, the tenacity to tackle healthcare delivery problems depends on collaboratively building upon the strengths, resources, and problem-solving abilities that prevail in Nigeria (Harrison 2016; Morrison et al. 2013). There is no doubt that using the principles of strategic doing to create new public management structures, clusters, and values could enable the country to accomplish its superb affordable healthcare goals for all citizens.

Future research should investigate what can be done by the Federal and State governments in Nigeria to prevent healthcare professional workers from migrating to other the country in the future. While efforts aimed at strengthening the health systems can be productive, promoting health workforce retention will be difficult if many of those enrolled in the educational programs never had the intention of practicing locally.

References

Abang M. (2019). Nigeria's medical brain drain: Healthcare woes as doctors flee (April 8). https://www.aljazeera.com/indepth/features/nigeria-medical-brain-drain-healthcare-woes-doctors-flee.190407210251424.html. Accessed September 13, 2024.

Abimbola S., Okoli U., Olubajo O., Abdullahi M., Pate M. (2012). The midwives service scheme in Nigeria. *PLOS Medicine*, DOI: 10.1371/journal.pmed.1001211. Accessed November 9, 2024.

Abimbola S., Olanipekun T., Schaaf M., Negin J., Jan., Martiniuk A. L. (2017). Where there is no policy: Governing the posting and transfer of primary healthcare workers in Nigeria. *International Journal of Health Planning Management*, 32(1): 492508.

Abimbola J.M, Makanjuola A.T, Ganiyu S.A, Babatunde U. M. M, Adekunle D. K, Olatayo A. A. (2016). Pattern of utilization of ante-natal and delivery services in a semi-urban community of North-Central Nigeria. *Journal of Africa Health Science*, 16(4): 962–971.

Abimbola S., Negin J., Martiniuk A. L., Jan S. (2017). Institutional analysis of health system governance. *Health Policy Plan*. 32(9):1337–1344. DOI: 10.1093/heapol/czx083.

Adegboyega K. and Abdulkareem S. B. (2012). Corruption in the Nigerian public healthcare delivery system. *Sokoto Journal of the Social Sciences*, 2(2): 98–114.

Adeloye D, David R.A, Olaogun A. A, Auta A, Adesokan A, Gadanya M, Opele J. K, Owagbemi O, Iseolorunkanmi A. (2017). Health workforce and governance: the crisis in Nigeria. *Human Resources Health*, 12;15(1):32–51.

Agbedia C. (2012). Re-envisioning nursing education and practice in Nigeria for the 21st century. *Open Journal of Nursing*, 2(3), DOI: 10.4236/ojn.2012.23035.

Akinyandenu O. (2013). Counterfeit drugs in Nigeria: A threat to public health. *African Journal of Pharmacy*, 7(36): 2571–2576.

Akinyemi O, Atilola O. (2013). Nigerian resident doctors on strike: insights from and policy implications of job satisfaction among resident doctors in a Nigerian teaching hospital. International Journal of Health Planning and Management. 28(1):e46–61.

Akinwumi, A. F., Esimai, O. A., Arije, O. et al. (2023). Preparedness of primary health care facilities on implementation of essential non-communicable disease interventions in Osun State South-West Nigeria: a rural–urban comparative study. *BMC Health Service Research*, 23, 154–169.

Akinwumi A. O. (2015). Psychological analysis of employees of the same gender, job cadre across ethnic groups in Nigerian organizations. https://jpbs.thebrpi.org/vol-3-no-1-june-2015-abstract-12-jpbs. Accessed November 9, 2024.

Akinwumi A. O., Fagbemi T., Oladele T. C., John S. A. S., Soladoye A. (2023). Contributory pension scheme and economic growth in Nigeria. *Journal of Business Development and Management Research*, 4(7), 33–50.

Alubo O., Zwandor A., Jolayemi T., Omudu E. (2002). Acceptance and stigmatization of PLWA in Nigeria. *AIDS Care*. 14(1): 117–120.

Asakitikpi A. E. (2019). Healthcare coverage and affordability in Nigeria: An alternative model to equitable healthcare delivery.

Ayodele J., Underwood M., Goldstone K., Agogo E. (2024). Enhancing trust and transparency for public health programs. DOI:10.1016/b978-0-323-90945-7.00008-7. Accessed November 9, 2024.

Awwire E., Okumagba M. T. (2020). Medical education in Nigeria and migration: A mixed-methods study of how the perception of quality influences migration decision making. *MEdEdPublish*, 1(7): 1–23.

Balogun J. A. (2022). The organizational structure and leadership of Nigeria healthcare system. In The Nigerian Healthcare System. Springer, Cham. 87–115.

Christian Connection for International Health (2021). Faith-based health system in Nigeria. https://www.ccih.org/wp-content/uploads/2017/09/HSS-FBO-Report-Nigeria.pdf. Accessed October 31, 2024.

Chukwuma J. N. (2024). Implementing health policy in Nigeria: The basic health care provision fund as a catalyst for achieving universal health coverage? *Development and Change*, 54(6): 1480–1503.

Cole B. Wilhelm M., Long P. V., Fielding J. E., and Kominski G. (2004). Prospects for Health Impact Assessment in the United States: New and Improved Environmental Impact Assessment or Something Different? *Journal of Health Politics, Policy and Law*, 29(6): 1154–1186.

Denhardt R., Denhardt J. and Blanc T. (2014). *Public Administration: An Action Orientation*. Boston, MA: Wadsworth/Cengage Learning.

Dibie R. (2018). *Business and Government Relations in Africa*. New York: Taylor and Francis/ Routledge Press.

Dibie R. (2022). Healthcare policy and administration Nigeria: A critical analysis. *The Journal of African Policy Studies*, 28(1): 101–139.

Dibie R., and Dibie J. (2017). Analysis of the paralysis of government leadership in Sub-Saharan Africa. *Africa's Public Service Delivery and Performance Review*, 5(1): 150–167.

Dibie R., Edoho F. M. and Dibie J. (2018). Business and government partnership in Nigeria. In *Business and Government Relations in Africa*, edited by Robert Dibie. New York: Routledge Press, pp. 99–131.

Dibie R. and Quadri M. O. (2019). Reinventing E-governance policy in local governments in Southern Nigeria. *The Journal of African Policy Studies*, 25(1): 1–30.

Duvivier R., Burch V. C, and Boulet J. R. (2017). A comparison of physician emigration from Africa to the United States of America between 2005 and 2015. *Journal of Human Resource Health*, 15: 41–76.

Emerson K. (2018). Collaborative governance of public health in low- and middle-income countries: lessons from research in public administration. *BMJ Global Health*, 3:e000381.

Enabulele O., Enabulele J. E. (2016). Nigeria's National health act: An assessment of health professionals' knowledge and perception. *Nigeria Medical Journal*, 57(5):260–265.

Enabulele J., Enabulele O., Nwashilli N. (2016). Knowledge of hospital emergency unit staff about the first-aid management of traumatic tooth avulsion in a tertiary hospital in Nigeria. https:// ecronicon.net/assets/ecde/pdf/ECDE-05-0000155.pdf. Accessed November 9, 2024.

Ezeonnwu C. (2013). Nursing education and workforce development: Implications for maternal health in Anambra State, Nigeria. *International Journal of Nursing and Midwifery* 5(3):35–45.

Federal Ministry of Health Nigeria (2007). *Traditional Medicine for Nigeria Policy*. Abuja, Nigeria: Government Press.

Federal Ministry of Health Nigeria (2018). *Second National Strategic Health Plan*. Abuja, Nigeria.: Government Press.

Federal Ministry of Health Nigeria (2014). *National Policy on Food Safety and Implementation Strategy*. Abuja, Nigeria: Government Press.

Federal Ministry of Health Nigeria (2015). *National Quality Assurance Policy for Medicine and Other Health Products*. Abuja, Nigeria: Government Press.

Federal Ministry of Health Nigeria (2016). National Healthcare policy. https://www.health.gov. ng/doc/National-Health-Policy-2016-21032019.pdf. Accessed September 7, 2023.

GlobalEdge (2022). Nigeria: Economy. https://globaledge.msu.edu/countries/nigeria/economy. Accessed September 12, 2024.

Harrison J. P. (2016). *Essentials of Strategic Planning in Healthcare*. (Second Edition). Chicago, IL: Health Administration Press.

Healthy people (2020). Healthy people.gov. https://www.healthypeople.gov/2020/leading-health-indicators/2020-lhi-topics/Clinical-Preventive-Services. Accessed December 15, 2023.

Holsinger J. W. and Calton E. L. (2018). *Leadership for public health: Theory and practice*. Chicago, IL: Health Administration Press.

ljazeera.com (2020). Nigerian doctors strike over lack of Private Practice Employment welfare concerns. https://.aljazeera.com/news/2020/06/nigerian-doctors-strike-lack-ppe-welfare-concerns-200615084342885.html. Accessed March 10, 2024.

International Trade Administration (2023). Nigeria country commercial guide. https://www. trade.gov/country-commercial-guides/nigeria-healthcare. Accessed March 6, 2024.

KPA (2024). Major challenges in the healthcare sector in Nigeria. https://kpakpakpa.com/ major-challenges-in-the-healthcare-sector-in-nigeria/. Accessed March 9, 2024.

Li C., Lalani F. (2020) The COVID-19 pandemic has changed education forever. this is how. https://www.weforum.org/agenda/2020/04/coronavirus-education-global-covid19-online-digital-learning. Accessed November 5, 2024.

Lohr K. N., Vanselow N. A., Detmer D. E. (1996). *The Nation's Physician Workforce: Options for Balancing Supply and Requirements.* Washington DC: National Academies Press.

Mclaughlin C. P. and Mclaughlin D. (2008). *Healthcare Policy Analysis: An Interdisciplinary Approach.* Boston: Jones and Bartlett Publishers.

Morrison E. (2013). Strategic Doing: A New Discipline for Developing and Implementing Strategy within Loose Regional Networks. Paper presented at the Australian-New Zealand Regional Science Association International Annual Conference, 3–6 December. (December). University of Southern Queensland, Hervey Bay, Queensland.

Odusote O. (2017). Exodus of doctors from Nigeria had reached an alarming proportion and called for improved health sector funding to discourage it. Today Nigeria Newspaper (November 16). News Agency of Nigeria. https://theeagleonline.com.ng/exodus-of-doctors-has-reached-alarming-proportion-nma/. Accessed September 11, 2024.

Office of Disease Prevention and Health Promotion (ODPHP) Report. (2020). Healthy People 2020. https://health.gov/our-work/national-health-initiatives/healthy-people/healthy-people-2020. Accessed September 12, 2024.

Office of the Assistant Secretary for Health (OASH). Report (2020). Healthy People 2020. https://odphp.health.gov/our-work/national-health-initiatives/healthy-people/healthy-people-2020. Accessed November 9, 2024.

Oloribe O. O., Udofia D., Oladipo O., Ishla T. A., Taylor-Robinson S. D. (2018). Healthcare workers industrial action in Nigeria: A cross-sectional survey of Nigerian physicians. *Human Resource Health* 16(1), 54–71.

Omoluabi E. (2014). Needs assessment of the Nigerian health sector. Abuja: International Organization for Migration Report (May), pp. 50–62.

Onyemelokwe C. (2023). In review: The healthcare framework in Nigeria. https://www.lexology.com/library/detail.aspx?g=f7abcd92-4099-4e27-ac2d-72247820c7ee. Accessed March 6, 2024.

Otte C., Katja W., Linn K., Steffen R., Francesca R., Dominique P., Kim H. (2015). Cognitive function in older adults with major depression: Effects of mineralocorticoid receptor stimulation, 69(1): 120–125.

Otte C., Wingenfeld K., Kuehl L. K., Richter S., Regen F., Piber D., Hinkelmann K. (2015). Cognitive function in older adults with major depression: Effects of mineralocorticoid receptor stimulation. *Journal of Psychiatric Research,* 69(1): 120–125.

Petterson A. (2018). *Africa and Global Health Governance: Politics and International Structures.* Baltimore. MD: John Hopkin University Press.

Peterson M. C. (2006). The Blue-Sky Initiative: A Description and a Challenge. Presentation at the Washington Health Legislative Conference.

Reddy S. K. (2016). Global burden of disease study (2015). *The Lancet Journal,* 388(10053): 1448–1449.

Rowitz L. (2009). *Public Health Leadership: Putting Principles Into Practice.* (Second Edition). Boston, MA: Jones and Bartlett Publishers.

Salami B., Dada F. O., Adelakun F. E. (2016). Human resources for health challenges in Nigeria and nurse migration. *Olicy, Politics, & Nursing Practice,* 17(2): 76–84.

Salaudeen A. (2018). Why are medical doctors leaving Nigeria? Development: (October 17).

Sama M. and Nguyen V. (2008). *Governing Health Systems in Africa.* Dakar, Senegal: Council fr the Development of Social Science Research in Africa (CODERIA).

Senkekubuge F., Modissenyane M., and Bishaw T. (2014). Strengthening health systems by health sector reforms. *Global Health Action*, 7: 23568. DOI: 10.3402/gha. v7.23568. [PubMed]. Accessed September 19, 2020.

Severe Malaria Observatory (2022). Nigeria Health System. https://www.severemalaria.org/ pays/nigeria/nigeria-health-system. Accessed March 6, 2024.

Shafritz, J. M., Russell E. W. and Borick C. P. (2011). *Introducing Public Administration*. (Seven Edition). Boston, MA: Longman Press.

Sotunde O., Iliyasu Z., Idon P. I., Ikusika F., Ibrahim U., Soyoye O., Alalade O. (2023). Pattern and severity of dental caries among adults in an urban population in Northwest Nigeria. *Nigerian Medical Journal*, 64(2):220–226.

Sotunde A., Ukomadu A., Ohuocha C., Heinrich M., Merriman J. (2020). Nigeria doctors strike for better benefits during corona crisis. Reuters. https://www.reuters.com/article/ us-health-coronavirus-nigeria-healthcare/nigeria-doctors-strike-for-better-benefits-during-coronavirus-crisis-idUSKBN23M1BZ. Accessed March 10, 2024.

United States Department of Health and Human Services (2020). Centers for Disease Control and Prevention, National Center for Health Statistics. Healthy People Final Review. Hyattsville (MD): NCHS; 2012. http://www.cdc.gov/nchs/healthy_people/hp2010/hp2010_final_ review.htm. Accessed December 15, 2020.

Welcome M. O. (2011). The Nigerian health care system: Need for integrating adequate medical intelligence and surveillance systems. *Journal Pharm Bioallied Science*, 3(4): 470–478. DOI: 10.4103/0975-7406.90100.

World Bank (2023). Health indicators: Nigeria country policy and institutional assessment. ocuments1.worldbank.org/curated/en/163861595588370916/pdf/. Accessed January 23, 2024.

World Bank Indicators (2023). Nigeria. https://databank.worldbank.org/reports.aspx?source=2 &country=NGA. Accessed November 9, 2024

World Economics (2023). Nigeria's Gross Domestic Product (GDP). https://www.worldeconomics. com/Country-Size/Nigeria.aspx. Accessed March 11, 2024.

World Health Organization (2006). The World Health Report: Working together for health. WHO. https://iris.who.int/handle/10665/43432. Accessed November 10, 2024.

World Health Organization (2016). *Global Health Workforce Alliance Geneva: World Health Organization*. Nigeria.

Chapter Twelve

SUSTAINABILITY OF HEALTH POLICY IN RWANDA

Robert Dibie, Lusanda Juta, and Raphael Dibie

Introduction

This chapter examines the nature of health policies in Rwanda and how the nation's government has been effective in improving mobility, and mortality rates over the past two decades. It argues that there is a need for policymakers in other African countries to acknowledge the complexity and dynamics of the health system factors that may affect the fabric of their respective societies and culture of good healthcare delivery management. The research method used for collecting data for this chapter includes the review of secondary data from government documents from the World Health Organization and several academic journals. The research analysis reveals that enhancing the healthcare delivery system in Rwanda will require shifting resources such as funds and political commitment to address the needs of the citizens of the country. The Republic of Rwanda has effectively formulated and implemented healthcare policies to accomplish the highest percentage of enrolment into the health insurance system in the African continent. The finding of the research analysis also reveals that a vibrant community health insurance system, universal health coverage, and enhanced health workers' capacity as well as high-quality assurance mechanism and managerial skills, which were adopted, constitute the major factors that have contributed to the nation's remarkable healthcare delivery accomplishments. The research also reveals that a universal health system could be a prominent political and most compatible coalition ideology that other African nations could use to shape their social protection and health delivery system. This is because some of the administrative and intervention techniques, which were implemented, require more comprehensive and holistic techniques. Thus, it is paramount for health administrators and policymakers as well as workers to be mindful of the complexity of health systems and the dynamics of any society or nation that may be planning to adopt such health insurance scheme. Some recommendations were provided on how to galvanize the culture of performance management in the health sector of Rwanda.

Brief History of Rwanda

The Republic of Rwanda is a country located in the Great Rift Valley of Central Africa. The country is regarded as a landlocked nation because it does not have access to the Atlantic Ocean. The Republic of Rwanda is located around the African Great Lakes region and Southeast Africa. The nation is also located less than 15 degrees south of the Equator (De Baets 2015; Rwanda, Brief History of the Country 2022; Twagilimana 2007). Rwanda practices a democratic system of Government. In 2000, Paul Kagame officially became the President of Rwanda after many years of ethnic and political crises between the majority Hutu and the minority Tutsi ethnic groups in the country (Farmer et al. 2013; Uvin 1999a).

Edouard Ngirente is the current Prime Minister. The capital of the nation is Kigali. The country's population in 2022 is estimated to be 13.25 million people (Government of Rwanda 2022).

Rwanda became an independent country in 1962. Before the nation gained independence, it was under the colonial administration of Germany and subsequently Belgium. It was during the Berlin conference in Germany between 1884 and 1885 that the Rwandan kingdom's territory was allocated to Germany as part of her colonial East Africa territory (De Baets 2015; Matfess 2015). According to Jefremovas (1995) Maron (2009) and Twagilimana (2007), the Rwanda kingdom was part of the German East Africa from 1897 to 1918. Furthermore, Rwanda became a Belgian trusteeship under a League of Nations mandate after the Second World War ('Hintjens 2001; Jefremovas 1995). The discriminatory practice during Belgium's trusteeship and colonial administration was such that the Tutsi minority was recognized as superior to the Hutu in respect of appointment into senior leadership positions (Uvin 1999b).

The act of discrimination against the Hutu galvanized serious tensions and conflicts between Tutsi and Hutu (Maron 2009; Twagilimana 2007). The German government that colonialized the Rwanda territory did not promote democracy, rather it allowed the traditional rulers of the Tutsi minority ethnic group to coordinate the affairs of the territory even though the Hutu ethnic group of people were in majority (Rwanda: A Brief History of the Country 2022; Matfess 2015). In addition, the Belgian colonial administration favored Tutsis over Hutus using racist beliefs to justify their discriminatory practices (Jefremovas 1995; Maron. 2009; History.com Editors 2009; Uvin 1999a). Unfortunately, these discriminatory practices were promoted due to the perception that the Tutsis tribal people have a different bone structure, including thinner noses and higher cheekbones. They were assumed to have come from European or North African descendants, unlike the Hutus, who were shorter, had wider noses, and therefore determined to be from African descendants (Maron 2009; History.com Editors 2009; Twagilimana 2007; Uvin 1999a).

Further, the Belgian colonial administration adopted the divide-and-rule concept. This allowed them to rely on indirect rule by Tutsi elites (Newburg 1995; Uvin 1995). The nature of their divide-and-rule initiative included the introduction of ethnic identity cards, which solidified the identities of Hutu and Tutsi, which had previously preferred traditional social status and wealth (Alluri 2009; Uvin 1999a).

Twagilimana (2007) and Historyworld (2022) described how the Belgium colonial administrators introduced ethnic conflict into a social structure where ethnicity previously did not exist (Twagilimana 2007). In 1933, the people of the Hutu ethnic group were subjected to forced labor by the Tutsi ethnic group. About 14% of Tutsi people were made to supervise the majority Hutu ethnic group, which constituted 85% of the population. The third ethnic group was the Twa with a population of 1% (Historyworld 2022; Newbury 1995; Vansina 2004).

Melvern (2000) and Newbury (1995) contended that because of pressure to decolonize Rwanda. Tension started to escalate in the 1950s. Belgian colonial authorities dropped their support for the minority Tutsi group. Subsequently, a revolution, by the majority Hutu population in 1959, led to violent upheaval. This forced many Tutsis to flee the country (History.com Editors 2009). In addition, after attaining independence from Belgium in 1962, a Hutu president was put into place, and violence against Tutsi remained commonplace for several years (Historyworld 2022, Melvern 2000; Newbury 1995).

The outcome of the election that was conducted in 1960 resulted in a victory for Grégoire Kayibanda, one of Hutu's ethnic leaders to lead a provisional government for the interim period to independence in 1962 (Historyworld 2022). A few years after independence in Rwanda, there was a coup within the Hutu regime. One of the outcomes of the coup was the removal of President Kayibanda in 1973 by a group of army officers. The Hutu tribe's military officer planned the coup and replaced President Kayibanda with Major-General Juvénal Habyarimana (Historyworld 2022; History.com Editors 2009). During his term in office, Major-General Habyarimana's government reinforced anti-Tutsi and pro-Hutu sentiments. His approach to governance galvanized another wave of violence directed at the Tutsi (Mamdani 2002; Newbury 1995; Sullivan 1994; Twagilimana 2007). He was reported to have made an egregious mistake by formulating a discriminatory law in 1986 that banned the return of Tutsi refugees in neighboring countries such as Uganda, Central African Republic, Tanzania, Democratic Republic of Congo (former Zaire), and Kenya (Historyworld 2022; Uvin 1999a). After Major-General Habyarimana realized his mistakes, he signed a peace treaty with the Rwanda Patriotic Front in August 1993 at a peace meeting in Tanzania. This treaty allowed the right for the return of all Rwanda's refugees. The treaty also propelled the merging of the Rwanda Patriotic Front with the national army, as well as the transitional period leading up to elections and a democratic government (Alluri 2009; De Baets 2015; Historyworld 2022; Mamdani 2002; Twagilimana 2007).

One of the major accomplishments of President Habyarimana's administration in Rwanda includes the promulgation of a constitution in 1978. Under the provision of this new constitution, the president played the role of head of state and head of government (Booth & Golooba-Mutebi 2012; Newbury 1995; Sullivan 1994). President Habyarimana also proposed the revision of Rwanda's constitution in 1991 that transformed the single-party state to a multiparty participation government (Maron 1994; Melvern 2004; Jefremovas 1995; Historyworld 2022). Furthermore, his accomplishment includes the replacement of the unicameral National Development Council in 1994 with a Transitional National Assembly. These changes were added to the 1995 Constitution of Rwanda. Unfortunately, President Juvénal Habyarimana's plane was shot down on April 6, 1994 (Maron 1994; Melvern 2004). The President of Burundi was also a passenger in the same plane that crashed because of a rocket attack just before landing at the Kigali airport in Rwanda (Alluri 2009; Jefremovas 1995; Maron 1994). Because of the sudden death of President Habyarimana, a rampage of genocide erupted in Kigali the nation's capital city. Radical armed mobs from the army, national police, and militias attacked and murdered Hutu political moderates in the capital city, including the Prime Minister, Agathe Uwilingiyimana (Jefremovas 1995; Maron 1994). It was also reported that *militia* groups of all kinds moved quickly to remove any possibility of dissent, and by the next morning, on April 7, 1994, the genocide was underway (History.com Editors 2009; Rwanda History 2009; Twagilimana 2007). Between April and July 1994, about 800,000 Rwandans were slaughtered. The weapons used in Rwanda's genocide was the local machete, which was normally used for agriculture. The United Nations peace-keeping forces, which were present in Rwanda, were powerless and could not intervene. According to Historyworld (2022) and History.com Editors (2009), the genocide ignited several weeks of intense massacres. The killings of more than one million people are estimated (Maron 1994; Twagilimana 2007). In addition, over 150,000 to 250,000 women were also raped (Maron 1994; Newbury 1995; Twagilimana 2007). In addition, members of the presidential guard started killing Tutsi civilians in a section of Kigali near the airport (Newburg 1995). The rampage after the sudden death of President Habyarimana, and the genocide that followed led to human disaster, as about two million refugees fled to the Democratic Republic of Congo, Burundi, and Tanzania (Gatehouse 2014). The Rwandan citizens, who fled the nation, were in most part more Hutus than people from the Tutsi ethnic groups. These citizens of Rwanda were all determined to escape from the Rwanda Patriotic Front (RPF) members that resumed their military campaign a day after the assassination of President Habyarimana (Booth & Golooba-Mutebi 2012; Newbury 1995; Sullivan 1994). The incident of the genocide also created a major healthcare delivery crisis in Rwanda.

Healthcare Challenges after the Rwanda Genocide

The genocide that took place in Rwanda in 1994 has been described as a profoundly serious humanitarian disaster and public health crisis (Overseas Development Institute 2011; Yarlagadda 2022). One of the consequences of the genocide was the death of over one million citizens and residents of the country (Lordos et al. 2021). The nation's government and health system totally collapsed. The majority of the citizens of the country suffer from mental health syndromes. In addition, many thousand residents of Rwanda were injured and displaced from their homes. Many women in the country were also raped (United States Agency for International Development 1996; Yarlagadda 2022). One of the most painful incidents was that children were separated from their parents. Many of the population of Rwanda also fled to neighboring countries for safety or were displaced from their homes.

In addition, the health infrastructure and human capital were completely destroyed. Thousands of Rwanda's citizens who were injured had no hospitals or clinics where they could seek treatment because more than 87% of the health facilities in Rwanda were destroyed during the civil war (Overseas Development Institute 2011). The devastating impact of the genocide made physicians and nurses flee the country for their safety. Because of the lack of physicians and nurses in the country, the healthcare system totally collapsed (Overseas Development Institute 2011; United States Agency for International Development 1996). It is also estimated that more than 83% of the healthcare workforce were killed in the mix of the genocide (United States Agency for International Development 1996; Yarlagadda 2022). Moreover, other healthcare services such as vaccinations, preventive healthcare practices, and prenatal care were totally interrupted. The lack of these healthcare services in Rwanda was also reported to have major psychological as well as serious mental health issues that made some people in the country commit suicide (Lordos et al. 2021; Overseas Development Institute 2011; United States Agency for International Development 1996; Yarlagadda 2022).

In an effort to restore the devasted healthcare system in the country, the Republic of Rwanda Government enacted a new policy in 1995 to facilitate the reconstruction of the health system. Subsequently, the United Nations agencies; the United States Agency for International Development (USAID), the International Red Cross committee, and many foreign donor agencies started stepping in to help Rwanda rebuild its destroyed healthcare system (Iyer et al. 2018; Yarlagadda 2022). By the year 2001, a major step had been taken to help the nation to rebuild its destroyed health system (The DHS Program 1997). Remarkably, trained health professionals, medicines, supplies, and equipment were also donated to the government of Rwanda. In addition, these foreign agencies worked diligently to help Rwanda start rebuilding its basic curative services and restore damaged water and sanitation systems (Overseas Development Institute 2011; United States Agency for International Development 1996; Yarlagadda 2022).

The Republic of Rwanda Government also adopted a new restructuring and decentralizing management healthcare system. Furthermore, district health officers were appointed and mandated to operate in providing health services to well-defined populations in either urban or rural regions all over Rwanda (Overseas Development Institute 2011; The DHS Program 1997; United States Agency for International Development 1996).

In addition, it has been reported that brain-drain incidents has negatively affected the ability of the Government of Rwanda to retain many of its highly qualified doctors (United States Agency for International Development 1996; World Bank indicators 2022). Although, the country has been training medical doctors and paramedical personnel as physiotherapists, radiologists, anesthesiologists, midwives, laboratory technicians, and dental technicians. Yet, it has not produced enough graduates to meet the local capacity needed (Ministry of Health Rwanda Health Performance Report 2017–2019).

Water and sanitation are considered human rights because a lack of clean water could lead to exposure to communicable and noncommunicable diseases in any country including Rwanda. In the past 15 years, universal access to safe water, sanitation, and hygiene (WASH) services has been a major priority of the Government of Rwanda (Republic of Rwanda Ministry of Health Report 2017–2019). In the past 5 years, 57% of the population has access to safe drinking water that is within 35 minutes of their house. During the same period, 64% of the citizens have access to toilets or sanitation systems that keep human waste out of contact with members of their community (Mason 2020; Umuhoza et al. 2022).

Despite this improvement, there seems to be a major disparity between the wealthy and poor citizens of Rwanda. On the one hand, 74% of the poorest households have toilets. On the other hand, 94% of the richest family have their own toilets. Another area of major improvement in the country is that about 5% of the households in the country have access to wash their hands with soap (UNICEF 2020). It has also been reported that international nongovernmental organizations have provided sources of clean water supply to over 650,000 people in the rural regions of Rwanda.

Major Health Policies Enacted by the Government of Rwanda

The Republic of Rwanda's healthcare system has tremendously improved after the genocide incident in 1994. It was reported that in 1996 Rwanda had about 112 doctors, 742 nurses, 77 laboratories, and 7 pharmacists, however since then the nation has had sensational transformation (Karim et al. 2021; Iyer et al. 2019; Word Health Organization, 2017). A recent report from the World Health Organization (2021) indicates that there are now over 1,350 physicians, 95,551 nurses, and over 21,826 hospitals in Rwanda (Karim et al. 2021; the Republic of Rwanda Ministry of Health 2018; Uwayezu et al. 2020; WHO 2020).

The Government of Rwanda has been classified as one of the most advanced nations in the African continent because of its foremost introduction of the Universal Health Insurance scheme (Nyandekwe et al. 2020). This is because the nation has made major advancements in the healthcare system for its citizens and economic development for almost 20 years to enhance its capability to provide effective healthcare for all its citizenry. It has also made public health insurance mandatory for all the citizens of Rwanda.

The Government of Rwanda has also enacted the Community-Based Health Insurance in 1999. The Community-based insurance scheme was especially enacted to be available to all noninsured citizens of the country who were mostly poor and reside in the rural areas of the nation. The community-based insurance is also locally called *Mutuelles* (Iyer et al. 2018; Ryamukuru et al. 2022). According to Iyer et al. (2018), Ndagijimana et al. (2019), and Karim et al. (2021), the government of Rwanda has accomplished exponentially in implementing its universal health coverage and community-based health insurance schemes. It is estimated that the nation has increased the number of its citizens that have enrolled in the community-based health insurance program from 7% in 2003 to over 74% in 2013 (Ndagijimana et al. 2019; Karim et al. 2021). In addition, Rwanda's universal health insurance model coverage has increased from 13% to over 84% in 2012. Meanwhile, it is estimated that the overall healthcare insurance program **coverage** constitutes about 6%–10% of the nation's population (Karim et al. 2021; Mason 2020; UNICEF 2022). Table 1 shows the types of health policies that the Republic of Rwanda has developed over the past 20 years.

Table 1 Types of Health Policy Enacted by the Government of Rwanda

	Title of Health Policy	Year Enacted	Goal of Health Policy
1	National Policy for the Control of HIV	2005	Control the treatment and minimize the spread of HIV
2	National Policy on Tuberculosis	2005	Enhance the treatment of Tuberculosis
3	National Medical Laboratory Policy	2005	Provide highly equipped laboratory facilities to help doctors provide good treat to their patients
4	National Financial Policy	2006	Effective management of the medical budget for all the hospitals in the country
5	National Pharmaceutical Policy	2006	Management of the importation of drug and their distribution to hospitals and medical centers in the country
6	Behavioral Change and Communication Policy	2006	Promote best practices in wellness to all citizens of Rwanda
7	Blood Transfusion Policy	2006	Establish criteria for collecting and distributing blood all over the country.
8	National Policy on Health Assurance	2007	Provide assurance to citizens on how to receive affordable healthcare
9	National Nutrition Policy	2007	Promote good eating habits as well as best practices of how citizens could eat hearty diet.
10	Environmental Health Policy	2008	Regulate water and air quality, food safety, waste disposal, occupational health, and injuries
11	Community Health Policy	2008	Promote primary care in communities where health equity is limited by socioeconomic factors.
12	National Policy for Child Health	2009	Regulate the care of children
13	National Policy on Traditional Medicine	2010	Promote beliefs of incorporating plant, animal, and mineral-based medicines,
14	National Policy for Palliative Care	2010	Increase access to high-quality palliative care for all people living with serious illness
15	National Health Promotion Policy	2010	Enhance citizens to change their behavior and attitudes in making healthy choices.
16	National Health Insurance Policy	2010	Is a policy that the government acted to guarantee that every person is covered for basic healthcare in the country.
17	Community-Based Health Insurance	2010	Health insurance mandates community members to pool funds to offset the cost of healthcare.
18	National Mental Health Policy	2011	Making access to mental health affordable

(Continued)

Table 1 (*Continued*)

	Title of Health Policy	Year Enacted	Goal of Health Policy
19	National Adolescent Sexual and Reproductive P and Right Policy	2011	Create awareness of Adolescent Sexual and Reproductive Health and Rights in the country
20	Human Resources for Health Policy	2011	Ensure the recruitment of qualified medical practitioners in the country.
21	Rwanda Family Planning Policy	2012	Provide female citizens the options from among a wide array of contraceptive methods
22	Medical Research Center Policy	2012	Supports health research studies that aim to deliver the practice and best patient
23	Health Sector Research Policy	2012	Enhance health research so that they can perform at the highest quality
24	Health Sector Sharing and Confidentiality Policy	2012	Provide a set of rules that limits access to information discussed between a person and their healthcare practitioners.
25	Pre-hospital Emergency Care Policy and Legal Framework	2012	Enhance the provision of initial emergency medical services at the scene of disaster.
26	National Food and Nutrition Policy	2014	Enhance sustainable food and nutrition security to eliminate malnutrition and to have a well-nourished and healthy population.
27	Noncommunicable Disease Policy	2015	Prevent conditions that are not caused by an acute infection, result in long-term illness, and often create a need for long-term treatment and care.
28.	National Community Health Policy	2015	Enhance health services that are delivered to communities outside major hospitals and clinics
29	Health Sector Policy	2015	Laws, regulations, and decisions implemented within society to promote wellness and ensure that specific health goals are met
30	Health Financing Sustainability Policy	2015	A good health financing system raises adequate funds for health so that people can equitably benefit from needed *healthcare*
31	National Pharmacy Policy	2016	Encompasses the research, production, distribution, disposal, and indications of any medications or drugs.
32	National Policy for Traditional Complementary and Alternative Medicine	2017	Increasing popularity of traditional and complementary medicine

Source: Government of Rwanda Ministry of Health Report (2017–2019).

Since 1994 when Rwanda recovered from the genocide incident, the government of the country has enacted several health policies to address the nation's health challenges. These health policies were formulated as well as implemented to respond to the citizens' healthcare needs (Republic of Rwanda Government 2005).

The Republic of Rwanda government enacted a Community Health Policy in 2008 with the goal to strengthen the healthcare delivery system as well as improve the quality of life of citizens of the country in various communities (Republic of Rwanda Government 2008). Before the enactment of the 2008 community health policy, there were major disparities in the administration of healthcare in the rural regions of Rwanda. The National Community Health Policy of 2008 was introduced to enhance the effectiveness of policies that were previously implemented in the country are (1) the National HIV/AIDS Policy of 2005; (2) the National Nutrition Policy of 2005; (3) the National Family Planning policy of 2005; and (4) the Reproductive Health Policy of 2003 (Iyer et al. 2018; the Republic of Rwanda Government 2008).

The above domestic health policies and the Rwanda Ministry of Health, Food and Drug Authority, Rwanda Biomedical Center, physicians, and nursing personnel as well as other international private and religious medical organizations play a key successful role in the healthcare delivery system in the country. There is no doubt that the Government of Rwanda has incrementally formulated and implemented sustained health policies that have galvanized the pace to substantially increase affordable healthcare and life expectancy in Rwanda (Iyer et al. 2018; Nyandekwe et al. 2020).

Apart from enacting sustainable health policies and specifying the new role of the Ministry of Health, Faith-based institutions, private for-profit, and nongovernment organizations are also actively involved in the delivery of healthcare services in both the urban and rural regions of the country (UNICEF 2022a). The combination of these types of healthcare coverage is further enabled by the Rwandan governance structures that were established at the national, province, district, and sub-district levels in the nation (Republic of Rwanda Ministry of Health Report 2019). The decentralized structure is related to how funding for healthcare delivery and health systems are distributed to all the district levels to ensure the success of both the universal healthcare scheme and the community-based insurance policies that have been adopted by the Government of Rwanda.

Traditional Medicine in Rwanda

As part of the affordable healthcare strategy, the Government of Rwanda enacted a National Traditional Complementary as an alternative medicine policy in 2017. This policy initiative was complementary to the government's desire to also regulate the practice of traditional medicine practice and the safety of the citizens Republic of Rwanda Ministry of Health Report 2019. Sick people are more likely to consult traditional practitioners as their modern healthcare providers, depending on the nature of the problem. To improve the quality of home deliveries, the Ministry of Health has developed programs to improve the network and skills of Traditional Birth Attendants (TBAs) (Republic of Rwanda Ministry of Health Report 2019). A training program was implemented in four pilot districts (Byumba, Cyangugu, Gikongoro, and Gitarama) to train 1,200 TBAs (Overview of the Health System in Rwanda 2020; UNICEF 2022b). The currently trained TBAs have also received basic equipment and supervision from government agencies. There are also plans put in place by the Ministry of Health to expand traditional attendants training programs to other districts in the country as the needs become very necessary (Overview of the Health System in Rwanda 2020).

Administration of Health Services

The Ministry of Health coordinates the administration of the health system in Rwanda. The Ministry of Health's goal is to provide access and affordable health to all the citizens of Rwanda. In the process of performing this mandate, the Ministry is also engaging in preventive, rehabilitative, and curative healthcare services to all the citizens and residents of the country Republic of Rwanda Ministry of Health Report 2019. The responsibility of the Ministry of Health also covers all health institutions or organizations in both the private and public sectors of Rwanda (Republic of Rwanda Ministry of Health Report 2019). In addition to the services provided by the Ministry of Health, other agencies also provide special services to enhance the healthcare system in the country (UNICEF Report 2021–2022). Further, the nation's Biomedical Center also plays a key role in the effective implementation of health programs. The role of the center includes disease prevention and improving research, as well as fostering the provision of health treatment to the general population of the country. The public health infrastructure constitutes 64% of all the health facilities in the country. While the private sector owns just 28% (the Republic of Rwanda Government 2001; UNICEF 2022b).

The health system in the Republic of Rwanda is divided into three service segments: (1) the central level; (2) the intermediate level; and (3) the peripheral level. The *central level* is organized into three levels, with each level having a defined technical and administrative platform called a minimum package of activities. In addition, the central level is associated with the five national referral hospitals. The major responsibility of the *central level* is the development of health policy and the overall strategic and technical framework within which health services are provided (Government of Rwanda, Ministry of Health Report 1995–2001). The *central level* is also responsible for monitoring and evaluating operational programs and managing the referral as well as the Teaching Hospitals. The teaching hospitals include Rwanda Military Hospital, Butare University Teaching Hospital, King Faisal Hospital, and Ndera Neuropsychiatric Hospital. These hospitals provide training for medical doctors as well as conduct medical and health science research in Rwanda (Ministry of Health, Health Sector Performance Report 2017–2019).

The *intermediate level* consists of 11 provincial hospitals. They are managed under health, gender, and social affairs guidelines. Some of these hospitals are being upgraded to minimize the increase in the demand for services at the national referral hospitals. It should be noted that the Public Health Department of Kigali City is also at the intermediate level (Ministry of Health, Health Sector Performance Report 2017–2019).

The *peripheral level* consists of an administrative office and district health offices. There are 36 district hospitals and 499 health centers at the peripheral level (Ministry of Health, Health Sector Performance Report 2017–2019). In addition, every district has an administrative office, a district hospital, and primary healthcare facilities (health centers). According to the Ministry of Health, Health Sector Performance Report (2017–2019), the main function of district hospitals is to care for patients referred by a primary-level facility. Furthermore, it is estimated that the peripheral level had 365 health facilities at the end of 2001; 252 were health centers while 113 were health posts and dispensaries. Although curative and rehabilitative care are the principal functions of the hospital, the hospitals are also responsible for supporting preventive and promotional activities within the catchment area (Ministry of Health, Health Sector Performance Report 2017–2019).

Analysis of Rwanda's Health System

The goal of this chapter is to analyze the nature and effectiveness of health policies in Rwanda and how the nation's government has been effective in improving mobility, and mortality rates over the past two decades after the genocide incident. The research method used for data analysis includes content analysis of the Republic of Rwanda Government policy documents, UNICEF Rwanda health budget brief, World Bank indicators and reports, World Health Organization reports, Rwanda Ministry of Health reports, United Nations Children's Fund reports, academic journals, and World Development indicators.

Rwanda's new health policy was influenced by many international dimensions with respect to important international policies and commitments guiding Rwanda's health policy are the Abuja Declaration of 2001, the African Health Strategy (2007–2015), the Paris Declaration (2005), the Accra Agenda for Action (2008), and more recently and the Rio Political Declaration on Social Determinants of Health 2011 (Rwanda, Ministry of Health 2015; Umuhoza et al. 2022).

The Community-based health insurance, which was adopted by Rwanda in 1999–2000, has been argued to be a vehicle for the establishment of University Health Insurance (Chemouni 2018; Sayinzoga and Bijlmaker 2016; Snogo 2016). What really galvanized the success of both the community-based health insurance and universal health insurance schemes in Rwanda? Some scholars argued that the success of these two health insurance schemes mostly depended on the signed performance contract by senior health administrators with the President of Rwanda (Guichaoua 2020; Sanogo et al. 2019). The performance contract with the President of Rwanda is the major mechanism. The performance contract stipulates a certain target which is determined at the beginning of each year. Failure to accomplish such a target could lead to the redeployment of the Major (Sayinzoga & Bijlmaker 2016; Umuhoza et al. 2022). Furthermore, the variation of performance could result in the earning of a lower salary (Expert Financial 2022; Guichaoua 2020; Sayinzoga & Bijlmaker 2016).

According to the UNICEF Report (2021–2022) and United Kingdom Development Initiatives (2013), foreign assistance contributes to the health expenditure in Rwanda.

This money comes from donors in American and European countries. Furthermore, Rwanda's Ministry of Health budget has increased incrementally from 282.3 billion FRW in 2020–2021 to FRW 733.1 in 2021–2022 (UNICEF Report 2021–2022). This means that there was a nominal increase in budget of 33.6% in Rwanda in 2021–2022. As part of the nation's commitment to affordable healthcare, the Government of Rwanda spent 16.5% of its total budget on healthcare in the fiscal year 2015/2016 of the nation. It has been reported that the health budget for that year and subsequent years surpassed the 15% that was required by the Abuja International Declaration of Health (Ministry of Health Rwanda 2016; Ministry of Health Kigali 2015). While the Government of Rwanda spent 11.2% of its GDP on the health sector in 2014–2015, the total public sector expenditure on public healthcare was 9.9%. During the same budget period, the out-of-pocket expenditure was 8.8% (Expert Financial 2022; Republic of Rwanda Ministry of Health 2017–2019).

Rwanda spent 6.41% of its GDP on health in 2019. However, two years later, the funds allocated to the health sector account for 43.2% down from 51.4% of the budget in 2020/2021. It should be noted however that domestic resources increased from FRW 145.1 billion in 2020/2021 to FRW 162.7 billion in 2021/2022. During the same period, the external funds donated to Rwanda increased from FRW 137.2 billion in 2020/2021 to FRW 214.3 billion in 2021/2022. The COVID-19 pandemic that occurred in 2020/2021 and the associated emergency in Rwanda could explain why the nation's budget increased in the same period. Foreign funding also increased during the COVID-19 pandemic period as well Condo et al. 2020; Expert Financial 2022; WHO Africa 2020). It is important to note that the success of the Government of Rwanda's health system depends on foreign donors. This reliance on foreign donors could create a serious predicament for the country if the money stops flowing in. According to Dibie (2022), if African nations continue to succumb to this type of dependency trap, they might be exposing their citizens to another form of neocolonialism. Table 2 shows the indicators of doctors and other qualified health professionals in Rwanda.

In the past 10 years, the Government of Rwanda and its private sectors partners in healthcare have been working diligently to address the major challenges of the ratio of one physician to over 10,000 citizens. This major gap in health workforce is because of the high turnover and limited career development, has posed major healthcare challenges in the country. It has also been reported that Rwanda has a nationwide inadequacy of physicians, nurses, and health facilities' managers with sufficient experience to respond to the needs of both the administrative structures and health workers (Overview of the Health System in Rwanda 2020; World Bank Group 2022; World Bank Indicators 2022).

This problem is more acute at the periphery level, where operational management and delivery of health services occur. The Ministry of Health, Rwanda Health Performance Report (2017–2019) indicated the continuous effort of the government to increase qualified health professionals. The major Teaching Hospital and Universities, including the Polytechnic regional centers, have been training the health workforce in the country. Between late 2019 and 2022, there were more than 1,492 doctors in Rwanda. This means that there is currently one doctor to more than 8,294 patients.

Table 2 Economics and Health Indicators in Rwanda

No.	Major Indicators in Rwanda	Explanation
1	Population	13.8 million (2022)
2	Gross domestic product (GDP)	US$10.59 trillion (2020)
3	Current health expenditure (% of GDP)	7.32 (2020)
4	Physicians/doctors per 1,000 people	0.1 (2019)
5	Nurse/midwives per 1,000 people	0.9 (2021)
6	Hospital beds per 1,000 people	1.6 (2007)
7	Birth attended by skilled health personnel	2,889
8	Population using at least basic drinking water service	65% (2022)
9	Population using at least basic sanitation	94% (rich people) 74% (poor people)
10	Population of people having electricity	52,6% (2021)
11	Population practicing open defecation	2% (2022)
12	Population using safely managed drinking water service	57%
13	Common disease in Rwanda	Lower respiratory infections; neonatal disorders; stroke; tuberculosis; ischemic heart disease
14	Life expectancy in 2019 at birth for females	68 years (2021)
15	Life expectancy in 2021 at birth for males	64 years (2021)
16	Mortality rate for female adults (per 1,000 people)	27 (2021)
17	Mortality rate for male adults (per 1,000 people)	277 (2021)
18	Mortality rate for infants (per 1,000 people)	33 (2021)
19	Poverty head count ratio at $2.15 a day (2017 PPP (% of population)	52% (2016)
20	Incidence of malaria (per 1,000 population at risk)	126.3 (2021)
	Multidimensional poverty head count ratio (% of total population)	28.7% (2016)
21	Tuberculosis incidence (per 100,000 people)	58 (2021)
22	HIV/AIDS prevalence adults (% ages 15–49)	2.6% (2021)

Source: United Nations Human Development Programme (2020). Human Development Report. https://hdr.und.or/en/2020-report. Accessed December 23, 2022. Republic of Rwanda Ministry of Health (2017–2019), Rwanda Health Sector Performance Report. Kigali: Government of Rwanda Ministry of Health.

There are also 10,409 nurses. This also means that there is one nurse to 1,420 patients. In addition, there are 1,562 midwives in the country. This is an indication to the fact that there is one midwife to 2,889 patients. Unfortunately, the government of Rwanda has not been able to accomplish the World Health Organization standard of one doctor to serve 1,000 patients (Ministry of Health, Rwanda Health Performance Report 2017–2019; World Bank Indicators 2022). In addition, substantial progress has been accomplished in childbirth attendance by skilled health staff in Rwanda. For instance, in the year 2020, births attended by skilled health staff for Rwanda was 94.2%. It has also been reported that births attended by skilled health staff of Rwanda increased from 26.7% in 2000 to 94.2% in 2020 growing at an average annual rate of 26.26% (World Data Atlas 2020; UNICEF 2020; World Health Organization 2021).

The quality of healthcare services in the Republic of Rwanda is constantly and regularly monitored through the following mechanisms: (1) Health facilities accreditation; (2) Performance-based financings; and (3) Integrative supportive supervision. The National Policy for Quality and Accreditation and Hospital Rwanda Accreditation Standards are major instruments that are used for the regulation of quality of health services in the country (Government of Rwanda Ministry of Health Report 2017–2019). To ensure high quality of health services, accreditation standards are developed, disseminated, and implemented in all public hospitals. There are also quality assurance boards, which were established in each health facility, all over Rwanda. To incrementally enhance quality in 2006, the Ministry of Health established accreditation programs in the Butari University Teaching Hospital, King Faisal Hospital, and the Kigali University Teaching Hospital (Government of Rwanda Ministry of Health report 2017–2019; Sayinzoga & Bijlmakers 2016). In addition, the Government of Rwanda enacted the Laboratory Accreditation Act in 2009. Following this health quality policy, the Ministry of Health of Rwanda launched the National Healthcare Accreditation Standards that included an accreditation performance toolkit, as well as surveyor and facilitator manual in 2012. To strengthen the already established accreditation method, in the year 2013, the Ministry of Health of Rwanda decided to connect performance-based financing to accreditation (Expert Financial 2022).

The health infrastructure and information technology are other areas where the Government of Rwanda had made substantial changes. This is because with an improved information technology infrastructure in the country, health facilities are expected to function faster as expected. Also, the provision of specialized services at secondary and tertiary levels could be adequate. It has been argued that information technology is a key mechanism for strengthening emergency and pre-hospital services (Rwanda Health Management Information System Manual 2013). Umuhoza et al. (2022) contend that since 2011, the Republic of Rwanda Government has adopted open-source software called DHIS2 for data collection and disease surveillance.

According to Cunningham et al. (2012), it is critical to communicate the benefits of evidence-based practice. Without a vibrant information system, hospital, health centers, and medical staff cannot effectively engage in such communication. This practice has enabled health institutions at both the central, and local clinics to collect and promote best practices in healthcare service delivery as well as strategic planning in the sector (Iyer et al. 2018; Rwanda Health Management Information System 2013). Therefore, the introduction of health information system has enabled health reports to be sent on a case-by-case basis through web-based system daily, weekly, monthly, and quarterly (Iyer et al. 2018; Rwanda Health Management Information System 2013; UNICEF 2022a).

The practice of using information system in health has also enhanced the ability of the Ministry of Health in Rwanda to monitor and study the nature and quality of treatment that are been offered. Furthermore, information technology has propelled research skills among physicians, nurses, and health laboratories in the country. According to Iyer et al. (2018), the Rwanda Ministry of Health also experienced some setbacks in the process of rolling its national community health database (Nshimyiryo et al. 2020; Sanogo et al. 2019; Woldemichael et al. 2019). Table 3 shows an assessment of the Rwanda's Health Polices.

During the past 10 years, international organizations such as UNICEF and WHO, have worked with over 30 districts in Rwanda to build facilities for household to use for hygienic and latrine purpose (UNICEF 2022). Despite these water and sanitation initiatives, the people in Rwanda are still engaging in open defecation in bushes, on beaches, fields, forests, open bodies of water, and solid waste disposal areas are reported to be about 1.96% of the population (World Bank Trading Economics Report 2022).

Table 3 Assessment of the Rwanda Health Policies Implementation

Assessment Factors	Implementation Action	Effective or Not Effective
Leadership and Governance	• Excellent Political commitment • Strong leadership and evidence-based health polices	• Particularly good • Good annual Performance evaluation of health professionals, Mayors, and health administrators
Qualified Health Professionals	• The ratio of one doctor to 8,000 patient is too high. • The ratio of one nurse to 1,420 is too high. • Provide incentive to discourage brain drain of qualified health professionals	• Need improvement • Effective in urban regions
Health Information Technology System	• Investment in health information system • Developed research skills of its health workforce. • Train more Rwanda health professionals on how to information technology and data management	• Currently effective but need incremental training of health workforce workers

(*Continued*)

Table 3 (*Continued*)

Assessment Factors	Implementation Action	Effective or Not Effective
Health Financing and Budget	• 6.41 % of GDP budget is still below the 15% of GDP recommended • Stop depending too much on foreign donors • Rwanda should their funding for health	• Currently effective but need to be less dependent on foreign donors overall
Health Quality	• Increase in life expectancy. • Health facilities accreditation • Performance-based financings • Integrative supportive supervision • Adoption of accreditation standards • Training accreditation surveyors and felicitators	• Currently effective
Health Administration	• Decentralized system • National referral hospitals • Intermediary level • Peripheral levels	• More effective in the urban than rural regions
Health Insurance	• Community-based health insurance • Universal Health Care	• More effective in the urban than rural regions
Water and sanitation	• 57% of the population have access safe drinking water • 74% of the poorest households have toilets • 1.96% of the citizens engaging in open defecation	• More effective in the urban than rural regions

Conclusion

The chapter has examined the health policies that the Republic of Rwanda had adopted since 1994 in order to increase access sufficiently and effectively to healthcare services for all its citizens by removing financial predicaments. The chapter fills the gap in the literature by providing several evidence on how political commitment, ethical and servant leadership commitments and equity driven policies could be effective mechanisms for achieving better healthcare services for all the people in Rwanda.

There is no doubt that affordable healthcare system is human right. The community-based insurance and universal healthcare policies enacted in Rwanda are commendable initiatives. The government has accomplished significant improvement in many key areas. The enactment and implementation of both community-based insurance and universal healthcare are good schemes that have contributed to the nation's higher life expectancy in the past decades. The factors that have contributed to the success of the adopted two schemes are the ability of the government to extend the coverage in both urban and rural regions of the nation, as well as healthcare service quality.

The evidence provided in this chapter shows that investment in information technology system is essential for evaluating and refining public policies effectively. Other Africa's low-income nations that are serious about their sustainable health development and the right attainment to an affordable healthcare system for their citizens should adopt the same model. On the one hand, appropriate national policies and professionally managed institutions are essential mechanisms to accomplish good economic development. The adoption of sustainable policies are factors in reducing unemployment and poverty in most African countries by 2040. Rwanda's political commitment to healthcare has tremendously increased life expectancy for both women and men in the country.

The analysis in this chapter reveals that strong ethical leaders, appropriate public and private investment in the health sectors, and information technology system could be good strategies to accomplish universal health coverage. Furthermore, equity-driven economic development policies and the appropriate use of foreign aid to invest in local capacity building could help other African nations just as it did in Rwanda to accomplish greater healthcare system. There is also the need to realize that strong leadership and political commitment are central to effective universal healthcare. Healthcare policies are designed to provide solutions to current challenges in the health delivery system.

In addition, the analysis also reveals that the mechanism needs to uplift the healthcare services in the country. It requires appropriate healthcare professionals, data indicators, education and training of more healthcare workforce, and the use of comparative strategic benchmarks. Furthermore, the health initiatives are required to improve patient's health services which include improving communication and the use of enhanced information technology system.

The nation's Food and Drug Administration officers should effectively engage in training doctors, nurses, and midwives on how to detect and monitor inappropriate dispensing of fake drugs in both the pharmaceutical stores and hospitals. The quality and safety of the country's healthcare delivery system should be a priority for all people, healthcare professionals, financing priority, and performance management systems employed in the nation for the Rwanda health policy goals to be accomplished.

References

Alluri R. M. (2009). The role of tourism in post-conflict peacebuilding in Rwanda. https://www.files.ethz.ch/isn/111583/wp2_2009.pdf. Accessed December 27, 2022.
Booth D., and Golooba-Mutebi F. (2012). Developmental patrimonialism? The case of Rwanda. *African Affairs London*, 111(444): 379–403.

Chemouni B. (2018). The political path to universal health coverage: Power, ideas, and community-based health insurance in Rwanda. *World Development*, 106: 87–98.

Condo J., Uwaizihiwe J. P., and Nasazimana S. (2020). Learn from Rwanda's success in tracking COVID-19. *Nature*, 581: 384–389. DOI: 10.1038/d41586-020-01563-7.

Cunningham C., Henderson J., Niccols A., Dobbins M., Sword W., Chen Y. et al. (2012). Preferences for evidence-based practice dissemination in addiction agencies serving women: A discrete-choice conjoint experiment. *Addiction*, 107: 1512–1524.

Cunningham F. C., Ramuthgala G., Pumb J., Georgious A., Westrook J. L., Braitwaiste J., (2012). Health professional networks as a vector for improving healthcare quality and safety: A systematic review. *British Medical Journal Quality Safety*, 21(3): 239–249.

De Baets A. (2015). Post-conflict historical education moratoria: A balance. *World Studies in Education*, 16(1): 15–37.

Development Initiates (2013). Instatement to end poverty. United Kingdom: Development Initiatives, 254–255 and 278–279. (2013). United.

Dibie R. (2022). Healthcare Policy and Administration in Nigeria." *The Journal of African Policy Studies*. 28(1): 101–139.

Expert Financial (2022). Overview of Healthcare in Rwanda. https://expatfinancial.com/healthcare-information-by-region/african-healthcare-system/rwanda-healthcare-system/. Accessed January 3, 2023.

Farmer P. F., Nutt C. T., Wagner C. M., Sekabaraga C. et al. (2013). Reduced premature mortality in Rwanda: lessons from success. *BMJ* 346: f65 doi: 10.1136/bmj.f65.

Gatehouse G. (2014). Patrick Karegeya: Mysterious death of a Rwandan exile. In BBC News March 26, 2014. http://www.bbc.com/news/world-. Accessed December 28, 2022.

Government of Rwanda (2022). Health development initiative: Annual report. https://hdirwanda.org/wp-content/uploads/2021/04/2022-Annual-Report_Final-Compressed.pdf. Accessed September 14, 2024.

Guichaoua A. (2020). Counting the Rwandan victims of war and genocide: Concluding reflections. *Journal of Genocide Research*, 22(1): 125–141.

Hintjens H. M. (2001). When identity becomes a knife, Reflecting on the genocide in Rwanda. *Ethnicities*, 1(1): 25–55.

History.com Editors (2009). Tutsi in Rwanda. https://www.history.com/topics/africa/rwandan-genocide. Accessed September 27, 2023.

Historyworld (2022). History of Rwanda. https://www.historyworld.net/history/Rwanda/769. Accessed November 9, 2024.

Iyer H. S., Chukwuma A., Mugunga J. C., Manzi A., Ndayizigiye M., and Anand S. (2018). Comparison of health achievements in Rwanda and Burundi. *Health and Human Right Journal*, 20(1): 199–211.

Jefremovas V. (1995). Acts of human kindness: Tutsi, utu and the genocide. *Issue: A Journal of Opinion*, 23(2): 28–31.

Karim N., Jing L., Lee J. A., Kharel R., Uwamahoro D., Nahayo E., Lubetkin D., Clancy C. M., Biramahire J., Aluisio A. R., Ndebwanimana V., and Clancy C. (2021). Lesson learned from Rwanda: Innovative strategies for prevention and containment of Covid-19. *Annals of Global Health*, 87(1): 23, 1–9.

Lemarchand, R. (2024, May 7). History of Rwanda. Encyclopedia Britannica. https://www.britannica.com/topic/history-of-Rwanda. Accessed September 14, 2024.

Lordos A., Ioannou M., Rutembesa E., Christoforou S., Anastasiou E., Björgvinsson T. (2021). Societal healing in Rwanda: toward a multisystemic framework for mental health, social cohesion, and sustainable livelihoods among survivors and perpetrators of the genocide against the Tutsi. *Health Human Rights*, 23(1): 105–118.

Mamdani M. (2002). *When Victims Become Killers: Colonialism, Nativism, and the Genocide in Rwanda*. Princeton, N.J.: Princeton University.

Maron J. (1994). What led to the genocide against the Tutsi in Rwanda? https://humanrights.ca/story/what-led-genocide-against-tutsi-rwanda. Accessed September 27, 2023.
Mason E. (2020). Universal health coverage: How Rwanda is moving forward with healthcare for all. https://www.innovationsinhealthcare.org/universal-health-coverage-how-rwanda-is-moving-forward-with-healthcare-for-all/. Accessed January 4, 2023.
Matfess H. (2015). Rwanda and Ethiopia: Developmental authoritarianism and the new politics of African strong men. *African Studies Review*, 58(2): 181–204.
Melvern L. (2004). *Conspiracy to Murder: The Rwandan Genocide*. London and New York, NY: Verso. ISBN 978-1-85984-588-2.
Melvern L. (2000). (8, illustrated, reprint ed.). London United Kingdom: Zed Books.
Ministry of Health Rwanda (2016). Rwanda Health Resource Tracker 2015–2016. https://www.moh.gov.rw/fileadmin/user_upload/Moh/Publications/Reports/HRTT_Report.pdf. Accessed November 10, 2024.
Ministry of Health Rwanda (2017). Health Performance Report 2017–2019. https://www.moh.gov.rw/fileadmin/user_upload/Moh/Publications/Reports/FINAL_Annual_Report_2017-2019_02062020.pdf.
Ndagijimana D., Mureithi C., and Njau-Ngomi N. (2019). Quality and safety management of healthcare services delivery among public hospitals in Rwanda: A cross-sectoral survey. *International Journal of Translational Medical Research and Public Health*, 3(2): 95–106.
Newbury C. (1995). Ethnicity and the politics of history in Rwanda. *Africa Today*, 45(1): 7–24.
Nshimyiryo A., Kirk C. M., Sauer S. M., Ntawuyirusha E., Muhire A., Sayinzoga F., Hedt-Gauthier B. (2020). Health management information system (HMIS) data verification: A case study in four districts in Rwanda. *PLoS One*, 15(7):e0235823.
Nyandekwe M., Nzayirambaho M., and Baptiste-Kakoma J. (2020). Universal health insurance in Rwanda: Major challenges and solutions for financial sustainability case study of Rwanda community-based health insurance part 1. *Pan-African Medical Journal*, 37(55): 1–37.
Overseas Development Institute (2011). *Rwanda's Progress in Health: Leadership, Performance, and Insurance*. Westminster, London United Kingdom: ODI Publications.
Overview of the Health System in Rwanda (2020). https://dhsprogram.com/pubs/pdf/spa3/02chapter2.pdf. Accessed January 4, 2023.
Republic of Rwanda, Ministry of Health (2018). Fourth Rwanda Sector Strategic Plan July 2018–June 2014. https//npngti.com/wp-content/uploads/2018/06/Rwanda_Not-Health-Sector-Plan_2018-2024.pdf. Accessed January 7, 2023.
Republic of Rwanda Government. Ministry of Health Report (2017–2019). *Rwanda Health Sector Performance Report*. Kigali: Government Press.
Republic of Rwanda, Ministry of Health (2015). Health Sector Policy. REPUBLIC OF RWANDA (moh.gov.rw). Accessed November 9, 2022.
Republic of Rwanda Government (1997a). *Ministry of Health Report*. Government Press Kigali.
Republic of Rwanda Government (1997b). *Ministry of Health Report*. Government Press Kigali.
Republic of Rwanda Government (2001). *Ministry of Health 1995–2001 Report*. Government Press Kigali.
Republic of Rwanda Government (2005). Rwanda's Health Sector Policy. https://www.uhc2030.org/fileadmin/uploads/ihp/Documents/Country_Pages/Rwanda/HealthSectorPolicy.pdf. Accessed January 4, 2023.
Republic of Rwanda Government (2008). National Community Health Policy. https://www.Advancingpartners.org/sites/default/files/projects/policies/chp_rwanda_2008.pdf. Accessed January 3, 2023.
Rwanda History (2009). https://www.africa.upenn.edu/NEH/rwhistory.htm. Accessed December 28, 2022.
Rwanda History (2022). Histiryworld. http://www.historyworld.net/wrldhis/plaintexthistories.asp?historyid=ad24#ixzz7oyC4iwEX. Accessed December 30, 2022.

Rwanda Social Security Board (2018). *Community Base Health Insurance. Fiscal Year 2016–2017 Annual Report.* Kigali, Rwanda. Government Press.

Republic of Rwanda, Ministry of Health Report (2019). Rwanda Health Sector Performance Report 2019–2020. https://www.moh.gov.rw/fileadmin/user_upload/Moh/Publications/Reports/Health_sector_performance_Report_FY_2019-2020.pdf. Accessed September 14, 2024.

Ryamukuru D., Mukantwari J., Munyaneza E., Twahirwa T. S., Bagweneza V., Nzamukosaha A., Musengamna V., Nyirasebura D., and Omondi L. (2022). *Rwanda Journal of Medical Sciences*, 5(2), 233–245.

Rwanda Health Management Information System Manual (2013). https://msh.org/wp-content/uploads/2014/12/ihssp_techbr2_final_ webv.pdf. Accessed November 9, 2024.

Sanogo T. (2019). Does fiscal decentralization enhance citizens' access to public services and reduce poverty? Evidence from Côte d'Ivoire municipalities in a conflict setting, *World Development*, 113(1): 204–221.

Sanogo N. A., Fantaye A. W., Yaya S., (2019). Universial health coverage and facilitation of euitable access to care in Africa. *Front Public Health*, 7(102): 1–17.

Sayinzoga F., Bijlmakers L. (2016). Drivers of Improved health sector performance in Rwanda: A qualitative view from within. *BMC Health Services Research*, 16(123).

Sullivan R. (1994). "Juvenal Habyarimana, 57, Ruled Rwanda for 21 Years". *The New York Times.* ISSN 0362-4331. Retrieved February 19, 2020.

The DHS Program (1997). Overview of the health system in Rwanda. https://dhsprogram.com/pubs/pdf/spa3/02chapter2.pdf. Accessed September 26, 2023.

Turshen M. and Twagiramariya C. (1998). 'Favors' to give and 'Consenting' victims: The sexual politics of survival in Rwanda, in *What Women Do in Wartime: Gender and Conflict in Africa 101*, Meredith Turshen & Clotilde Twagiramariya eds., Zed Books.

Twagilimana A. (2007). *Historical Dictionary of Rwanda.* Metuchen, N.J.: Scarecrow Press, Page xliii.

Umuhoza S. M., Musange S., Nyandwi A., Gatome-Munyua A., Mumararungu A., and Hitimana R. (2022). Strengths and weaknesses of strategic health purchasing for universal health coverage in Rwanda. *Health System Reform*, 8(2): 1–59.

United States Agency for International Development (1996). Rebuilding postwar Rwanda: The role of the international community. https://www.oecd.org/derec/unitedstates/5018 94 61. Accessed September 26, 2023.

United Nations Children's Fund (UNICEF) (2022a). Health Budget Brief: Investing in Children's Health in Rwanda. https://www.unicef.org/esa/media/10131/file/UNICEF-Rwanda-2021-2022-Health-Budget-Brief.pdf. Accessed January 7, 2023.

United Nations Children's Fund (UNICEF) (2022b). Rwanda Water, Sanitation and Hygiene. https://www.unicef.org/rwanda/water-sanitation-and-hygiene. Accessed January 13, 2023.

UNICEF (2019). UNICEF Rwanda Ebola Situation Report. September 20, 2019. https://www.unicef.org/rwanda/sites/unicef.org.rwanda/files/2019-09/Ebola-sitRep-UNICEP-Rwanda-Sept-2019.pdf. Accessed January 16, 2023.

UNICEF (2019). Rwanda Country Office Annual Report. https://www.unicef.org/reports/country-regional-divisional-annual-reports-2019/Rwanda. Accessed November 10, 2024.

UNICEF (2020). UNICEF Situation Reports on COVID-19 in Rwanda. https://www.Unicef.org/rwanda/reports/2020-unicef-situation-reports-covid-19-rwanda. Accessed September 10, 2024.

UNICEF (2022a). Annual Report. https://www.unicef.org/reports/unicef-annual-report-2022. Accessed November 10, 2024.

UNICEF (2022b). Global Annual Results Reports. https://www.unicef.org/reports/global-annual-results-2022. Accessed November 10, 2024.

United Nations Human Development Programme (2020). National Human Development Report 2020: Rwanda. https://hdr.undp.org/content/national-human-development-report-2020-rwanda#:~:text=The%20Report%20is%20based%20on,must%20be%20tailored%20to%20citizens'. Accessed November 10, 2024.

Uvin P. (1995). Fighting hunger at the grassroots: Paths to scaling up. *World Development*, 23(6), 927–939.

Uvin P. (1999a). Ethnicity and power in Burundi and Rwanda: Different paths to mass violence. *Comparative Politics*, 31(3): 253–271.

Uvin P. (1999b). Development aid and structural violence: The case of Rwanda. *Development Journal* 42(3): 49–56.

Uwayezu M. G., Nikuze B., Fitch M. L. (2020). A focus on cancer care and the nursing role in Rwanda. *Can Oncal Nursing Journal*, 30(3): 223–226.

Vansina, J. (2004). *Antecedents to Modern Rwanda: The Nyiginya Kingdom*. Wisconsin: The University of Wisconsin Press. pp. 18–24.

Woldemichael A., Takian A., Akbari Sari A., Olyaeemanesh A. (2019). Inequalities in healthcare resources and outcomes threatening sustainable health development in Ethiopia: panel data analysis. *BMJ Open*. 9(1):e022923. DOI: 10.1136/bmjopen-2018-022923.

World Bank Group (2022a). The World Bank in Rwanda. https://www.worldbank.org/en/country/rwanda. Accessed September 14, 2024.

World Bank Indicators (2022b). World Development Indicators. https://databank.worldbank.org/source/world-development-indicators. Accessed November 10, 2024.

World Bank Trading Economics Report (2022). Rwanda, people at least basic sanitation. https://tradingeconomics.com/rwanda/people-using-basic-sanitation-services-urban-percent-of-urban-population-wb-data.html.

World Data Atlas (2020). Rwanda – Births attended by skilled health staff as a share of total number of births. https://knoema.com/atlas/Rwanda/topics/Health/Health-Service-Coverage/irths-attended-by-skilled-health-staff.

World Health Organization (2020). COVID-19 in Rwanda: A country response. July 20, 2020. https: www.who.int/nees/item/24-07-2019-who-applauds-rwanda-s-ebola-preparedness-efforts. Accessed January 16, 2023.

World Health Organization (2020). WHO's results in Africa July 2020 – June 2021. https://www.afro.who.int/sites/default/files/2021-08/016_WHO-AFRO_RD-Report-20-21_Ex-Summary_EN_0.pdf. Accessed November 10, 2024.

Yarlagadda S. (2022). Growth from Genocide: The stiry of Rwanda's healthcare system. https://hir.harvard.edu/growth-from-genocide-the-story-of-rwandas-healthcare-system/. Accessed September 26, 2023.

Chapter Thirteen

SIERRA LEONE HEALTHCARE SYSTEM AND SERVICES

Muriel Harris, Leonda Richardson, and Imisha Gurung

Introduction

The World Health Organization (WHO 2020) characterizes health equity as the absence of unfair and avoidable or remediable differences in health status among groups of people. This can be achieved when those with lower socioeconomic status do not face financial barriers or other obstructions such as language, culture, stigma, distance, and an overall dearth of resources (Orach & Garimoi 2009). People living in poverty are at a greater risk of death than their wealthier counterparts, largely because they lack access to public health initiatives like clean water, sanitation, food security, education, and economic opportunities (Peters et al. 2008). Disease-specific burdens also differ by socioeconomic status as people living in poverty are more likely to die from tuberculosis than those who have higher incomes.

The purpose of this chapter is to inform the readers about the challenges facing Sierra Leone's healthcare system. The chapter examines how the nation is characterized by a severe shortage of healthcare workers and providers in clinical medicine, nursing practice, general practice, and family medicine. It argues that health equity is achieved when everyone in Sierra Leone has access to the same level of healthcare. The chapter also discusses the health trends and debates over the last decade in Sierra Leone. It covers increasing the importance of healthcare systems to meet the population's needs to achieve health equity in the country. According to the World Bank (2019), Sierra Leone has one of the world's lowest life expectancies of 54.8 years, owing to high rates of infectious diseases such as malaria, tuberculosis, and HIV/AIDS. Malaria has historically been endemic in the country, accounting for approximately 40% of hospitalizations of adults and children, while a high prevalence of late diagnosis and undiagnosed tuberculosis cases has further strained the country's healthcare sector. Furthermore, women have been exposed to more health challenges, such as their efforts as primary caregivers during the Ebola pandemic, resulting in higher infections. Maternal and child mortality remain the highest in the world. Additionally, the country's mental healthcare services and rehabilitation are also underdeveloped, owing to the pressure to develop high quality physiological healthcare facilities but also the limited concern for the mental health needs of the society issues that require professional intervention, with many former child soldiers in the civil war turning to drugs and substance abuse as coping mechanisms for their traumatic experiences. The analysis conducted reveals that there is also a shortage of finance and human resources needed to maintain and run health facilities with a shortage of personnel numbers and as low as one doctor per 1,000 population in the nation (Rowe et al. 2018, Bitton, et al. 2019, Kaye et al. 2020). In addition, there are not enough medical professionals who are willing to work in rural areas (Bitton et al. 2019). The chapter also explores how the application and domains of healthcare are addressed in the country with respect to air quality, food safety, water disposal, occupational health, and sustained injuries of citizens and residents of the nation. One country in Sub-Sahara Africa facing tremendous healthcare system challenges is Sierra Leone. West Africa. Finally, some policy recommendations are provided.

Health Administration in Sierra Leone

The Sierra Leonean healthcare system which is managed by the Ministry of Health and Sanitation has been heavily understaffed and afflicted by a lack of medical equipment, poor accessibility to healthcare, and a healthcare personnel ratio falling below the Sub-Saharan average ratio of two workers per 10,000 people (Samura 2016; McPake, Dayal, and Herbst 2019; Wurie, Samai & Witter 2016; Woodward et al. 2018). The country has a decentralized two-tier healthcare structure that consists of the *peripheral*, and the *secondary* care levels (Caviglia et al. 2021; James et al. 2020; Sanny 2020; Vernooij, Koker & Street 2021).

The peripheral healthcare level consists of community health programs and dispensaries.

The peripheral healthcare level function as the primary source of public healthcare is further classified into three types of facilities, (i) the maternal and child healthcare health centers that aim to reach smaller communities of 400–2000 people; (ii) the community health posts; and (iii) the community health centers. Sierra Leone's universal healthcare policy aims to establish at least 149 health centers in each of the locations that constitute the 14 districts in the country (Gabani et al. 2024; Vaughan et al. 2015; Vernooij, Koker & Street 2021). Further, the peripheral healthcare level is subdivided into maternal and child health posts serving a population of 500–5000, Community Health Posts serving a population of 5000–10,000 staffed by State-Enrolled Community Health Nurses (SECHNs), and Community Health Centers (CHCs) at chiefdom level serving a population of 10,000–30,000 (Gabani et al. 2024; Robinson 2019).

The *secondary healthcare level* is also divided into 13 districts, each with a health management team that plans and trains communities while each district has about 45 peripheral care units with a minimum target of at least 100 healthcare specialists in each district (Gabani et al. 2024; Vaughan et al. 2015). In addition, Sierra Leone has 21 districts, and three referral hospitals that serve a population of 7.6 million citizens. While the *secondary level* includes regional-level and district-level hospitals, the *tertiary level* includes Connaught Hospital, Ola During Children Hospital, and Princess Christian Maternity Hospital (Gabani et al. 2024; Koka et al. 2016). There are also 45 private sector clinics and 27 private hospitals, mostly in the Freetown area. Some of the private health facilities are either for-profit or non-profit that are operated by faith-based organizations in Sierra Leone (Gabani et al. 2024; Robinson 2019).

Public–private collaborations have been vital in increasing healthcare training that has gradually increased healthcare awareness among the country's citizens (Hemingway et al. 2021; Kumar, Mostafa & Ramaswamy 2018). About 90% of medical care in Sierra Leone is provided through the assistance of foreign aid primarily through the United Kingdom and the United States government funding (Robinson 2019; WHO 2018), as well as, through nongovernmental organizations (NGOs), and nonprofit healthcare organizations (Jofre-Bonet & Kamara 2018; Kelly, Weiser & Tsai 2016). International NGOs such as UNICEF have been at the forefront of developing quality maternal healthcare in Sierra Leone. UNICEF funds the Sierra Leone National Reproductive, Maternal, Neonatal, Child, and Adolescent Health (RMNCAH) framework that reduced maternal and neonatal mortality by 90% between 2017 and 2021. The program involved funding to increase the number of special infant care units, and training programs targeting over 2,500 healthcare workers (including community health volunteers, traditional, public, and private healthcare) of levels I, II, and III natal, and infant care. Collaborative efforts have been adopted in developing Village Development Committees (VDCs) that aim to increase knowledge dissemination (Dreyfus et al. 2018) while also encouraging public participation in expressing their views, creating demand, and monitoring healthcare quality (Hemingway et al. 2021; James & Bah 2014; Vernooij, Koker & Street 2021).

Healthcare Challenges in Sierra Leone

In terms of service utilization, the most rapid increase in health expenditure in Sub-Saharan Africa was on services for children under five years old, which increased by 84.3% from 2000 to 2008 (Yunus, Hairi & Choo 2019). This might have been a result of government policies designed to ensure equity in access to healthcare and an effort to achieve Millennium Development Goal 4, which aims to reduce child mortality in developing countries (Kanu et al. 2014; Bloom et al. 2015; Strasser et al. 2016). However, there was a lack of resources prioritized toward other age groups such as the elderly, who have higher rates of morbidity and mortality due to chronic conditions (Adua et al. 2017; Tang et al. 2004). Often, older patients present with multiple issues in addition to their age-related diseases, which means that providers must address multiple complaints simultaneously, something that might be challenging, especially if they are inadequately trained or experience equipment/supply shortages (Adua et al. 2017; Narayan et al. 2018). Providing preventative care services (e.g., nutrition support and vaccinations) is also more complicated since most seniors live at home, where managing access to services can pose logistical challenges (Ansumana et al. 2020; Yunus, Hairi, & Choo, 2019). The issue of service delivery for this patient population is the challenge of defining what constitutes quality care for older persons (Bloom et al. 2015; Oleribeet et al. 2019; Pieterse 2016).

Utilization of healthcare services in Sierra Leone's societies is influenced by gender with women of lower socioeconomic status having less access to medical care than men of the same age and income level (Fang et al. 2016; Hoque 2016). Nonetheless, healthcare utilization is usually lower among men than women in Sierra Leone, a factor attributed to masculine norms that encourage men to show toughness, pain endurance, minimal contact, and negative attitudes toward professional healthcare services (Novak et al. 2019). In addition, gendered power dynamics in most households have left men controlling the family's healthcare services utilization, leading to more women being affected by the men's reluctance to access healthcare services (Harris et al. 2020; Novak et al. 2019). In addition, the disparity in utilization between men and women may result from factors that include provider's attitudes, human resource constraints due to a preference for males as health workers, and cultural barriers which prevent women from accessing prenatal care or having complete control over decisions surrounding their pregnancies (Adjiwanou, Bougma & LeGrand 2018; Oloyede 2017). This is particularly important because antenatal care has been shown to reduce mortality rates among mothers and children (Gajovic et al. 2019; Phull et al. 2021).

Gender norms also result in differences in health-seeking behavior: for example, male children receive better treatment during illness than female children (Fang et al. 2016), while women are less likely to seek proper medical care for symptoms such as abdominal pain (Carlson-March et al. 2022; James et al. 2018). Further, women's traditional gender roles give them more responsibilities than men within the family because they take care of children, the elderly, sick and disabled household members, and members of their families making it difficult to seek proper medical care (Gajovic et al. 2019; Jalloh et al., 2018). Gender inequality in Sierra Leone significantly influences different households' healthcare utilization (Cornish 2019). Delays in seeking healthcare services among men tend to increase their chances of developing more severe complications and combined with higher income levels among men, such factors make it more likely that men will receive higher in-patient admission rates than women for similar healthcare services (Harris et al. 2020; Percival et al. 2018). Factors such as women's economic empowerment and a free government sponsored healthcare program have increased healthcare access among women. However, in many Sierra Leonean societies, there is a belief that pregnancy and childbirth are typical conditions, preferring traditional health methods over any medical professional, and pregnant women are more likely to seek care from a traditional birth attendant than healthcare workers (Cornish et al. 2021 Hoque 2016; James et al. 2018). This is also true of other conditions and was evident during the Ebola epidemic when many sought traditional health methods initially.

There have been challenges in preserving positive attitudes toward healthcare workers in many African countries due to higher reported instances of unethical and unprofessional behavior such as discriminatory behavior toward patients (Elston et al. 2020; Woodward et al. 2018; Wurie, Samai & Witter 2016). As a result, rural areas experience the brunt of poor service delivery lowering the rating of healthcare practitioners (Johnson et al. 2020). Further, policies on rotation among healthcare workers between urban and rural areas are poorly followed with over 70% of the workforce serving mostly in urban areas (Wurie, Samai & Witter 2016 Johnson et al. 2020). People living in urban areas have better access to medical supplies and medical professionals than those in rural areas (Nathaniel-Wurie et al. 2012; Theuring, Koroma & Harms 2018). By 2017, the number of healthcare providers had risen to

9,000 although most of the increase consisted of community health volunteers (Barr et al. 2019; Goodyear-Smith et al. 2019; Pieterse & Lodge 2015). Seventy percent of the healthcare workers serve the urban areas while only 30% are in rural regions which make up 63% of the population (Hopwood et al. 2021; McPake, Dayal & Herbst 2019; Witter et al. 2018). With most healthcare workers concentrated in urban regions, there is an increased reliance on traditional healthcare among rural communities over an extended period (Jofre-Bonet & Kamara 2018; Kelly, Weiser & Tsai 2016).

The government's responsibility to protect and advance the interests of society includes the delivery of highquality healthcare. The government of Sierra Leone has taken multiple steps in enabling the delivery of healthcare services across the country (Government of Sierra Leone 2020; Johnson et al. 2021), most notably the Free Health Care Initiative (FHCI) in 2010 (Hopwood et al. 2021; Johnson et al. 2021, McPake, Dayal & Herbst 2019). FHCI was primarily developed to help increase the utilization of mainstream healthcare services while also bridging the effects of wealth inequality in access to healthcare for prenatal care and for children under five years (James & Bah 2014; Kamara et al. 2017; Sanny, 2020; Vernooij, Koker & Street 2021). The current model, however, favors the wealthy, highly educated, and people living in urban areas (Idriss et al. 2020; Jalloh et al. 2019; Kanu 2019).

In 2014, the government launched the Health Sector Recovery Plan 2015–2020 to improve universal access to quality and affordable healthcare. It launched the National Emergency Medical Service (NEMS) in 2019, aimed at facilitating emergency ambulance services designed to operate in out-of-hospital services, including accidents and childbirth (Caviglia et al. 2021; Li 2020). NEMS enabled better use of ambulances donated during the Ebola pandemic while improving the scope and breadth of healthcare services in the country (Li 2020). Jalloh et al. (2019) study exploring the impact of FHCI on maternal healthcare indicated a greater than 24% increase in antenatal care (ANC), postnatal care (PNC), and institutional delivery rates between 2008 and 2013. The government has also been involved in multiple international initiatives that aim to improve healthcare facilitation, including the updating of the 1978 Alma-Ata Declaration to the Astana Declaration of 2018 (Goodyear-Smith et al. 2019), and pledging to implement the sustainable development goals of 2014 (Ensor, Lievens & Naylor 2008; Goodyear-Smith et al. 2019; Pieterse & Lodge 2015). In adopting the Astana Declaration of 2018, Sierra Leone has been developing a more robust framework for primary healthcare (PHC) through initiatives such as community-based healthcare services and health promotion (Kahl 2018; McPake, Dayal & Herbst 2019) targeting key healthcare components such as preventive healthcare, pain management, rehabilitative, and palliative care (Ensor, Lievens & Naylor 2008; James et al. 2020; McPake, Dayal & Herbst 2019; Sanny 2020).

Providing affordable, accessible, and sustainable healthcare delivery to their citizens is best achieved through ensuring that there are enough human resources to train the people, financial allocation for public health services, maintaining quality equipment within public hospitals, and ensuring low-cost pharmaceuticals are readily available is a responsibility of governments (Bertone et al. 2018; Jofre-Bonet & Kamara 2018; Tsawe & Susuman 2020; Valtorta et al. 2018).

In addition, a lack of trust has had a negative influence on perceptions of the healthcare system. The 2014 Ebola outbreak in Sierra Leone with all 14 medical districts affected and a total of 14,122 reported cases and 3,955 deaths, was attributed to a weak health system and a lack of adequate infection control (IPC) (Jofre-Bonet & Kamara 2018; Sylvester et al. 2017, Theuring, Koroma & Harms 2018).

Data Analysis and Discussion

The purpose of this study was to assess perceptions of the healthcare system in Freetown, Sierra Leone, from the perspectives of a cross-section of adult residents. This initial study was conducted between summer of 2021 and 2023 to assess healthcare utilization, their trust in the government and administration related to healthcare, skills, and competencies of healthcare providers, availability, and affordability of services. The study included age, marital status, and level of education as factors that might impact those perceptions. The research questions for this study were as follows:

Research question 1: To what degree do respondents relate the lack of trust in the healthcare services in the country to corruption and unethical behavior of political and administrative leaders?

Research question 2: To what extent do respondents relate the competencies and skills of providers with medical treatment outcomes?

Research question 3: How does age relate to one's marital status?

- *Research question* 3.1: To what extent is age related to perceptions of the availability of emergency services?
- *Research question* 3.2: To what extent is age related to perceptions of medical treatment outcomes?

Research question 4: How do the characteristics of healthcare centers and providers impact the overall rating of healthcare services?

Research question 5: How do age, marital status, level of education, and gender impact the perception of affordability of healthcare services,

- *Research question* 5.1: How do age, marital status, level of education, and gender impact perception of satisfaction with healthcare services?

The target population for this study was residents of Sierra Leone. This convenience sample included individuals over the age of 18 living on the west side of the city. It was conducted during the COVID-19 epidemic. A survey instrument employed for this study assessed perceptions of healthcare utilization, access, policies, and health administration in Sierra Leone. The 40-item survey consisted of five sections: Section A consisted of demographic questions such as age, gender, marital status, and level of education. Section B contained questions that asked about the healthcare experience and perception of participants. Section C pertained to the governments' role in the affordability of healthcare delivery in Sierra Leone, and Section D asked about the condition of government hospitals. Lastly, Section E assessed perceived barriers to high-quality healthcare in Sierra Leone. Sections B through E included Likert scale questions that measured the level of agreement 1—strongly disagree, 2—disagree, 3—neither 4—agree, 5—strongly agree. In the analysis, due to the small sample size of the study, these categories were collapsed into three measurement levels reflect, disagree, neutral, and agree. Surveys were distributed to individuals who were 18 years and older, who were invited to participate. To protect participant identity and ensure the confidentiality of any identifying information, participants were also instructed not to provide any identifying information, such as their name on the survey.

Frequency statistics were run for each question to identify any missing data, duplicate questions, and categories with low frequencies. The "prefer not to answer" category for gender only included one case and question 14 was a duplicate of question 13, therefore they were removed from the dataset. Additionally, question 12 had to be reverse coded due to the wording of the question. The data cleaning process also included recoding each question category for ease of analysis. Question two, which assessed for age, originally included five categories (18–21 = 1, 22–30 = 2, 31–40 = 3, 41–50 = 4, and 50 and older = 5), this was recoded into two age groups: youth (18–30 = 1) and adult (30 and older = 2). Marital status was recoded from single = 1, married = 2, divorced = 3, and other = 4 to married and other = 2; divorced and single remained the same. Educational attainment originally included less than secondary school = 1, secondary school/BECE/WASSCE = 2, national diploma or vocational school = 3, bachelors/HND = 4, experts = 5, and Ph.D. = 6. These categories were recoded as secondary school or less = 1 and more than secondary school = 2.

Likert scale categories containing low frequencies were also merged and recoded. Disagree and strongly disagree were merged and recoded as 1, strongly agree and agree were merged and recoded as 2, neutral remained coded as 3. The Likert type categories for 3 questions (16–18) were recoded. Strongly agree/agree as yes, strongly disagree/ disagree as no, and neutral remained its own category. Furthermore, question five, "utilization of care," that assessed the frequency of visits (1–2 times = 1, 3–4 times = 2, 5–6 times = 3, and over 7 times a year = 4) and was recoded into a dichotomous variable with a rating of 1 being 1–2 times a year and a rating of 2 being 3 or more times a year and renamed. Question six assessed the overall rating of hospitals and health centers with the following categories: excellent = 1, particularly good = 2, good = 3, fair = 4, and poor = 5. These categories were recoded and merged as follows: undesirable = 0 (fair and poor) and desirable = 1(excellent, particularly good, and good).

Given the nature of the instrument, the primary data analytic procedures consisted of cross-tabulations. Logistic regression, which included Cox and Snell R-square values, was conducted for certain dichotomous outcome variables to predict the probability of the outcome based on selected predictor variables, as well as multinomial logistic regression to predict the probability of category placement on a dependent variable based on multiple independent variables. The primary variables included in the analysis were age, perception of extremely high medical treatment outcomes, lack of trust in the healthcare system, and overall rating of hospitals or health centers. Of the respondents who reported their gender 56.5% ($n=35$) were male and 42% ($n=26$) were female; one respondent preferred not to report their gender. In this study, 58% (*n*=36) of respondents reported being single and 42% (*n*=26) reported being married or "other" (Table 1). Forty-three percent (*n*=27) of the sample were 18–30 years old, and 56.5 (*n*=35) were 31 or older. The highest level of education was a diploma or vocational school, 32.5% (*n*=20). This was followed by a bachelor's degree/HND degree, 26% (*n*=16), and secondary school, 24% (*n*=15). Eight percent obtained either a master's or less than a secondary level of education.

Table 1 Perceptions of Healthcare Services, and Facilities

Survey Items	Disagree (%)	Neutral (%)	Agree (%)
Availability of services			
Hospitals and health centers in my COUNTRY do NOT provide emergency services	18 (29.5)	16 (26.2)	27 (44.3)
The hospitals provide X-rays, MRIs, and other diagnostic tests	32 (51.6)	9 (14.5)	21 (33.9)
Quality of facilities			
Hospitals and health centers in my CITY have modern equipment	38 (61.3)	14 (22.6)	10 (16.1)
Many government hospitals' buildings are mostly dilapidated	10 (16.9)	9 (15.3)	40 (67.8)
Many government hospitals have modern buildings and wards are kept exceptionally clean	50 (80.6)	3 (4.8)	9 (14.5)
Hospitals and mental health centers in my COUNTRY have constant electricity	45 (72.6)	7 (11.3)	10 (16.1)
Condition/quality of facilities			
Particularly good competencies & skills of medical providers in my CITY hospital	21 (34.4)	19 (31.1)	21 (34.4)
Doctors and nurses in my CITY hospitals are caring & friendly to their patients	21(33.9)	18 (29)	23 (37.1)
All doctors in the hospitals are specialists	44 (71)	7 (11.3)	11 (17.7)
Very few specialist doctors and hospitals in the country	5 (8.1)	0 (0)	57 (91.9)
Patient outcomes and trust			
Patients' medical treatment outcomes in hospitals in my COUNTRY are extremely high	17 (27.9)	8 (13.1)	36 (59)
Corruption and unethical behavior of political and administrative leaders	2 (3.3)	3 (4.9)	56 (91.8)
Lack of trust in the poor healthcare services in the country	4 (6.6)	3 (4.9)	54 (88.5)

Data were analyzed to assess the frequency distribution of each response category. The complete dataset consisted of 61–62 total responses for each item. The data show that individuals were more likely to report utilizing the healthcare services only 1 or 2 times per year and 90% of the respondents reported that the services were excellent, particularly. good, or particularly good. However, 41% of the respondents indicated that they could afford healthcare services and pay for their medication.

Descriptive analysis also provided data on the frequency of responses to questions selected for this study. Respondents provided responses to questions about the availability of services as well as the quality of the facilities and the medical personnel and their trust in the healthcare system. In this sample, almost 50% agreed that the country does not provide emergency services for its residents, and an equivalent number (50%) disagreed that it provides X-rays, MRIs, and other diagnostic tests. Many of the respondents reported on the poor condition of the hospitals (68%–80%), the lack of electricity (72%), and modern equipment (61%). Overall, respondents did not think the healthcare personnel were competent (34%) or caring toward their patients (34%). They (71%) believe that most of the doctors are specialists, however, they recognize that there are very few specialists and specialist hospitals in the country. They (88%) lack trust in the healthcare system and 92% reported that they recognize there is an elevated level of corruption and unethical behavior among political and administrative leaders. All these factors may lead to the perception among only 59% of respondents in this study who agreed that medical outcomes are extremely high. Almost 30% of respondents disagreed that medical outcomes were high.

The next section answers each of the research questions in turn.

Research question 1: To what degree do respondents relate the lack of trust in the healthcare services in the country to corruption and unethical behavior of political and administrative leaders?

Cross-tabulation shows that 85% of participants related their lack of trust in healthcare services to corruption and unethical behavior of political and administrative leaders as barriers to high quality healthcare (Table 2).

Furthermore, Chi-square tests show statistical significance at the $p < 0.05$ level (0.001), suggesting that respondents who agreed were 10.3 times more likely to relate corruption and unethical behavior of political and administrative leaders with a lack of trust in healthcare services than those who disagreed.

Table 2 Cross-tabulation of lack of trust in the healthcare services and corruption and unethical behavior

		Corruption and unethical behavior of political and administrative leaders			
		Disagree (%)	Neutral (%)	Agree (%)	Total
Lack of trust in the healthcare services in the country	Disagree	0	1 (1.7)	3 (5)	4 (6.7)
	Neutral	1 (1.7)	1 (1.7)	51 (85)	53 (88.4)
	Agree	1 (1.7)	1 (1.7)	1 (1.7)	3 (5.1)
Total		2 (3.4)	3 (5.1)	55 (91.7)	60 (100)

Research question 2: To what extent do respondents relate the competencies and skills of providers with medical treatment outcomes?

Twenty-eight percent of respondents linked extremely high medical treatment outcomes for hospitals in their country to providers having exceptionally good competencies and skills in their city. Respondents who agreed were 12.6 times and significantly ($p = 0.029$) more likely to relate competencies and stills of providers with medical outcomes (Table 3).

Given the distribution of the sample as well as the demographic distribution, of the population, age was used as the basis for understanding the difference in perceptions of youth compared with older adults.

Research question 3: How does age relate to one's marital status?

Regarding age and marital status respondents who identified as youth were more likely to report being single (37%), compared to those of age 31 and older (36%) that reported being married or "other."

Research question 3.1: To what extent is age related to one's perception of the availability of emergency services.

Age played a role in the perception of the availability of emergency services in this study. This is because (44% of the respondents indicated that the hospitals and health centers do not provide emergency. On the other hand, 26% of the respondents remained neutral. Adults of age 31 and over were more likely to believe that emergency services are provided. In this study, 21% of youth and 23% of older respondents agreed that emergency services are not provided while among the older respondents, almost one-third (24.5%) also disagreed (Table 4). The younger adults were also eight times more likely ($p = 0.019$) to believe that the country does not provide emergency services.

Research question 3.2: To what extent is age related to the perception of medical treatment outcomes?

Age played a role in the perception of medical treatment outcomes in this study. In a crosstabulation showing the perception of extremely high medical treatment outcomes in hospitals by age, fewer youth (18%) than adults (41%) agreed that patients' medical treatment outcomes in hospitals are extremely high. There was a significant difference ($p = 0.012$) in perception between youth and older adults.

Research question 4: How do the characteristics of healthcare centers and providers impact the overall rating of healthcare services?

Table 3 Cross-tabulation of Competencies and Skills of Providers and Medical Treatment Outcomes

		Competencies & skills of medical providers in my city hospital are particularly good		
		Disagree (%)	Neutral (%)	Agree (%)
Patients' medical treatment outcomes in hospitals in my country are extremely high	Disagree	6 (10)	7 (11.7)	4 (6.7)
	Neutral	6 (10)	2 (3.3)	0 (0)
	Agree	9 (15)	9 (15)	17 (28.3)
Total		21 (35)	18 (30)	21 (35)

Table 4 Cross-tabulation: Age and LOA Hospitals and Health Centers in Sierra Leone do NOT Provide Emergency Services

		Hospitals and health centers in my country do NOT provide emergency services		
		Disagree (%)	Neutral (%)	Agree (%)
Age	Youth: 18–30	3 (4.9)	10 (16.4)	13 (21.3)
	Adult: 31 and above	15 (24.6)	6 (9.8)	14 (23)
Total		18 (29.5)	16 (26.2)	27 (44.3)

Binary logistic regression was used for the analysis of overall rating, as the outcome variable and characteristics related to healthcare providers and health centers as predictors. None of the variables entered in this model expressed statistical significance. The Cox and Snell R-square shows the amount of variance in the dependent variable because of the independent variable. Therefore, for block 1, we see that 2.8% of the variance in the overall rating of hospitals and health centers can be explained by provider characteristics, and 14% of the variance in overall rating is explained by health center characteristics.

Research question 5: How do age, marital status, level of education, and gender impact perception of affordability of healthcare services?

For the multinomial logistic regression analysis, statistical significance was set as $p < 0.05$. The reference category for each multiple regression analysis was "yes" and affordability of afford healthcare services was the outcome variable. Age and level of education yielded statistically significant predictions regarding the affordability of healthcare services. Assessing the Likelihood Ratio Tests, the level of education and age both have a statically significant impact on the level of agreement to affordability of services ($p = 0.068$, $p = 0.002$). Youth were 76% ($p = 0.015$) more likely to report a "neutral" level of agreement with the ability to afford healthcare services as opposed to reporting "yes" Furthermore those with a secondary level of education or less were 2% ($p = 0.049$) more likely to select a "neutral" level of agreement with ability to afford healthcare services.

Research question 5.1: How do age, marital status, level of education, and gender impact perceptions of satisfaction with healthcare services?

For the variable satisfaction with the type of healthcare services provided, the Likelihood Ratio Tests show that the only variable with a statistically significant impact on the level of satisfaction with healthcare services provided is the level of education ($p = 0.017$). Respondents with a secondary education or less were 2.4% ($p = 0.008$) more likely to report dissatisfaction with healthcare services provided than to report satisfaction with healthcare services provided.

Health equity is achieved when everyone has access to the same level of healthcare. Thus, global health debates have focused increasingly on the importance of healthcare systems to meet the population's needs to achieve health equity. This study highlights the importance of achieving health equity but importantly the factors that could contribute to that outcome. It showed that most participants related a lack of trust in the healthcare services to corruption and unethical behavior of political and administrative leaders as barriers to high-quality healthcare. The perception of unethical and corrupt behavior leading to mistrust illustrated in this study is consistent with existing literature (Sylvester et al. 2017; Theuring, Koroma & Harms 2018; Yendewa et al. 2018; Vernooij Koker & Street 2021) and with citizens' experience of challenges and questionable charges and bribery (Sanny 2020). Other factors such as favoritism and poor management of facilities may account for the findings in this study, similar to those described by Wurie, Samai and Witter (2016).

Overall, respondents in this study were less likely to relate high medical treatment outcomes to providers although almost one-third did agree that they have particularly good competencies and skills which is consistent with findings by Johnson et al. (2020) and identified competence as a factor in health outcomes. Even aside from competency less than a quarter, found personnel caring and friendly which may be reflected in the poor working conditions in the healthcare sector (Deck 2018; Johnson et al. 2020). In addition, all respondents reported that there are very few specialists in the system. The perception of the respondents is the poor condition of the healthcare system that most described as deplorable and lacking electricity, modern buildings, and basic cleanliness. They also reported a lack of facilities for X-rays, MRIs, and other diagnostic services.

This sample was from a predominantly urban sector of the country although many may have settled in the city following the war and although almost 50% of respondents said they could afford healthcare services and medication and yet those were younger and had a lower level of education (less than secondary school), were less likely to be able to afford healthcare or find it satisfactory.

It is conceivable that older adults (>31 years) are more aware of the healthcare services. Individuals over 31 years compared to respondents 18–30 years old, were more likely to believe that patients' medical treatment outcomes in hospitals are extremely high (41% vs 18%). This could be because respondents 31 and older have higher levels of education, increasing their ability to access higher quality healthcare. Educational attainment as a social determinant of health (SDoH) is connected to access, delivery, quality of care, and satisfaction with care. Treacy, Bolkan, and Sagbakken (2018) note that less than 40% of patients are usually satisfied with the overall treatment and care they receive at their hospital in Sierra Leone.

Conclusion

This sample provided a high overall rating for the healthcare system, but the current study identified factors that could be used as a guide and foundation for intervening to improve the healthcare system in Sierra Leone as well as for future research. This study found that individuals who have less education are more likely to be dissatisfied as well as not be able to afford healthcare. Individuals who were younger and single were also less likely to utilize healthcare, but they were also more pessimistic about treatment outcomes. Individuals in this study lacked trust in the healthcare system that they related to corruption and unethical behavior and experienced a system that was not caring or friendly with few competent and skilled personnel. The importance of policies that address a myriad of factors to improve healthcare perceptions and reality cannot be understated based on the findings of this study and others that have been previously published.

While policies to improve healthcare facilities and services as well as provide competent skilled health personnel, it is also important to recognize that the Ministry of Health and Sanitation is severely understaffed with the healthcare personnel ratio falling below the two per 10,000 population, coupled with a lack of medical equipment and poor accountability (Samura 2016, McPake, Dayal & Herbst 2019, Wurie, Samai, & Witter 2016, Woodward et al. 2018).

Recent efforts to improve access to healthcare as well as the training of health personnel should improve what has been a less than acceptable healthcare system in the country (World Bank 2020; World Health Organization 2020). Public–private collaborations have been vital in increasing healthcare training that has gradually increased healthcare awareness among the country's citizens (Cornish et al. 2019; Hemingway et al. 2021; Kumar, Mostafa & Ramaswamy 2018). The Ebola Pandemic of 2014–2015 laid bare many of the inadequacies of the system, and the continually high maternal and child mortality continues to expose the need for strong policies that improve trust in the system, address corruption and mismanagement, and improve healthcare for all.

References

Adjiwanou, V., Bougma, M., & LeGrand, T. (2018). The effect of partners' education on women's reproductive and maternal health in developing countries. *Social Science & Medicine*, 197, 104–115.

Adua, E., Frimpong, K., Li, X., & Wang, W. (2017). Emerging issues in public health: A perspective on Ghana's healthcare expenditure, policies, and outcomes. *EPMA Journal*, 8(3), 197–206.

Ansumana, R., Bah, F., Biao, K., Harding, D., Jalloh, M. B., Kelly, A. H., Koker, F., Koroma, Z., Momoh, M., Rogers, M. H., Rogers, J., Street, A., Vernooij, E., & Wurie, I. (2020). Building diagnostic systems in Sierra Leone: The role of point-of-care devices in laboratory strengthening. *African Journal of Laboratory Medicine*, 9(2), 1029. DOI: 10.4102/ajlm.v9i2.1029.

Barr, A., Garrett, L., Marten, R., & Kadandale, S. (2019). Health sector fragmentation: Three examples from Sierra Leone. *Globalization and Health*, 15(1), 1–8.

Bertone, M. P., Wurie, H., Samai, M., & Witter, S. (2018). The bumpy trajectory of performance-based financing for healthcare in Sierra Leone: Agency, structure and frames shaping the policy process. *Globalization and Health*, 14(1), 1–15.

Bitton, A., Fifield, J., Ratcliffe, H., Karlage, A., Wang, H., Veillard, J. H., … & Hirschhorn, L. R. (2019). Primary healthcare system performance in low-income and middle-income countries: A scoping review of the evidence from 2010 to 2017. *BMJ Global Health*, 4(Suppl 8), e001551.

Bloom, D. E., Chatterji, S., Kowal, P., Lloyd-Sherlock, P., McKee, M., Rechel, B., … & Smith, J. P. (2015). Macroeconomic implications of population ageing and selected policy responses. *The Lancet*, 385(9968), 649–657.

Carlson-March, R., Aimone, A., Ansumana, R., Swaray, I. B., Assalif, A., Musa, A. (2022). Child, maternal, and adult mortality in Sierra Leone: Nationally representative mortality survey, 2018–2020. *The Lancet Global Health*, 10(1), E114–E123.

228TRANSFORMING HEALTHCARE IN AFRICA

Caviglia, M., Dell'Aringa, M., Putoto, G., Buson, R., Pini, S., Youkee, D., ... & Barone-Adesi, F. (2021). Improving access to healthcare in Sierra Leone: The role of the newly developed national emergency medical service. *International Journal of Environmental Research and Public Health*, 18(18), 9546.

Cornish, H., Walls, H., Ndirangu, R., Ogbureke, N., Bah, O. M., Tom-Kargbo, J. F., ... & Ranganathan, M. (2021). Women's economic empowerment and health related decision-making in rural Sierra Leone. *Culture, Health & Sexuality*, 23(1), 19–36.

Cornish H., Walls H., Ndirangu R., Ogbureke N., Bah O. M., Favour Tom-Kargbo J., Dimoh M., Ranganathan M. (2019). Women's economic empowerment and health related decision-making in rural Sierra Leone. *Culture, Health & Sexuality*. DOI: 10.1080/13691058.2019.1683229.

Deck, C., & Sheremeta, R. M. (2018). The tug-of-war in the laboratory. ESI Working Paper 18-21. Retrieved from https://digitalcommons.chapman.edu/esi_working_papers/275/. Accessed November 11, 2024.

Dreyfus, J., Gayle, J., Trueman, P., Delhougne, G., & Siddiqui, A. (2018). Assessment of risk factors associated with hospital-acquired pressure injuries and impact on health care utilization and cost outcomes in US hospitals. *American Journal of Medical Quality*, 33(4), 348–358.

Elston, J. W., Danis, K., Gray, N., West, K., Lokuge, K., Black, B., ... & Caleo, G. (2020). Maternal health after Ebola: Unmet needs and barriers to healthcare in rural Sierra Leone. *Health Policy and Planning*, 35(1), 78–90.

Ensor, T., Lievens, T., & Naylor, M. (2008). Review of financing of health in Sierra Leone and the development of policy options.

Fang, L. Q., Yang, Y., Jiang, J. F., Yao, H. W., Kargbo, D., Li, X. L., ... & Cao, W. C. (2016). Transmission dynamics of Ebola virus disease and intervention effectiveness in Sierra Leone. *Proceedings of the National Academy of Sciences*, 113(16), 4488–4493.

Gabani, J., Mazumdar, S., Hadji, S. B., Amara, M. M. (2024). The redistributive effect of the public health system: The case of Sierra Leone, *Health Policy, and Planning*, 39(1), 4–21.

Gajovic, G., Janicijevic, K., Andric, D., Djurovic, O., & Radevic, S. (2019). Gender differences in health care utilization among the elderly. *Serbian Journal of Experimental and Clinical Research*, 22(3): 195–203.

Goodyear-Smith, F., Bazemore, A., Coffman, M., Fortier, R. D., Howe, A., Kidd, M., ... & van Weel, C. (2019). Research gaps in the organisation of primary healthcare in low-income and middle-income countries and ways to address them: A mixed-methods approach. *BMJ Global Health*, 4(Suppl 8), e001482.

Government of Sierra Leone (2020). Government budget and statement of economic and financial policies for the financial year 2021. https://mof.gov.sl/documents/government-budget-and-statement-of-economic-and-financial-policies-for-the-financial-year-2021/. Accessed March 13, 2024.

Harris, D., Endale, T., Lind, U. H., Sevalie, S., Bah, A. J., Jalloh, A., & Baingana, F. (2020). Mental health in Sierra Leone. *BJPsych International*, 17(1), 14–16.

Hemingway, C. D., Jalloh, M. B., Silumbe, R., Wurie, H., Mtumbuka, E., Nhiga, S., ... & Pulford, J. (2021). Pursuing health systems strengthening through disease-specific programme grants: Experiences in Tanzania and Sierra Leone. *BMJ Global Health*, 6(10), e006615.

Hopwood, H., Sevalie, S., Herman, M. O., Harris, D., Collet, K., Bah, A. J., & Beynon, F. (2021). The burden of mental disorder in Sierra Leone: A retrospective observational evaluation of programmatic data from the roll out of decentralised nurse-led mental health units. *International Journal of Mental Health Systems*, 15(1), 1–27.

Hoque, M. R. (2016). An empirical study of mHealth adoption in a developing country: The moderating effect of gender concern. *BMC Medical Informatics and Decision Making*, 16(1), 1–10.

Idriss, A., Diaconu, K., Zou, G., Senesi, R. G., Wurie, H., & Witter, S. (2020). Rural–urban health-seeking behaviours for non-communicable diseases in Sierra Leone. *BMJ Global Health*, 5(2), e002024.

Jalloh, M. B., Bah, A. J., James, P. B., Sevalie, S., Hann, K., & Shmueli, A. (2019). Impact of the free healthcare initiative on wealth-related inequity in the utilization of maternal & child health services in Sierra Leone. *BMC Health Services Research*, 19(1), 1–15.

Jalloh, M. F., Li, W., Bunnell, R. E., Ethier, K. A., O'Leary, A., Hageman, K. M., … & Redd, J. T. (2018). Impact of Ebola experiences and risk perceptions on mental health in Sierra Leone. *BMJ Global Health*, 3(2), e000471.

James, P. B., & Bah, A. J. (2014). Awareness, use, attitude, and perceived need for Complementary and Alternative Medicine (CAM) education among undergraduate pharmacy students in Sierra Leone: A descriptive cross-sectional survey. *BMC Complementary and Alternative Medicine*, 14(1), 1–9.

James, P. B., Taidy-Leigh, L., Bah, A. J., Kanu, J. S., Kangbai, J. B., & Sevalie, S. (2018). Prevalence and correlates of herbal medicine use among women seeking Care for Infertility in Freetown, Sierra Leone. *Evidence-Based Complementary and Alternative Medicine*. 2018(1), 9493807.

James, P. B., Wardle, J., Steel, A., Adams, J., Bah, A. J., & Sevalie, S. (2020). Providing healthcare to Ebola survivors: A qualitative exploratory investigation of healthcare providers' views and experiences in Sierra Leone. *Global Public Health*, 15(9), 1380–1395.

Jofre-Bonet, M., & Kamara, J. (2018). Willingness to pay for health insurance in the informal sector of Sierra Leone. *PLoS One*, 13(5), e0189915.

Johnson, F., Hayton, J., Lowsby, R., & Harrison, H. L. (2020). Challenges to developing emergency services in Sierra Leone. *European Journal of Emergency Medicine*, 27(5), 321–322.

Johnson, O., Sahr, F., Begg, K., Sevdalis, N., & Kelly, A. H. (2021). To bend without breaking: A qualitative study on leadership by doctors in Sierra Leone. *Health Policy and Planning*.

Kahl, C. H. (2018). *States, Scarcity, and Civil Strife in the Developing World*. Princeton, NJ: Princeton University Press.

Kamara, S., Walder, A., Duncan, J., Kabbedijk, A., Hughes, P., & Muana, A. (2017). Mental health care during the Ebola virus disease outbreak in Sierra Leone. *Bulletin of the World Health Organization*, 95(12), 842.

Kanu, A. F. (2019). *Health System Access to Maternal and Child Health Services in Sierra Leone* (Doctoral dissertation, Walden University).

Kanu, J. S., Tang, Y., & Liu, Y. (2014). Assessment on the knowledge and reported practices of women on maternal and child health in rural Sierra Leone: A cross-sectional survey. *PLoS One*, 9(8), e105936.

Kaye, A. D., Okeagu, C. N., Pham, A. D., Silva, R. A., Hurley, J. J., Arron, B. L., … & Cornett, E. M. (2020). Economic impact of COVID-19 pandemic on health care facilities and systems: International perspectives. *Best Practice & Research Clinical Anaesthesiology*.

Kelly, J. D., Weiser, S. D., & Tsai, A. C. (2016). Proximate context of HIV stigma and its association with HIV testing in Sierra Leone: A population-based study. *AIDS and Behavior*, 20(1), 65–70.

Koka, R., Chima, A. M., Sampson, J. B. et al. (2016). Anesthesia practice and perioperative outcomes at two tertiary care hospitals in Freetown, Sierra Leone. *Anesthesia and Analgesia*. 123, 213–217.

Kumar, M., Mostafa, J., & Ramaswamy, R. (2018). Federated health information architecture: Enabling healthcare providers and policymakers to use data for decision-making. *Health Information Management Journal*, 47(2), 85–93.

Li, S., (2020). *Hope on Wheels: A First-of-its-kind National Emergency Medical Service (NEMS) in Sierra Leone*. The World Bank Group. https://blogs.worldbank.org/en/health /hope-wheels-first-its-kind-national-emergency-medical-service-nems-sierra-leone. Accessed September 14, 2024.

McPake, B., Dayal, P., & Herbst, C. H. (2019). Never again? Challenges in transforming the health workforce landscape in post-Ebola West Africa. *Human Resources for Health*, 17(1), 1–10.

Narayan, V., John-Stewart, G., Gage, G., & O'Malley, G. (2018). "If I had known, I would have applied": Poor communication, job dissatisfaction, and attrition of rural health workers in Sierra Leone. *Human Resources for Health*, 16(1), 1–11.

Nathaniel-Wurie, L., Martin, G., Cooper, G., De Bernier, G. L., Ajayi, T., Martineau, F., ... & Lako, S. (2012). PS33 health-seeking behaviour in the era of free healthcare in urban slums in Sierra Leone. *Journal of Epidemiol Community Health*, 66(Suppl 1), A51–A51.

Novak, J. R., Peak, T., Gast, J., & Arnell, M. (2019). Associations between masculine norms and health-care utilization in highly religious, heterosexual men. *American Journal of Men's Health*, 13(3), 1557988319856739.

Oleribeet, O. O., Momoh, J., Uzochukwu, B. S., Mbofana, F., Adebiyi, A., Barbera, T., ... & Taylor-Robinson, S. D. (2019). Identifying key challenges facing healthcare systems in Africa and potential solutions. *International Journal of General Medicine*, 12, 395.

Oloyede, O. (2017). Rural-urban disparities in health and health care in Africa: Cultural competence, lay-beliefs in narratives of diabetes among the rural poor in the eastern cape province of South Africa. *African Sociological Review/Revue Africaine de Sociologie*, 21(2), 36–57.

Orach, D., & Garimoi, C. (2009). Health equity: Challenges in low-income countries. *African Health Sciences*, 9(s2), S49–S51.

Percival, V., Dusabe-Richards, E., Wurie, H., Namakula, J., Ssali, S., & Theobald, S. (2018). Are health systems interventions gender blind? Examining health system reconstruction in conflict affected states. *Globalization and Health*, 14(1), 1–23.

Peters, D. H., Garg, A., Bloom, G., Walker, D. G., Brieger, W. R., & Hafizur Rahman, M. (2008). Poverty and access to health care in developing countries. *Annals of the New York Academy of Sciences*, 1136(1), 161–171.

Phull, M., Grimes, C. E., Kamara, T. B., Wurie, H., Leather, A. J., & Davies, J. (2021). What is the financial burden to patients of accessing surgical care in Sierra Leone? A cross-sectional survey of catastrophic and impoverishing expenditure. *BMJ Open*, 11(3), e039049.

Pieterse, P. M. (2016). "Free healthcare, free die": The efficacy of social accountability interventions in the health sector in Sierra Leone.

Pieterse, P., & Lodge, T. (2015). When free healthcare is not free. Corruption and mistrust in Sierra Leone's primary healthcare system immediately prior to the Ebola outbreak. *International Health*, 7(6), 400–404.

Robinson, C. (2019). Primary health care and family medicine in Sierra Leone. *African Journal of Primary Health Care & Family Medicine*, 11(1), 1–3.

Rowe, A. K., Rowe, S. Y., Peters, D. H., Holloway, K. A., Chalker, J., & Ross-Degnan, D. (2018). Effectiveness of strategies to improve health-care provider practices in low-income and middle-income countries: A systematic review. *The Lancet Global Health*, 6(11), e1163–e1175.

Samura, S. S. (2016). *The Impact of Free Healthcare on Hospital Deliveries in Sierra Leone* (Doctoral dissertation, Walden University).

Sanny, J. A., (2020). *Sierra Leoneans say Health Care Hard to Access, Beset with Corruption – Especially for the Poor*. The Africa Portal.

Strasser, R., Kam, S. M., & Regalado, S. M. (2016). Rural health care access and policy in developing countries. *Annual Review of Public Health*, 37, 395–412.

Sylvester, S. J., Hann, K., Denisiuk, O., Kamara, M., Tamang, D., & Zachariah, R. (2017). The Ebola outbreak and staffing in public health facilities in rural Sierra Leone: Who is left to do the job? *Public Health Action*, 7, 54. DOI: 10.5588/pha.16.0089.

Tang, N., Eisenberg, J. M., & Meyer, G. S. (2004). The roles of government in improving health care quality and safety. *Joint Commission Journal on Quality and Safety*, 30(1), 47–55.

Theuring, S., Koroma, A. P., & Harms, G. (2018). In the hospital, there will be nobody to pamper me": A qualitative assessment on barriers to facility-based delivery in post-Ebola Sierra Leone. *Reproductive Health*, 15(1), 1–9.

Treacy, L., Bolkan, H. A., & Sagbakken, M. (2018). Distance, accessibility, and costs. Decision-making during childbirth in rural Sierra Leone: A qualitative study. *PLoS One*, 13(2), e0188280.

Tsawe, M., & Susuman, A. S. (2020). Factors associated with the upsurge in the use of delivery care services in Sierra Leone. *Public Health*, 180, 74–81.

Valtorta, N. K., Moore, D. C., Barron, L., Stow, D., & Hanratty, B. (2018). Older adults' social relationships and health care utilization: A Systematic review. *American Journal of Public Health*, 108(4), e1–e10.

Vaughan, E., Sesay, F., Chima, A., Mehes, M., Lee, B., Dordunoo, D., & Sampson, J. (2015). An assessment of surgical and anesthesia staff at 10 government hospitals in Sierra Leone. *JAMA Surgery*, 150(3), 237–244.

Vernooij, E., Koker, F., & Street, A. (2021). Responsibility, repair, and care in Sierra Leone's health system. *Social Science & Medicine*, 114260.

Witter, S., Wurie, H., Namakula, J., Mashange, W., Chirwa, Y., & Alonso-Garbayo, A. (2018). Why do people become health workers? Analysis from life histories in 4 post-conflict and post-crisis countries. *The International Journal of Health Planning and Management*, 33(2), 449–459.

Woodward, A., Lake, E. G., Rajaraman, N., & Leather, A. (2018). Specialist training aspirations of junior doctors in Sierra Leone: A qualitative follow-up study. *BMC Medical Education*, 18(1), 1–15.

World Bank (2020). Poverty & Equity Brief. Africa Western & Central. Sierra Leone. https://databank.worldbank.org/data/download/poverty/987B9C90-CB9F-4D93-AE8C-750588BF00QA/SM2020/Global_POVEQ_SLE.pdf. Accessed March 12, 2022.

World Health Organization (2020). Sierra Leone biennial report. https://www.afro.who.int/sites/default/files/2022-10/WHO%20Sierra%20Leone_2020-2021_Biennial%20Report.pdf. Accessed September 14, 2024.

Wurie, H. R., Samai, M., & Witter, S. (2016). Retention of health workers in rural Sierra Leone: Findings from life histories. *Human Resources for Health*, 14(1), 1–15.

Yendewa, G. A., Poveda, E., Yendewa, S. A., Sahr, F., Quiñones-Mateu, M. E., & Salata, R. A. (2018). HIV/AIDS in Sierra Leone: Characterizing the hidden epidemic. *AIDS Reviews*, 20, 104–113.

Yunus, R. M., Hairi, N. N., & Choo, W. Y. (2019). Consequences of elder abuse and neglect: A systematic review of observational studies. *Trauma, Violence, & Abuse*, 20(2), 197–213.

Chapter Fourteen

HEALTH POLICY AND CHALLENGES IN SOMALIA

Yusuf Nur and Robert Dibie

Introduction

This chapter examines the health policies and physical infrastructure of healthcare delivery in Somalia. It argues that the humanitarian crisis because of the civil war in Somalia for many decades has negatively affected the formulation of policies and effective implementation of healthcare delivery in the country. In addition, the lack of a community healthcare approach has not been the center of healthcare delivery in Somalia. Thus, the nature of the healthcare needs of the citizens of the country has negatively affected the humanitarian crisis and economic development in the country. The research methods applied for this chapter involved using both questionnaire administration and semi-structured interviews to gain insights into the effectiveness of health policies as well as citizen perception of the healthcare delivery system in Somalia. Content analysis of World Health Organization, African Development Bank, and United Nations reports as well as United States Central for Disease Center (CDC) reports reviewed. Several academic journal articles were also reviewed. The finding of this research reveals that apart from the civil wars in Somalia, the healthcare delivery system in the country is severely affected by inadequate medical products, funding technology in the healthcare delivery system, inadequate health workforce, leadership, and lack of health delivery network in rural communities. In addition, poor government funding, lack of accountability or coordination in the way healthcare is delivered to citizens, and the challenges of insecurity, instability, and frequent confusion between local and international paradigms of health approaches have negatively affected the health delivery system in the country. Recommendations on how the government and private sectors could adopt a good steward leadership approach to effectively coordinate Somalia's health system's vision, direction, and policies to ensure vibrant basic healthcare services to all citizens soon are provided.

Brief History of Somalia

Democratic Republic of Somalia is a country in the northeastern Horn of the African continent. The nation has a boundary with Ethiopia in the west, and Kenya in the south. It also has a boundary with Djibouti and the Red Sea in the northwest. The Indian Ocean covers the south, east, and northeastern parts of Somalia. The current population of Somalia will be 17.5 million people in 2022 (World Bank Indicators 2023). In addition, the gross domestic product (GDP) of Somalia in 2022 was $8.18 billion (World Bank Indicators 2022). The Somalia Democratic Republic was granted independence by British and Italian colonial administrations and became a united Somalia nation on July 1, 1960.

The first settlers of the Somali region were ethnic Cushites people who migrated from the fertile lakes of southern Ethiopia (Healy & Bradbury 2010; Lewis 1965; Rose & Hullburd 1992). The original settlers were divided into various ethnic groups. These ethnic groups continue to exist in Somalia, Egypt, and Ethiopia in the northeastern part of Africa in present times. There are several archeological evidence that confirms that most of the coastline of present-day Somalia has been settled by the African people from the northeastern part of the continent since AD 100 (Lewis 1965; United Nations 2020b). The Somalis people also had contact with Arab traders traveling along the Red Sea and Indian Ocean. Further, the Somali people were one of the first people to convert to Islam. The Arabs established the city of Zeila now called Saylac along the Horn of Africa was a central trading hub until the seventeenth century, when Christians started to trade with the people of Somalia and Ethiopia (Lewis 1965). Somalia has long been an important center for commerce with the rest of the ancient world (Farah & Ruhela 1993; Lewis 1965; United Nations 2020).

During the Middle Ages Mogadishu, the current capital city of Somalia was known as one of the favorite party towns for Arab sailors in northeast Africa (Farah & Ruhela 1993; Lewis 1965).

Furthermore, in the ninth or tenth century, Somalis began pushing south from the Gulf of Aden coast. About this time, Arabs and Persians established settlements along the Indian Ocean coast (Ingiriis 2018; Lewis 1965; United Nations 2020). During the fifteenth and sixteenth centuries, Portuguese explorers attempted without success to establish Portuguese sovereignty over the Somali coast (Encyclopedia 2020; Farah & Ruhela 1993). In addition, between 1875 and 1910 Britain, France, and Italy made territorial claims of the peninsula Indian Ocean. Explorers from Britain started arriving in Somalia already and incrementally secured controlled the port city of Aden in Yemen, just across the Red Sea and wanted to control its counterpart, Berbera, on the Somali side (Encyclopedia 2020; Lewis 1965; United Nations 2020). According to the Ingiriis (2018) and the United Nations (2020), Red Sea was seen as a crucial shipping lane to British colonies in India, and they wanted to secure these major ports at all costs (Ingiriis 2018; United Nations 2020). Further, the British armed forces occupied Aden in 1839. In addition, they also developed an interest in the northern Somali coast. However, by 1874, Egyptians occupied several points on the shore, but their occupation was short-lived. The bilateral relationship between British and Somalia propel both nations to sign several protectorate treaties between 1884 and 1886 (Lewis 1965).

The British and Somali leaders signed a protectorate treaty. In addition, the Italian explorer expansion in Somalia began in 1885, when Antonio Cecchi, an explorer, led an Italian expedition into the lower Juba region and signed a commercial treaty with the sultan of Zanzibar (Lewis 1965; Encyclopedia 2020). The Sultan of Zanzibar also leased concessions along the Indian Ocean coast to Italy (Issa-Salwe 1996; United Nations 2020). According to Lewis (1965), Farah & Ruhela (1993), and the University of Central Arkansas (2023) between 1940 and 1941, the army of the Italian colonial administration briefly occupied British Somaliland but were soon defeated by the British, who conquered Italian Somaliland and reestablished their authority over the territory. Because of the outcome of World War II, the Italian hegemony of Somalia was short-lived, and Mussolini, the President of Italy, realized that there was no point in expanding his ambition in Somalia (Ingiriis 2018; Lewis 1965).

In 1959, the United Nations General Assembly resolved that Italian Somaliland would receive its independence in 1960 (Encyclopedia 2020; Lewis 1965). During this same period, Somalis in British Somaliland were also demanding self-government. As Italy agreed to grant independence on July 1, 1960, to its trust territory (Ingiriis 2018). Later that same year, the United Kingdom granted Somalia its formal protectorate independence on June 26, 1960. This gesture of the Italian and British colonial administration galvanized the two Somali territories to join to form a united Somali Republic on July 1, 1960. On July 20, 1961, the Somali people ratified a new constitution, drafted in 1960, and one month later Aden 'Abdullah Osman Daar was elected the nation's first president. (Encyclopedia 2020; Lewis 1965; Wikipedia 2023). Thus, the Somali Republic was formed by the union of Somalia, which previously had been under Italian administration as a United Nations trust territory, and Somaliland, which had been a British protectorate until June 26, 1960. In addition, despite the fact that Somalis had received their primary political education under British and post-war Italian tutelage, the virulently anti-imperialist parties rejected the European's advice whole cloth and threw their lot in with the Soviet Union and the People's Republic of China (Ingiriis 2018). By the middle of the 1960s, the Somalis had a formal military relationship with Russia whereby the Soviet Union provided extensive materiel and military training to the Somali armed forces (United Nations 2020).

Healy and Bradbury (2010) and Lewis (2015) contend that the collapse of the Somalis' state was the consequence of a combination of internal and external factors. According to the above historians, first, there were the legacies of European colonialism that divided the Somali people into five states (Healy & Bradbury 2010; Lewis 2015).

According to the United Nations (2020) just after gaining independence early 1960s, troubling trends began to emerge when the north started to reject referendums that had won a majority of votes, in favor of southern Somaliland. Further, Somalia's internal disputes were manifested outward in hostility to Ethiopia and Kenya, which they felt were standing in the way of a united greater Somalia government (Ingiriis 2018; United Nations 2020). Subsequently, election fraud from the displaced Somalia Youth League escalated more protests in the country. The protest gave the military juntas a reason to plan a coup. On October 15, 1969, a bodyguard killed President Shermaarke while Prime Minister Igaal was out of the country (Khayre 2016; Lewis 1965; United Nations 2020).

The military leaders dissolved parliament, suspended the constitution, arrested members of the cabinet, and changed the name of the country to the Somali Democratic Republic. Major General Jalle Mohamed Siad Barre, commander of the army, was named chairperson of a 25-member Supreme Revolutionary Council. Further, the new governing body, the Supreme Revolutionary Council (SRC), installed General Siad Barre as its president in November 1969 (Encyclopedia 2020). Vice-President Muhammad Ainanshe Guleid unsuccessfully attempted to overthrow General Barre on May 5, 1971 (University of Central Arkansas 2023). The Somali government suppressed a military rebellion led by Colonel Abdullahi Yusuf on April 9, 1978, resulting in the deaths of 20 government soldiers. In addition, government troops clashed with Somali Salvation Front rebels on July 2–3, 1980, resulting in the deaths of 72 active-duty soldiers (University of Central Arkansas 2023). The Chinese government agreed to provide economic assistance to the government on April 18, 1978. On October 26, 1978, 17 military personnel were executed for their involvement in the military rebellion. Some 200 individuals were killed during the crisis (ABC News 2001; Healy & Bradbury 2010; University of Central Arkansas 2023). Furthermore, legislative elections were held on December 30, 1979, and the Somali Revolutionary Socialist Party won 171 out of 171 seats in the People's Assembly. General Barre was elected president by the People's Assembly on January 26, 1980, for a second term as president. Government troops clashed with SSF rebels on February 8, 1980, resulting in the deaths of 52 military officers. Government troops clashed with SSF rebels on July 2–3, 1980, resulting in the deaths of 72 active duty soldiers (Ingiriis 2018). President Barre declared a state of emergency on October 21, 1980, and a 17-member Supreme Revolutionary Council took control of the government on October 23, 1980 (University of Central Arkansas 2023). Further, President Barre was reelected without opposition on December 23, 1986.

The next three decades resulted in notable improvements through the expansion of health facilities and mobile outreach services. Further, the nation has faced infectious military coups, war, murder, and a sequence of environmental and manufactured calamities since the late 1990s, resulting in a long, drawn-out, and thorough collapse state (ABC News 2001; Office of the Historian, United States Department of State 2023). As a result, of this political crisis, the healthcare system in Somalia is unstable, divided, and inadequate. In the 1970s, academic institutions upscaled their training of healthcare providers, who were then deployed across the healthcare system. During the same period, many senior Somali medical doctors underwent postgraduate studies at Italian universities and, after returning, engaged in academic teaching, training physicians, nurses, midwives, and a range of other health workers. Another milestone in building research capacity was the Swedish Government's support in the 1980s to the Somali National University, Mogadishu. This initiative helps to train about 23 Somali faculty members in master's or doctoral programs at Swedish universities (American Broadcasting News 2001; Bile et al. 2022).

Somalia inherited a weak post-colonial, healthcare system based on curing disease rather than preventing it, with most rural and nomadic populations having negligible access to essential healthcare services (Bile et al. 2022; Njoku 2013). The next three decades resulted in notable improvements through the expansion of health facilities and mobile outreach services (American Broadcasting News 2001). Further, the nation has faced infectious military war, murder, and a sequence of environmental and man-made calamities since the late 1990s. As a result, the healthcare system is unstable, divided, and inadequate. Aid workers are frequently attacked because they perform life-saving humanitarian work (Aljazeera News 2016; Bile et al. 2022; Khayre 2016).

The civil war, which broke out in the 1990s, led to tragic disruptions to the health system in the long term, due to a protracted complex emergency accompanied by famines and population displacement (Omer et al. 2018; Said 2021). The transition to recovery of health-system organization, regulation, and workforce development began in the 2010s with the institution of a transitional federal government, creating opportunities to initiate the pursuit of universal health coverage (United Nations 2020a). During this recovery phase, around 25 academic institutions with undergraduate medical or health courses and a few master's training courses were operationalized, and steps were taken to revive collaboration with Swedish universities.

Health Challenges in Somalia

The Somalia health system has incrementally improved from what it used to be after three decades of wars and political instability. However, there continue to be significant challenges in both the provision of health services and enabling access to the services (Gele 2020; Jeene 2017). Somalia's health system remains weak (Morrison & Malik 2023). The United Nations (2020b) reports that one-fifth of the population in Somalia still lacks access to healthcare, which continues to pose severe challenges to the population's health in both urban and rural communities in the country. The nature of limited government or publicly funded hospitals and clinics, the only healthcare alternative in the country has been a highly priced privately operated health facility (United Nations 2020a).

Access to healthcare is also a major challenge because the majority of the privately operated health facilities are in major towns, leaving the poor majority in the rural areas, out of affordable healthcare services (Farah et al. 2022; Gele 2020; Qayad 2008; WHO 2021).

According to the World Health Organization Report (2021b) after 30 years of instability, Somalia's health system is among the most fragile in the world. Somalia's health outcomes are lower when compared to neighboring countries in northeast Africa. The poor health delivery system is basically due to lagging health facilities, non-available health workers, and high-quality health awareness education (Knofczynski 2017; World Health Organization 2023a). The severe impact of the COVID-19 pandemic between 2019 and 2022 in Somalia has really buttressed the gaps in maternal and child health services and high fertility rates of women in the country (Abdirahm et al. 2021; Mohamed et al. 2022).

The current health sector human resource challenges in the Federal Republic of Somalia include a shortage in the training and production of qualified health workers; the difficulty in realizing the desirable workforce skill mix; the lack of uniform standards for workforce training curricula, and educational programs (Ibrahim et al. 2022; Tran et al. 2021). In addition, the biggest predicament that led to the shortage of health workers in Somalia is the civil war (International Committee of the Red Cross 2022). Because of the war most of the prominent doctors and nurses fled the country.

According to Ibrahim et al. (2022), some physicians were also victims of the war. Some scholars contend that in 2004, it was estimated that there were about 250 physicians and 360 nurses in Somalia, however during the civil war more than 350 doctors and over 500 nurses fled the country for their safety (Humanitarian Program Circle 2023; Muchena 2021; Somalia, Ministry of Health, and Human Services 2014a; Qayad 2008). According to an Amnesty International Report (2021), in 2017, Somalia had a ratio of one surgeon per 1,000,000 people. Only an estimated 15% of people have access to medical care in rural areas due to lack of enough physicians. Between 2018 and 2022, the ratio of physicians has remained stagnant at 0.023 physicians to 1,000 and 0.112 nurses to 1,000 people (Farah et al. 2022). Another issue that has contributed to the flight of doctors and nurses from Somalia is the very low salary that they are paid (Ibrahim et al. 2022).

Although physicians are now allowed to operate their own private clinics the question of the affordability of paying high out-of-pocket fees for treatment by poor rural populations has also limited access to healthcare (Ahmed et al. 2020; Farah et al. 2022). Other challenges include no clear medical workforce certification and accreditation systems, and inadequate teaching facilities. There are also other healthcare challenges such as ineffectively harmonized salaries and incentives as well as poor working environments that have a major bearing on the quality of service delivery, performance, motivation, and retention of the health workforce (Farah et al. 2022; Gele 2020). The abduction of health workers also constitutes another critical challenge in healthcare delivery in Somalia (Ahmed et al. 2020; Humanitarian Program Circle 2023; Gele 2020).

The Federal Democratic Republic of Somalia tends to experience limited availability of medications. Because of the lack of an appropriate supply of drugs physicians are reported to prescribe inappropriate treatment with what they have instead of waiting forever for the supply to arrive at an indefinite date or time (Osman 2022). This major challenge has only led to a high rate of death in both urban and rural regions of the country (Ibrahin 2022). Further, most of the generic drugs in the nation are from unknown manufacturers or counterfeit (Yenet et al. 2023). In addition, ambulance services are not available in the rural regions of Somalia. It is only in the nation's capital that you can find some ambulance services. However, in other bigger cities, ambulance services are not reliable. The Somalia Red Crescent Society has been reported to provide some limited emergency ambulance services mostly in the bigger cities (United States Department of State 2023).

The Federal Republic of Somalia is reported to have one of the highest mental health predicaments in the world (Abdillahi et al. 2020; Ibrahim et al. 2022). The civil war that took place in the country has resulted in a devasting impact on the citizens of the country. Ibrahim (2021) contends that conflict-related trauma, poverty, unemployment, and rampant substance abuse have escalated mental health predicaments and severe humanitarian crises in Somalia. Some scholars contend that Somali women and men endured torture, rape, or mental health pains that were widely used as a means of terrorizing the population into submission (Samartzis & Talias 2020; Schuchman & McDonald 2004). According to Maruf (2023), World

Health Organization (2017) nearly 40% of the population in Somalia has a mental or psychological disorder (Maruf 2023). To compound this problem, there are inadequate mental health services in Somalia. Currently, only 5%–10% of the primary healthcare centers in the country can offer mental health services to the population that needs mental healthcare (Maruf 2023). The low-capacity psychiatric clinics. According to the World Health Organization (2021) report, the lack of treatment increases the burden of illness in terms of mortality, morbidity, stigma, and discrimination (Ibrahim 2022; Samartzis & Talias 2020).

According to World Bank Indicators (2022), the Federal Republic of Somalia has been spending an average of just 1.24% in 1998 and 1.26% in 1999 of its GDP every year for the past few years of its health system (Country Economy 1999). This amount is far below the 15% Abuja Declaration of 2001 target set by African Union countries. Currently, there is limited investment in the health sector, with Somalia's health spending below 5% of its GDP (World Bank Indicators 2022). This predicament has exacerbated the inequitable access to available essential health services in the nation.

Many scholars contend that access to healthcare remains dangerously low in the Democratic Republic of Somalia (Farah et al. 2022; Dalmar et al. 2017; Mohamud 2021). As of April 2022, the nation only had one government hospital that is in the country's capital city, Mogadishu (Oyella 2022). Because of the shortage of functional hospitals and clinics, the population of the country often must seek healthcare services at a private healthcare facility (Ahmed et al. 2022; Oyella 2022).

In addition to other factors, lack of adequate immunization and inadequate access to quality healthcare facilities, medications, and life-saving medical supplies has constituted one of the major causes of children's high mortality for children between the ages of one to six months in Somalia (Bilal 2023). Furthermore, the United Nations Children's Fund officer in Mogadishu, Somalia contends that 4 in 100 Somali children die during the first month of life, 8 in 100 before their first birthday, and 1 in 8 before they turn five. This accounts for more than 60% of the under-five deaths in the country. In addition to this, 1 in 20 women aged 15–49 die due to pregnancy- or birth-related complications every year (Bilal 2023). These health predicaments facing innocent children in Somalia could have been avoided if there were effective emergency services, reachable access to healthcare services, and medical information technology systems in the country.

Poor infrastructure has negatively affected the health delivery system in Somalia (Amnesty International 2022; Muchena 2021). On the other hand, civil war, constant al-Shabab insurgency, as well as pervasive government corruption constrain investment and development to provide equitable healthcare for people living in both the urban and rural of the country (Morrison & Malik 2023). In addition, challenges of natural hazards including drought and seasonal flooding, all contribute to damage and destruction of the ecosystem in the country (Humanitarian Program Circle 2023; Morrison & Malik 2023). Further, Somalia is characterized by poor access to clean water, proper sanitation, and solid waste management leading to negative impacts on the health and welfare of Somalis as well as the economy (Humanitarian Program Circle 2023; Muchena 2021).

TRANSFORMING HEALTHCARE IN AFRICA

Types of Health Policies

The health policy development process in any democratic country envisages the scaling up of government leadership, management, health workforce, and service delivery capacity, while sustaining health partners in both the public and private sectors support (Dibie 2022). In the care of the Federal Republic of Somalia, several years of civil war affected the democratic process that could positively enable the formulation of public policies. Although health system financing constituted a major challenge during the civil war and just after the end of the crisis averting the transitional funding gap has also negatively affected the policy-making process. Below are some of the major health policies that have been enacted by the Federal Republic of Somalia.

Federal Government of Somalia Health Sector Strategic Plan 2020–2026: The goal of the National Health Sector is to adopt new strategies to address the emerging healthcare challenges in the country. The strategic was adopted after critically analyzing the strengths and weaknesses as well as outcomes of the previous health plan for 2013–2016 and 2017–2021. Some of the other goals of the National Health Strategic Plan 2020–2026 include strengthening the capacity of health decision-makers' ability to share strategic directions for health system development in the country (Federal Government of Somalia 2021). The new strategic plan also requires strengthening the training of the healthcare workforce in accredited institutions as well as in-service training (Federal Government of Somalia 2021). It is also anticipated that the new National Strategic Plan could galvanize the promotion of best practices in the use of resources to improve the health condition and access to better health of the citizens of Somalia (Federal Government of Somalia 2021).

Somali Medicines Law and Drug Act (2019): The goal of this health policy is to establish a strong supply chain system, which will be pivotal for sustainable and equitable recovery of the health system from the convergence of crises the country is facing. Currently, Somalia neither have a vibrant drug regulatory system nor a pharmaceutical product evaluation and registration agency. The nations also do not have any established mechanism to administer the regulation of import and export control, licensing and inspection of pharmaceutical products, and post-marketing surveillance. It is anticipated that the new Medicine Law and Drugs Act will enhance the medicine regulatory authority and supply chain system to promote sustainable and equitable access to safe drug supply in Somalia (Federal Government of Somalia 2014b; World Health Organization 2023).

Somalia National Medicine Act of 2014: The goal of this policy is to develop the pharmaceutical services in the country using available resources to meet the requirements of the entire population in the prevention, diagnosis, and treatment of disease using efficacious quality, safe, and cost-effective essential medicines and medical supplies, and rational use of drugs by prescriber, dispensers, and consumers in Somalia. In addition, the National Medicine Act of 2014 was expected to strengthen the efficiency of the pharmaceutical supply chain system to ensure sustainable and equitable access to and availability of affordable and good-quality essential medicines (Federal Government of Somalia. 2014a; World Health Organization 2023).

Somalia Health Policy Act of 2014: The goal of this policy is to enhance the shared commitment to the post-conflict health development principles of enhanced levels of accountability, reaffirmation of the EPHS program implementation, and strengthening the decentralization and participation processes. It will also aim at scaling up local interventions, promoting human resource and leadership development, building effective partnerships, and integrating the ongoing targeted humanitarian support to the currently pursued health system development (Federal Government of Somalia 2014b). The health policy of 2014 was expected to establish a roadmap for the launching of universal health coverage (UHC) and the accomplishment of the health-related Millennium Development Goals (MDGs) (Federal Government of Somalia 2014b). In addition, the policy strategically incorporates a commitment to expand basic health, nutrition, hygiene, and water and sanitation services to all geographical areas (Federal Government of Somalia 2014b).

Mental Health Policy of 2012: The goal of this policy is to set out plans to develop and organize mental health services, including the development of community-based services, training, research, and legislation. However, due lack of funding and political will, the policy remains only on paper and is yet to be implemented (Federal Government of Somalia 2012; Ibrahim et al. 2022).

Nature of Health Administration in Somalia

The administration of the health system in Somalia comprises five levels and the private sector health providers. The levels are (1) Community (The Primary Health Unit). (2) Health Center Primary/MCH Health Unit; (3) Referral Health Center; (4) Regional Hospital; and (5) The Ministry of Health. The Ministry of Health in Somalia coordinates all the activities of the above administrative levels. The Ministry of Health also has 18 administrative regions. medical officers in each of the administrative regions that report to the curative services department. In addition, the Ministry of Health is responsible for the population of over 17 million people in Somalia. Currently the primary health center (level 1) and health center (level 2) report to their district health officer (level 3), who along with the hospital director reports to the regional health officer (level 4). The above multilevel facility's four structures were recently supplemented by a community-based program (Somalia Ministry of Health, and Human Services 2014).

The *primary or community health administration level* are healthcare facilities that are located in rural geographical regions. The health facilities at this level tend to promote preventive and simple curative healthcare services (Somalia Ministry of Health, and Human Services 2014). Whenever there are special initiatives to promote nutrition education or dispense immunization at the primary level more health workers are temporarily deplored to the rural region (Somalia Ministry of Health, and Human Services 2014).

The next health administration level is the *health center.* The health centers are operated by qualified midwives and nurses. One of the major functions of the health center is the provision of basic emergency obstetric care to sick people who visit the center for treatment (Somalia Ministry of Health, and Human Services 2014).

The health center also has a number of delivery beds for the purpose of emergency obstetric care for women. In addition, the health center level also provides few maternal and child healthcare services at the district level because most of the facilities do not have the technical capacities (Somalia Ministry of Health and Human Services 2014).

The Referral Health Center or the District Hospital is the third level of the health administration system in Somalia. According to the Somalia Ministry of Health, and Human Services (2014) report, the referral or district hospitals are required to provide very crucial referral support functions that include comprehensive emergency obstetric care services, implying. This is because referral district hospitals tend to be more equipped with comprehensive emergency obstetric or child delivery care than the lower health center and primary levels. It is estimated that the referral or district hospitals serve a population of 100,000 people each year (Somalia Ministry of Health, and Human Services 2014).

Regional Hospitals are the highest health level of facilities in Somalia. The regional hospitals are mandated to provide specialist services to all their patients. Services at the regional hospitals are performed by highly qualified and mid-level health professionals and paramedic staff (Somalia Ministry of Health, and Human Services 2014). The regional health level has semi-independent management from the regional medical officers who work under the directives and authority of the national public healthcare coordinators (Somalia Ministry of Health, and Human Services 2014; Qayad 2008). The Ministry of Health staff clinic, hospitals, health posts, and vertical programs are all involved in projects dealing with tuberculosis, malaria, and schistosomiasis, as well as the programs on immunization in all regions in the country (Bilal 2023; Federal Government of Somalia 2020; Hassan & Filiz 2022).

Because of the political crisis and the disparities in the government's own health facilities, there has been a major increase in private health sectors in Somalia. The types of private sector healthcare providers include (a) private-for-profit, (b) private-not-profit, and (c) traditional health facilities (Ahmed et al. 2020). Although the private sector health providers tend to work as referral points for beneficiaries from government and nongovernmental-operated health facilities in the country, there is a major concern that the private sector remains unregulated (Ahmed et al. 2020; Bilal 2023). Further, traditional, spiritual, and herbal medicine practices often delay the utilization of modern health services needed to provide faster cures (Ibrahim et al. 2022; Qayad 2008; World Health Organization 2023b).

Data Analysis and Discussion

The goal of this chapter is to analyze the effectiveness of health policy and the healthcare delivery system in the Federal Republic of Somalia. The data used for the analysis of healthcare policy effectiveness were derived from both primary and secondary sources. The primary research involves the administration of a questionnaire to 150 respondents. One hundred and twenty-one or 86.7% of respondents returned their completed questionnaire. The questionnaire respondents constitute 50.4% female and 49.6% men. In addition, 40% of the respondents had visited a hospital or clinic to receive treatment at least twice a year. Another 33% had also visited a hospital or clinic between 3 and 4 times recently to receive treatment. While 21% of the respondents visited 5–6 times a year and 6% also visited the hospital more than 7 times during the same period.

The secondary research methods adopted include the review of the Federal Republic of Somalia Government's Ministry of Health and Human Service Reports, World Health Organization Reports, United Nations Human Development Index Annual Report, Center for Disease Control, and United States Agency for International Development, academic as well as professional journals articles. Data were analyzed using SPSS to determine the effectiveness and challenges facing the health policy and quality of the healthcare delivery system in the Federal Republic of Somalia Government.

Table 1 analyzes the nature of healthcare delivery and health policy in the Federal Republic of Somalia Government. The result of the questionnaire reveals that 73.6% of the respondents agree that political leaders and rich citizens of Somalia country prefer to seek healthcare services in foreign nations due to lack of trust in Somalia's healthcare system. Furthermore, 70.3% of the respondents agree that there is a lack of effective health policy implementation or regulation in the country. On one hand, 70.9% of the respondents indicated the corruption and unethical behavior of political and administrative leaders in government negatively affects the health system's funding in the country. On the other hand, 67.5% reported that the lack of appropriate funding for the healthcare system in Somalia has negatively affected the quality of healthcare delivery in the country. While 63.6% of the respondents agree that hospitals and health centers in the city that they live in constantly have electricity, 16.6% of the respondents disagree that there was no constant electricity in the hospital in their rural township.

Furthermore, 68.6% of the questionnaire respondents reported that the Federal Republic of Somalia's Government does not promote equity in the delivery of healthcare to underserved citizens in the country. In addition, 59.6% disagree that the Government of Somalia is effectively regulating medical professional licensing and disciplinary boards.

Another 45.8% of the respondents stated that government payment of low salaries to doctors and nurses has encouraged their migration to foreign countries. While 40.3% disagree that low salaries for doctors and nurses were not the reason for their migration. Other factors such as the civil war and poor working conditions could be major factors that propel the migration of the health professional workforce from Somalia. Further, 41.3% of the questionnaire respondents indicated that most hospitals in Somalia do not have modern medical equipment. It should be noted that 45.5% of the respondents stated that they can afford to pay for their healthcare treatment and medication costs without government subsidies. While 33% reported that they cannot afford to pay for their healthcare treatment.

Despite the poor state of healthcare in rural regions in Somalia, 42.1% of the respondents indicated that the healthcare provided by doctors in their city in Somalia is highly commendable. Table 2 provides a summary of the economic and health indicators of the Federal Republic of Somalia.

Table 1 The Nature of Healthcare Delivery and Policy Effectiveness in Somalia

Questions	Strongly Agree	Agree	Neutral	Strongly Disagree	Disagree	Agree %	Disagree %
1 Healthcare provided by doctors in my city is highly commendable	6.6%	35.5%	28.9%	8.3%	20.7%	42.1%	29%
2 Most hospitals in my country do not have modern equipment	9.9%	31.4%	26.4%	6.6%	25.6%	41.3%	32.2%
3 I can afford my healthcare treatment and medication costs without government subsidies.	15.7%	29.8%	21.5%	16.5%	16.5%	45.5%	33%
4 Most rural public hospitals in my country do not have specialist doctors and nurses.	4.3%	28.9%	10.7%	12.4%	5%	33.2%	17.4%
5 Government pay of low salaries to doctors and nurses has encouraged their migration to foreign countries.	15.1%	30.3%	14.3%	17.6%	22.7%	45.8%	40.3%
6 Lack of effective health policy implementation or regulations	39.7%	30.6%	9.1%	11.6%	70.3%	70.3%	20.7%
7 Government promotes equity in the delivery of healthcare to underserved citizens in the country.	5%	9.1%	17.4%	36.4%	32.2%	14.1%	68.6%
8 Political leaders and rich citizens of my country prefer to seek healthcare services in foreign nations.	46.3%	27.3%	14%	5.8%	6.6%	73.6%	12.4%
9 Government is effectively regulating medical professional licensing and disciplinary boards	9.1%	14%	17.4%	29.8%	29.8%	23.1%	59.6%
10 Hospitals and health centers in my city have constant electricity.	21.7%	42.5%	19.2%	5.8%	10.8%	63.5%	16.6%
11 Lack of appropriate funding for the healthcare system in my country.	28.3%	39.2%	15%	6.7%	10.8%	67.5%	17.5%
12 Corruption and unethical behavior of political and administrative leaders in government negatively affect the health system's funding.	41.7%	29.2%	15.8%	8.3%	5%	70.9%	13.3%
Mean						49.3%	30.1%

Source: Derived from Field research in Somalia between 2020 and 2023.

Table 2 Economics and Health Indicators of Somalia

No.	Major Indicators in Ghana	Explanation
1	Population	17.5 million (2022)
2	Gross domestic product (GDP)	US$8.13 billion (2022)
3	Current health expenditure (% of GDP)	1.26 (1999); 1.24 (1998)
4	Nurses and midwives per 1,000 people	0.112 (2022)
5	Physicians/doctors per 1,000 people	0.023 (2022)
6	Population using safely managed drinking water service	0.1% (2014)
7	People using safely managed sanitation services (% of population)	44% (urban); 21% (rural) (2020)
8	People practicing open defecation (% of the population)	23% (2020)
9	Common disease	HIV/AIDS, tuberculosis, cardiovascular diseases, malaria, neonatal disorders and malnutrition, mental health, schistosomiasis, and leprosy
10	Life expectancy at birth for females	57 years (2021)
11	Life expectancy at birth for males	55 years (2021)
12	Mortality rate for female adults (per 1,000 people)	295 (2021)
13	Mortality rate for male adults (per 1,000 people)	381 (2021)
14	Mortality rate for infants (per 1,000 people)	71 (2021)
15	Tuberculosis incidence (per 100,000 people)	250 (2021)
16	Population living below income poverty line PPP $1.90 a day	No data reported
17	Population in multidimensional handout poverty (%)	No data reported
18	Contribution deprivation in health to multidimensional poverty	No data reported
19	Infants lacking immunization for measles (% of one-year old)	42% (2021)
20	Malaria incidence (per 1,000 people at risk)	63.3% (2021)
21	HIV/AIDS prevalence of adults (% ages 15–49)	0.1% (2021)

Source: World Bank Indicators (2022). United Nations Human Development Program Index (2022); World Health Organization (2023).

The Federal Republic of Ghana currently spends an average of 1.26% of its GDP on healthcare in the past two years due to the negative impact of the civil war over the past two decades. However, the nation's GDP in 2022 was US$8.13 billion (World Bank Indicators 2022; United Nations Human Development Program Index 2022).

In 2022, the ratio of one doctor to 1,000 people in Somalia was 0.023. While the ratio of one nurse or midwife to 1,000 people in Somalia was 0.112. These indicators show that a country like Somalia with 17.5 million people is experiencing a serious shortage of health workers. This shortage of the health workforce in the country might lead to other ramifications. Further, the population using safely managed drinking water services in the country constituted just 0.1% in 2014. The number of people using safely managed sanitation services in 2020 was 44% in the urban regions and 21% in the rural regions. In addition, the number of people practicing open defecation constituted 23% of the population in 2020 (World Bank Indicators 2022).

According to the World Health Organization (2023) report, most of the common communicable and noncommunicable diseases in the Federal Republic of Somalia are HIV/AIDS, tuberculosis, cardiovascular diseases, malaria, neonatal disorders and malnutrition, mental health, schistosomiasis, and leprosy. These diseases are also associated with poor personal hygiene and environmental sanitation, chronic illnesses, human behavior, and infections due to a lack of basic health services such as obstetric and preventive services (World Health Organization 2023). Further, the Humanitarian Program Circle (2023) reported that approximately 6.7 million people living across the Federal Public of Somalia have increased and more severe health needs, an increase of 11% from 2022. According to Humanitarian Program Circle (2023), this increase is due to the ongoing drought, conflicts, and insecurity in the country. Thus, ongoing, and rising food insecurity and lack of safe water contribute to increased morbidity and mortality and increased risk of disease outbreaks (World Health Organization 2023). Furthermore, the violent mass casualty events in Somalia have constantly led to increased deaths and a growing number of complex trauma cases among many adults and children living in the country. Furthermore, about 64% of the population in the Federal Republic of Somalia is confronted with a lack of access to functional health facilities near where they live (Humanitarian Program Circle 2023). In addition, 27% of the estimated 13 million non-displaced persons live in urban areas, while an estimated 61%t of the population in the country need health services that they might not afford to pay out-pocket for. An estimated 35% of the non-displaced people in Somalia live in rural regions and need health assistance that is very far from where they live and there is no modern form of transportation to easily get access to hospitals or clinics (Morrison & Malik 2023).

The life expectancy at birth for females living in the Federal Republic of Somalia is reported to be 57 years in 2021, while the life expectancy of males is 55 years in 2021 (World Bank Indicators 2022; United Nations Human Development Program Index 2022). Further, the mortality rate for female adults per 1,000 people was 295 in 2021, while the mortality rate for male adults per 1,000 people was 381. Unfortunately, the mortality rate for infants per 1,000 people was 71 in 2021. In addition, the tuberculosis incidence per 100,000 people in Somalia was 250 in 2021 (World Bank Indicators 2022; United Nations Human Development Program Index 2022).

Conclusion

The chapter has examined the nature of health policies and the challenges of healthcare delivery in Somalia. It argues that now that there are no wars in Somalia, the government of the nation must endeavor to improve its health sector. This is because appropriate investment in the health sector could spell over or propel long-term benefits toward the country's economic growth and development. In addition, good investments in healthcare are likely to increase life expectancy and productivity, resulting in growth in GDP as well as social and economic development in the country (Dibie 2018; Nur 2018; World Health Organization 2021a).

To improve health outcomes with limited available resources, targeted, cost-effective investments in health services are critical. This would include a package of high-impact, cost-effective interventions that target the primary burdens of disease—family planning; maternal health and newborn health; malaria; HIV/AIDS; immunization; and child health, with nutrition. The government should use any gains from debt relief to increase health budgets significantly and progressively from the 2% pre-COVID-19 allocation with the aim of ultimately hitting the 15% of the annual budget in line with the Abuja Declaration, which it has signed up to (Amnesty International 2021).

The government must be mindful that without an adequate healthcare workforce, drugs, and other medical supplies there can be no healthcare system. It should be noted that local production of drugs could enhance the self-sufficiency of medicine and the avoidance of dependency. Increasing the salary and benefits and providing better working conditions for medical doctors and nurses could help to retain them from living in Somalia for foreign countries. Further, adopting performance-related rewards would appeal to doctors, nurses, and other health workforce personnel who are looking for a competitive advantage in a disjointed environment such as the Federal Republic of Somalia.

In addition, efforts to translate traditional medicine and the use of plants should be galvanized by investing in research that is associated with medicinal plants as well as sources for materials that could propel local production of drugs in the country. Thus, the government and its Ministry of Health and Human Services should formulate health policies that could ensure the citizens' right to access adequate health facilities wherever they live across the country. Collaboration with foreign healthcare providers and organizations to seek more funding and modern health equipment is paramount for the future success and economic development of Somalia. Furthermore, collaboration with international institutions to build teaching and research universities in the country could revamp the training of physicians and nurses in Somalia. This set of health workforce development training in the country could propel adequate and equitable high-quality healthcare treatment for citizens living in urban and rural areas in the country.

Future strategic plans in Somalia should explore not only universal health insurance, but more efforts should also be made to privatize the healthcare system in the country in the near future. The benefit of privatization of the health system in any country includes an opportunity for the private sector to contribute more funding for building modern health infrastructure as well as enhancing medical equipment in the country. Furthermore, promoting healthy behavior is another strategy that could be used by the government to galvanize safe and healthy lifestyles and social services.

Finally, adopting more use of medical information technology could enhance the management of the health systems in Somalia. This is because the use of modern information technology could make it very easy to communicate and transfer patients medical records, conduct data analysis, conduct fast treatment payment, X-ray, scanning, digital therapeutic treatment, data-driven capacity, health diagnosis, wearable devices, telehealth, telemedicine, and radiographic analysis. In addition, information technology can be used as a mechanism for digital solutions that could enhance people to better manage their healthcare. All these benefits of information technology could enhance the management of the health systems in Somalia. Furthermore, information technology will also facilitate better communication between the federal and state levels sharing of data as well as developing an effective regulatory framework that is very crucial for improving the healthcare system in the country.

References

Abdillahi F. A., Ismail E. A., Singh S. P. (2020). Mental health in Somaliland: A critical situation. *BJ Psychology International*, 17(1): 11–14.

Abdirahman Elmi M., Hashi A. O., Dahir U. M., Abdirahman A. A., Romo Rodriguez O. E. (2024). Electronics in healthcare: adaptation and challenges of digital records in Somali hospitals, SSRG *International Journal of Electronics and Communication Engineering*, 11(9): 1–10.

Ahmad, M., Ahmed, I., Jeon, G. A. (2022). Sustainable advanced artificial intelligence-based framework for analysis of COVID-19 spread. *Environment, Development and Sustainability*. DOI: 10.1007/s10668-022-02584-0.

Ahmed Z., Ataullahjan A., Gaffey M. F. et al. (2020). Understanding the factors affecting the humanitarian health and nutrition response for women and children in Somalia since 2000: A case study. *Conflict Health*, 14(35): 1–19.

Aljazeera News (2016). Somalia: The forgotten story. https://www.aljazeera.com/program/al-jazeera-world/2016/11/2/somalia-the-forgotten-story. Accessed September 15, 2023.

American Broadcasting Corporation (ABC) News (2001). Somalia timeline: October 25. https://abcnews.go.com/International/story?id=80454&page=. Accessed November 10, 2024.

Amnesty International (2021). Amnesty International Report 2021/22: The state of the world's human rights. https://www.amnesty.org/en/documents/pol10/4870/2022/en/#:~:text=The%20　Amnesty%20International%20Report%202021,in%20the%20corridors%20of%20power. Accessed November 11, 2024.

Amnesty International (2022). Amnesty International Report 2022/23: The state of the world's human rights. https://www.amnesty.org/en/documents/pol10/5670/2023/en/#:~:text=10%2F5670%2F2023-,Amnesty%20International%20Report. Accessed October 31, 2022.

Bilal N. K. (2023). Somalia health: every child has the right to survive and thrive. https://www.unicef.org/somalia/health. Accessed September 13, 2023.

Bile K., Warsame M., Ahmed A. D. (2022). Fragile states need essential national health research: The case of Somalia. https://www.thelancet.com/journals/langlo/article/PIIS2214-109X(22)00122-X/fulltext#back-bib2. Accessed September 13, 2023.

Country Economy (1999). Somalia: Government health expenditure. https://countryeconomy.com/government/expenditure/health/Somalia. Accessed September 15, 2023.

Dalmar A. A., Hussein A. S., Walhad S. A. et al. (2017). Rebuilding research capacity in fragile states: The case of a Somali–Swedish global health initiative. *Global Health Action*. 101348693.
Dibie R. (2018). *Business and Government Relations in Africa*. New York: Routlege Press.
Dibie R. (2022). Healthcare policy and administration in Nigeria: A critical analysis. *The Journal of African Policy Studies*, 28(1): 70–101.
Encyclopedia (2020). History of Somalia. https://www.nationsencyclopedia.com/Africa/Somalia-HISTORY.html#ixzz8DJOrjkJK.
Farah A. M, Ruhela S. P. (1993). *Somalia: From the Dawn of Civilization to the Modern Times*. India: Vikas Publishing House PVT LTD.
Farah A. A., Sh-Ahmed A. M., Hersi I. M., Swed S., Sharif-Ahmed E. M., Hasan M. M., Motawea K. R., Ahmed S. M. A., Shoib S. (2022). Double burden on health services in Somalia due to COVID-19 and conflict. *Annals of Medicine and Surgery (London)*, 79: 103968. DOI: 10.1016/j.amsu.2022.103968.
Federal Government of Somalia (2012). *Mental Health Policy. Ministry of Health and Human Services*. Mogadishu: Government Press.
Federal Government of Somalia (2020). The Somalia national medicine policy. https://moh.gov.so/en/wp-content/uploads/2020/07/Somalia-National-medicine-policy-2014.pdf. Accessed March 14, 2024.
Federal Government of Somalia (2021). *Somalia Health Sector Strategic Plan 2020–2026. Ministry of Health and Human Services*. Mogadishu: Government Press.
Federal Government of Somalia, Ministry of Health, and Human Services (2014a). *Somalia Health Policy: The Way Forward*. Mogadishu, Somalia: Government Press.
Federal Government of Somalia, Ministry of Health, and Human Services (2014b). *Somalia Health Policy: The Way Forward*. Mogadishu, Somalia: Government Press.
Gele A. (2020). Challenges facing the health system in Somalia and implications for achieving the SDGs. *European Journal of Public Health*, 30(5): 1–13.
Hassan K. I., Filiz E. (2022). Impact of Covid-19 pandemic on health system in Somalia. *Selcuk Soglik Dergisi*, 3(2): 192–204.
Healy S., Bradbury M. (2010). Endless war: A brief history of the Somalia conflict. https://www.c-r.org/accord/somalia/endless-war-brief-history-somali-conflict. Accessed August 30, 2023.
Humanitarian Program Circle (2023). Humanitarian needs overview Somalia. https://crisisresponse.iom.int/sites/g/files/tmzbdl1481/files/appeal/documents/20230208_Somalia%20_HNO_2023.pdf. Accessed September 16, 2023.
Ibrahim M. (2021). COVID-19 in Africa one year on: Impact and prospects. https://mo.ibrahim.foundation/sites/default/files/2021-06/2021-forum-report.pdf. Accessed November 11, 2024.
Ibrahim O. A., Belley-Côté E. P., McIntyre W. F. (2022). Letter by Ibrahim et al Regarding Article, "Anterior-Lateral Versus Anterior-Posterior Electrode Position for Cardioverting Atrial Fibrillation." *Circulation*. 145(21):e1056. DOI: 10.1161/CIRCULATIONAHA.122.059061.
Ingiriis M. H. (2018). *From Pre-Colonial Past to the Post-Colonial Present: The Contemporary Clan-Based Configurations of State Building in Somalia*. London, England: Cambridge University Press.
International Committee of the Red Cross (2022). ICRC health response in Somalia. https://www.icrc.org/en/document/icrc-health-response-somalia. Accessed September 14, 2023.
Issa-Salwe, Abdisalam M. (1996). *The Collapse of the Somali State: The Impact of the Colonial Legacy*. London: Haan Associates. pp. 34–35.
Jeene H. (2017). Strengthening affordable access to quality essential medicines in the private health sector of Somalia. https://www.researchgate.net/publication/318015862. Accessed September 20, 2023.
Khayre A. A. M., (2016). Somalia: An overview of the historical and current situation. https://ssrn.com/abstract=2771125 or http://dx.doi.org/10.2139/ssrn.2771125. Accessed September 19, 2024.
Knofczynski A. (2017). Improving response to common diseases in Somalia. https://borgenpproject.org/response-common-diseases-in-Somalia/. Accessed September 16, 2023.
Lewis I. M. (1965). The Modern History of Somaliland: From Nation to State. F. A. Praeger. p. 37.

Lewis I. M. (2015). *The Modern History of Somalia.* Boulder, CO: Westview Press.

Maruf H. (2023). Study: Somali people highly traumatized' after years of conflict. https://www. voanews.com/a/somali-people-highly-traumatized-after-years-of-conflict/6923368.html. Accessed September 20, 2023.

Mohamud K. B. (2021). Somali Health Action Journal–A collaborative venture for health research and development. *Somali Health Action Journal.* DOI: 10.36368/shaj.vli1.262

Mohamed K. B., Emmelin M., Freij L. et al. (2022). Who published what on Somali health issues? Forming the policy for SHAJ through a bibliometric study. *Somali Health Action.* DOI: 10.36368/shaj.v2i1.281.

Morrison J., Malik S.M. M. R. (2023). Population health trends and disease profile in Somalia 1990–2019, and projection to 2030: ill the country achieve sustainable development goals 2 and 3? *BMC Public Health,* 23(1):66–79.

Muchena D. (2021). Amnesty International's Director for East and Southern Africa. https:// www.icrc.org/en/document/icrc-health-response-somalia. Accessed September 14, 2023.

Njoku R. C. (2013). *The History of Somalia.* Santa Barbara, CA: Greenwood Press.

Nur, Y. (2018). *Business and Government Relations in Somalia. In Business and Government Relations in Africa edited by Robert Dibie.* New York: Routledge Press, pp. 147–161.

Office of the Historian, United States Department of State (2023). A guide to the United States' History Recognition, Diplomatic, and Consular Relations, by country, since 1777: Somalia. https://history.state.gov/countries/somalia. Accessed September 14, 2023.

Omer A. I., Ali F. A., Mohamu'd A. O., Osman S. M., Ibrahim M. A. (2018). Perceived quality of tuberculosis treatment services from patient perspectives in selected Tb management units, Mogadishu-Somalia. *Somali Journal of Medicine & Health Sciences,* 3(1): 1–14.

Osman A. N. (2022). Somalia's healthcare system: The current landscape and the solutions we need. https://www.garoweonline.com/en/opinions/somalia-s-healthcare-system-the-current-landscape-and-the-solutions-we-need. Accessed September 20, 2023.

Oyella S. (2022). Somalia: UN expert warns health care standards "dangerously low. https:// www.ohchr.org/en/press-releases/2022/04/somalia-un-expert-warns-health-care-standards-dangerously-low. Accessed September 13, 2023.

Qayad M. G. (2008). Healthcare services in transitional Somalia: Challenges and Recommendations. https://digitalcommons.macalester.edu /cgi/viewcontent.cgi?article=1069&context=bildhaan. Accessed September 19, 2024.

Said, A. et al. (2021). One more of life's difficulties: the impacts of Covid-19 on livelihoods in Somalia. Retrieved from Supporting Pastoralism and Agriculture in Recurrent and Protracted Crises: https://www.sparc-knowledge.org/news-features/features/one-more-lifes-difficulties-impacts-covid-19-livelihoods-somalia.

Samartzis L, Talias M. A. (2020). Assessing and improving the quality in mental health services. *International Journal of Environmental Research and Public Health.* 17(1):249. DOI:10.3390/ ijerph17010249.

Schuchman D. M., McDonald C. (2004). Somali mental health. *Bildhaan: An International Journal of Somali Studies.* https://ethnomed.org/resource/somali-mental-health/. Accessed September 19, 2023.

Steele C. M., Peladeau-Pigeon M., Barbon C. A. E., Guida B. T., Namasivayam-MacDonald A. M., Nascimento W. V., Smaoui S., Tapson M. S., Valenzano T. J., Waito A. A., Wolkin T. S. (2019). Reference values for healthy swallowing across the range from thin to extremely thick liquids. *Journal of Speech, Language, and Hearing Research.* 62(5):1338–1363.

Somalia Ministry of Health, and Human Services (2014). The Somalia National Medicine Policy. https://moh.gov.so/en/wp-content/uploads/2020/07/Somalia-National-medicine-policy-2014.pdf. Accessed October 31, 2024.

Tran N. T., Mayers J., Malilo B., Chabo J., Muselemu J., Riziki B., Libongo P., Shire A., Had H., Ali M., Kahow M. H., Adive J. E., Gabru B., Monaghan E., Morris C. N., Gallagher M., Jouanicot V., Pougnier N., Amsalu R. (2021). Strengthening health systems in humanitarian settings: Multi-stakeholder insights on contraception and postabortion. *Care rogram in the Democratic Republic of Congo and Somalia*, 2(1). https://www.frontiersin.org/journals/global-womens-health/articles/10.3389/fgwh.2021.671058/full Accessed September 19, 2023.

United Nations Human Development Program Index (2022). Human development report. https://hdr.undo.org/en/2022-report. Accessed September 16, 2023.

United Nations (2020a). Permanent mission of the Somali Republic to the United Nations. https://www.un.int/somalia/somalia/country-facts. Accessed September 14, 2023.

United Nations (2020b). Inter-agency group for child mortality estimation. child mortality Estimates: 2020. https://childmortality.org/data/Somalia. Accessed September 19, 2023.

United States Department of State (2023). Somalia health. https://travel.state.gov/content/travel/en/international-travel/International-Travel-Country-Information-Pages/Somalia.html. Accessed September 20, 2023.

University of Central Arkansas (2023). Somalia 1960 to present. https://uca.edu/politicalscience/home/research-projects/dadm-project/sub-saharan-africa-region/somalia-1960-present/. Accessed September 15, 2023.

Wikipedia (2023). History of Somalia. https://en.wikipedia.org/wiki/history_of_Somalia. Accessed September 14, 2023.

World Bank Indicators (2022). Somalia. https://data.worldbank.org/indicator/NY.GDP.MKTP.CD.Locations=CM Accessed September 16, 2023.

World Health Organization (2021a). Somalia economic update: Investing in health to anchor growth. https://www.worldbank.org/en/country/somalia/publication/somalia-economic-update-investing-in-health-to-anchor-growth. Accessed September 13, 2023.

World Health Organization (2021b). Investing in mental health in Somalia: Harnessing community mental health services through task shifting. http://www.emro.who.int/images/stories/somalia/documents/policy_brief_mental_health.pdf?ua=1. Accessed September 21, 2023.

World Health Organization (2023). Somalia country data. https://www.who.int/data/gho/data/countries/country-details/GHO/somalia?countryProfileId=79e4cda0-11b1-4806-9c63-d40904289ced. Accessed August 16, 2023.

World Health Organization (WHO) (2023a). WHO in Somalia: Essential medicines and pharmaceutical policies. https://www.emro.who.int/somalia/priority-areas/essential-medicines-and-pharmaceutical-policies.html. Accessed September 21, 2023.

World Health Organization (2023b). WHO helps Somalia establish a functional medical supply chain as part of resilience-building for the health system. https://www.emro.who.int/somalia/news/who-helps-somalia-establish-a-functional-medical-supply-chain-as-part-of-resilience-building-for-health-system.html. Accessed September 19, 2023.

Yenet A., Nibret G., Tegegne B. A. (2023). Challenges to the availability and affordability of essential medicines in African countries: A scoping review. *Clinicoecon Outcomes Research*, 13(15):443–458.

Chapter Fifteen

HEALTH POLICY ANALYSIS IN SOUTH AFRICA

Kealeboga Maphunye and Robert Dibie

Introduction

This chapter examines the nature of health policy and the challenges of healthcare delivery in South Africa. It argues that although the government of South Africa has been preparing to adopt universal health coverage that could ensure access to affordable healthcare, the challenges of racial and economic disparities in the country may prevent the attainment of the proposed goal of the policy initiatives. Further, since 1994, the government of South Africa has enacted health policies such as the National Health Policy, and National Health Insurance Policy and has recently proposed to formulate Universal Health Coverage without focusing on how to de-escalate the challenges of mixed success. Thus, equitable, affordable, and high-quality health coverage cannot be accomplished in the future without solving the current healthcare disparities predicament. The research method adopted for this research involved interviews and the administration of a questionnaire to 1,648 respondents such as public sector staff, nongovernmental organizations employees, traders, academic staff, law enforcement personnel, unemployed citizens, and community and provincial health practitioners. Interviews with 273 respondents, including officials of public and private sectors as well as foreign NGO stakeholders were conducted. The secondary research methods adopted included the review of the reports of the National Department of Health in South Africa, the World Health Organization white papers, the United Nations Human Development annual report, the Center for Disease Control, and academic as well as professional journal articles. Data were analyzed using SPSS to determine the effectiveness and challenges facing the health policy and quality of the healthcare delivery system in South Africa. The finding of this research reveals that despite the new policy initiatives adopted by the government of South Africa, health services are still falling below the basic standards of patients' expectations because they are highly fragmented with discriminatory effects and disparities between urban and rural regions. Moreover, there are glaring differences even between urban and peri-urban areas that are usually attributed to South Africa's apartheid-derived racial and socioeconomic inequalities. In addition, improvement initiatives were not able to produce the expected high-quality healthcare services that citizens or patients desired due to a lack of resources, and enough trained medical doctors as well as avoidable errors, shortage of resources in medicine and medical technology, and poor record keeping. It is recommended that decentralization policies must be implemented cautiously after confirmation that there is sufficient managerial capacity at district or provincial levels. Further, senior health officials and physicians must be held accountable (i.e., consequence management) when they fail to deliver quality healthcare as required by their job description in the country.

Brief History of South Africa

The Republic of South Africa is a country on the southernmost tip of the African continent. The nation has boundaries with countries such as Botswana to the north, and Lesotho, the enclave territory next to the southwestern province of South Africa called the Free State. Further, Mozambique and Swaziland are to the southeast, while the Republic of Namibia is to the northwest. The Republic of South Africa also has a boundary with the Democratic Republic of Zimbabwe to the northeastern (GlobalEdge 2022). The southern and eastern parts of South Africa are bordered by the Indian Ocean, while the southwestern part of the country has a boundary with the Atlantic Ocean (Dibie 2018; GlobalEdge 2023). The ecosystem of the country is unique in that it has a plateau covering the largest part of the land. The unique plateau which covers most parts of the eastern part of South Africa extends downwards from a height of more than 8,000 meters to about 2,000 meters in the sandy Kalahari Desert (Britannica 2022; British Broadcasting Corporation Report 2022). In addition, the Western Cape offers several internationally renowned beaches, lush winelands around Stellenbosch and Paarl, craggy cliffs at the Cape of Good Hope, forest and lagoons along the Garden Route, and the city of Cape Town, beneath the flat-topped Table Mountain (GlobalEdge 2022).

The nation now called South Africa has a very interesting history before it became a republic that now practices a democratic system of government. The current territory called South Africa was known as the Union of South Africa by British colonies of the Cape and Natal, the Boer republics of Transvaal, and Orange Free State (British Broadcasting Corporation Report 2022). Consequently, in 1910, two formal British colonies namely the Cape and Natal, and the Boer Republic of Transvaal and Orange Free State consolidated to become the Union of South Africa. Further, in 1934, the status of the Union Act was enacted by the parliament to constitute it as a new sovereign independent country.

Further, in 1948, a policy of apartheid that separated the original Black citizens and white owners of the nation was promulgated when the White National Party (NP) took over the governance of the former colony called the Union of South Africa. As a result of the separateness policies adopted by the White National Party to discriminate against the original black owners of the nation, health, education, social welfare, water, and sanitation including virtually all private and public services were racially segregated, with black people receiving the worst treatment at the bottom of the country's White, Colored, Indian, and Black population classification system. Subsequently, 70 black demonstrators were brutally killed in a black township (an area demarcated for the black population in apartheid South Africa) called Sharpeville in 1960 (British Broadcasting Corporation Report 2022). This brutality was also visited upon black communities in Langa, Nyanga (near Cape Town), including Cato Manor near Durban (Natal). Unfortunately, another 600 black citizens of South Africa were killed in clashes between them and white security forces in Soweto. Because of the brutal killing that took place in South Africa, many world leaders and the United Nations declared apartheid as a Crime Against Humanity in 1966 (Davids et al. 2005; Mandela 2013).

The world leaders condemned the apartheid regime and placed sanctions on the leaders and economy of the country. Through international pressure and internal resistance by the oppressed black population, such actions forced the white regime to engage in negotiations to bring apartheid to an end between 1991 and 1994 (British Broadcasting Corporation Report 2022). In April 1994, the negotiations ended, and the first nonracial and truly democratic election was conducted for the first time with an oversight role by international election observers (Dovlo 2009). In addition, the formation of a government of national unity under President Nelson Rolihlahla Mandela's leadership was adopted (Britannica 2022, Mandela 2013).

In 1989, the former President of South Africa FW De-Klerk promulgated a liberalized reforms policy that included the lifting of the ban on the African National Congress, Pan-African National Congress including several formerly outlawed anti-colonial and anti-apartheid organizations, and the release of all political prisoners including Nelson Mandela after serving 27 years in jail for protesting against the apartheid that was practice by the Dutch White colonial regimes (1948–1994). During Nelson Mandela's 27 years imprisonment, it was reported that he rejected at least three conditional offers of release (Mandela 2013). He constantly engaged in various political and anti-apartheid talks to end white minority rule in South Africa. In addition, in 1991, Mandela was unanimously elected ANC President to replace his ailing friend, Oliver Tambo. Further, due to his diligent campaign to end the apartheid regime in South Africa, Nelson Mandela and former apartheid President FW de Klerk jointly won the Nobel Peace Prize in 1993. A year later, Mandela and millions of previously disenfranchised black South African citizens were allowed to vote for the first time in their lives on April 27, 1994 (Mandela 2013). History was made when Nelson Mandela was inaugurated as the first black South African democratically elected President on May 10, 1994, after decades of white rule. What is unique about President Mandela is that, unlike other African leaders, he stepped down after one term (four years) as President of his country. In addition, he forgave his political enemies when he agreed to work with them to form an inclusive Government of National Unity. After President Mandela stepped down from his position, he went on to establish the Nelson Mandela Children's Fund in 1995 (Mandela 2013) and the Nelson Mandela Children's Hospital. After a trailblazer leader's values and accomplishments, President Mandela died in December 2013 at his home in Johannesburg (Mandela 2013).

The current president of South Africa is Cyril Matamela Ramaphosa. President Ramaphosa, Mandela's third successor, was elected president by the parliament of the country in February 2018 after his predecessor Mr. Jacob Zuma (Mandela's second successor) resigned because of corruption allegations and several lawsuits (British Broadcasting Corporation Report 2022).

In addition, the Republic of South Africa is endowed with many human, natural, and mineral resources. In 1867, diamonds were discovered in the Kimberley region and subsequently, the Kimberley mines started producing 95% of the world's diamonds. Subsequently, in 1886, one of the world's largest gold deposit regions was discovered in the Witwatersrand region (present-day Johannesburg). The South African five major gold mines include the Driefontein Mine, the Kloof gold mine: the Impala Gold Mine, the South Deep Gold Mine, and the Tshepong Gold Mine (GlobalData 2022). Further, South Africa also has five major coal mines, the Grootgeluk mine located in Limpopo, the New Vaal mine located in the Free State, Wolvekrans Middelburg complex mine, the Syerfontein mine and the Kriel mine (Mining Technology 2022). According to the British Broadcasting Corporation Report (2022), these mineral resources became the trajectory of South Africa's dynamic economic development, major industrial sectors, health system, and avenue for international trade.

Adverse Effects of the Apartheid Regime on Healthcare

The oppression of the black citizens and the original owners of the South African land as well as the massive killing of indigenous people whenever they protested the apartheid regime did not resonate well with the rest of the world. The brutality that took place led to several protests in many countries (Davids et al. 2005; Mandela 2013). Black people in the United States, Canada, Brazil, and Western European countries also protested and called for their respective nations' governments to sanction the white apartheid regime in South Africa. Because of the constant high levels of protests around the world against the South African government's apartheid policies in the 1960s, 1970s, and 1980s, several sanctions were imposed on the white government of South Africa by the international community (Mandela 2013). The government of South Africa was also expelled from international organizations (British Broadcasting Corporation Report 2022). Many multinational companies also divested their operations and businesses in South Africa because of the oppressive apartheid policies of the countries against their black citizens (Baker et al. 2010; Maphumulo & Bhengu 2019).

The healthcare system during the apartheid regime discriminated against not only the black people in the country, but citizens of mixed race, and Indians as well (Baker et al. 2010). Baker et al. (2010) and Chassin and Loeb (2013) contend that the South African white apartheid government created 10 ethnic territories in which the black citizens were segregated. Further, each of these 10 Bantustan ethnic territories had their health departments that were poorly funded and equipped. The discriminatory disparities between hospitals and health clinics in white towns and black territories with respect to funding, medical equipment, infrastructure, and workforce led to very poor healthcare services and an unnecessarily high death rate of black citizens (Baker et al. 2010; Maphumulo & Bhengu 2019). To further compound the healthcare problems, there was an unequal distribution of doctors and nurses in the white towns during the apartheid regime compared to the black territories (How South Africa stumbles on health care for all 2017). These malicious practices caused black people in South Africa to suffer from mental and physical exhaustion as well as deterioration of medical conditions and sometimes death (Chassin & Loeb 2013; Maphumulo & Bhengu 2019; Twala 2014). Moreover, the health conditions of Black, and Indian people were relatively poor compared to those experienced by Whites, who continuously enjoyed the greatest slice of the health and other public service budgets in the country.

Major Health Policies Enacted in South Africa

The South Government of South Africa's Constitution stipulates the obligation of the government to provide affordable healthcare for all its citizens (Maphumulo & Bhengu 2019). During the past 30 years (1994–2024), the healthcare system has incrementally improved in respect of safety, equality of delivery, and access to a wider group of citizens unlike four decades ago during the apartheid regime (Pauw 2022; Maphunye 2006).

The provision of healthcare and the implementation of laws and regulations governing health practices in South Africa is the function of both the National Department of Health and provincial governments (Dibie 2022). The health policies that have been enacted in the country are assigned to the National Ministry of Health for the purpose of issuing and promoting compliance with all policies. The National Department of Health provides the guidelines and the implementation procedures for all health policies that are enacted by the National Health Council of South Africa (Republic of South Africa, National Department of Health Annual Report 2021–2022).

Table 1 shows the most important health policies that the Government of South Africa has enacted since 1994.

Table 1 Major Types of Health Policy Enacted in South Africa

	Title of Health Policy	Year Enacted	Goal of Health Policy
1	Medicines and Related Substances Act	1965	Provides for the monitoring, evaluation, investigation, inspection, and control of medicines
2	Occupational Diseases in Mines and Works Act	1973	Responsible for the payment of benefits to workers and ex-workers in controlled mines suffering from cardiopulmonary diseases because of work exposures.
3	Health Professions Act	1974	Regulates the health professionals registered under the Health Professions Act.
4	Pharmacy Act	1974	Regulates the pharmacy profession with registered pharmacy professionals and pharmacies as well as ensuring good pharmacy practice.

(Continued)

Table 1 (*Continued*)

	Title of Health Policy	Year Enacted	Goal of Health Policy
5	Dental Technicians Act	1979	Regulates the professions of dental technicians and dental technologists
6	Allied Health Professions Act	1982	Regulates allied or complementary health professors facing within the mandate of the council.
7	National Policy for Health Act	1990	Enhanced healthcare standards and provide adequate healthcare for all citizens regardless of their race in South Africa
8	South African Medical Research Council	1991	Mandated to improve the health and quality of life through research, development, and technology transfer
9	Occupational and Safety Act	1993	Promote the safety and health of workers at the workplace in South Africa
10	Primary Health Care Act	1994	Promote the goal of delivering healthcare sufficiently to all citizens in urban and rural
11	Medical Schemes Act	1998	Regulates the Medical Scheme Industry
12	National Health Laboratory Service	2000	Provides cost-effective laboratory services to all public sector healthcare providers
13	National Health Act	2003	Monitors and enforces the compliance of health establishments with the prescribed norms and standards of healthcare.
14	Nursing Council Act	2005	Regulates the nursing profession by establishing and maintaining nursing education and training as well as practice standards
15	Traditional Health Practitioners Act	2007	Regulates traditional health practice and traditional health practitioners including students engaged in learning traditional health practice in South Africa
16	National Health Insurance	2019	Improving access to quality healthcare and creating public funds for all health services

Sources: Republic of South Africa, National Department of Health Annual Report (2021–2022). Pretoria, Townland 351-JR: Government Press.

The Republic of South Africa's Constitution contains the Bill of Rights, which mandates the government to ensure the rights of all citizens to have access to healthcare services in the country (Republic of South Africa, National Department of Health Annual Report 2021–2022; Stewart & Wolvardt 2019). These multiple policies also entail the guidance and mandates that were given to the National Department of Health to enforce the implementation of almost all the healthcare policies in the country (Laitinen et al. 2019; Malema & Muthelo 2018). Many scholars contend that the Government of South Africa has accomplished many of its healthcare policy goals (Columbia Public Health 2023; Hlafa et al. 2019; Malakoane et al. 2020; Stewart & Wolvaardt 2019). It should be noted however, that despite the strategic national health policies enacted it was mostly at the provincial and municipal levels of government that implemented the health policies in the country (Maphumulo & Bhengu 2019; Pauw 2022).

While the National Health Policy was enacted in 1994 to provide healthy lifestyles for all citizens of South Africa, the healthcare provision was divided between the private and public sectors. According to the South African National Treasury Report (2021), the government often allocates about 12% of its GDP to the private sector which supports just 16% of the population, while the public sector provides healthcare for the remaining 84% of the citizens of the country that rely on the poorly managed health system (Burger & Christian 2018; Mitchel et al. 2020; National Treasury 2021; World Bank Indicators 2023). To correct the current challenges in the health system in South Africa, the national government is proposing to formulate a National Health Insurance in 2026 (Conmy 2018; South Africa Government 2023; Michel et al. 2019).

Health Administration in South Africa

The health system in South Africa constitutes both the private and public sectors (Government of South Africa 2022; Michel et al. 2019). It is reported that the public sector provides about 86% of the health services to the citizens of the country while the private sector covers the remaining 14% (Government of South Africa 2016). Further, the public and private sectors of the health system are divided along socioeconomic classifications (Malakoane et al. 2020). On the other hand, the poor and those who cannot afford to pay for health insurance normally seek healthcare from public health hospitals and clinics (Stewart & Wolvaardt 2019). Unfortunately, these disparities in health delivery in the country contribute to the difference in the quality of healthcare between services provided by both the private and public sectors (Stewart & Wolvaardt 2019; Zwarenstein 1994).

The National Department of Health manages the administration of the public health system. Further, the nation's governance is divided into nine provincial governments. Each of the provinces has its own Department of Health that engages in the delivery of healthcare. The nine provincial departments of health are mandated to engage in the promotion of preventive health services, as well as healthy lifestyles (Britnell 2015; Hlafa et al. 2019; Stewart & Wolvaardt 2019).

The public health system in South Africa is divided into three subsectors: (a) the primary sector; (b) the secondary sector; and (c) the tertiary sector. The *primary sector* constitutes over 2,300 clinics. According to the Government of South Africa report (2022), the tertiary sector provides health services to citizens in various locations. The tertiary sector is managed by different provincial health departments that are supervised by the National Department of Health (Britnell 2015; Malakoane et al. 2020).

The *second-tier sector* is the secondary or district hospitals. They are bigger in nature in all their operations than what is available at the primary tier (Government of South Africa, National Department of Health 2021, Michel et al. 2019). Unlike the primary tier sector, the district tier could conduct patient tests and some level of procedures. The district tiers also have specialist doctors and nurse practitioners who could support physicians perform medical procedures.

The tertiary sector hospitals are much bigger in nature than the primary and district clinics and hospitals. Their infrastructure is huge hospitals and operates with advanced technology and research centers (Britnell 2015). The nature of the kind of health services that they provide requires the tertiary hospital to be fully staffed by specialist doctors who perform major surgeries (Maphumulo & Bhengu 2019; Michel et al. 2019). In addition, some of the major challenges in the implementation of the healthcare policies in the country are affiliated with the difference in approach to management as well as the caliber of leadership approach in both the public and private sectors in the country (Stewart & Wolvaardt 2019).

The Government of South Africa through its National Department of Health subsidizes the public health system in the country. It is reported that the public health system tends to be unfunded by the government (Burger & Christian 2018; Michel et al. 2019; Muller 2020). Further, the larger regional hospitals are under the administration of the various provincial health departments. There are also smaller primary care clinics and hospitals that are managed at the municipal government level in South Africa (Burger & Christian 2018; Pauw 2021).

According to Michel et al. (2019) and Stewart and Wolvaardt (2019), while the public sector management of the health system has been characterized as having poorly skilled managers the (usually white-dominated) private sector has embraced competent and highly professional health specialists. Bureaucratic idiosyncrasy which allows nurses to be clinical managers instead of specialist doctors, has constituted a model that puts political patronage about human rights to better healthcare in South Africa (Crush & Tawodzera 2014; Stewart & Wolvaardt 2019. Since 1994, the Republic of South Africa's Government has used structural intervention, legal, and social programs, and fiscal and monetary policies to galvanize the redistribution and healthcare delivery initiatives in the country (Bloch 2010; Government of South Africa report 2022; Pauw 2022; Stewart & Wolvaardt 2019).

Traditional Medicine

In addition to the primary tier, district tier, and tertiary sectors the Republic of South Africa Government recognizes the vitality of traditional medicine. Historically most people in rural areas who could not afford the cost of modern healthcare depended on traditional medicine. Because this historical practice of healthcare provided my traditional healer the Government of South Africa enacted the Traditional Health Practitioners Act of 2007 (Republic of South Africa, National Department of Health Annual Report 2021–2022). It is estimated that over 80% of the population of South Africa depends on the services of traditional medicine practitioners in one form or the other (Michel et al. 2019).

The common treatments provided by traditional healers in the country include chiropractic medicine, homeopathy, naturopathy, and osteopathy. Further, licensed traditional healers are required to have specified qualifications from the government agency that regulates the group (Pauw 2022). Those who seek treatment from traditional healers must pay out of pocket for their respective treatment (Maphumulo & Bhengu 2019; Ned et al. 2017; Zubane 2011). In addition, the provisions of the Traditional Health Practitioners Policy of 2017 seem not to be appropriate for the more formalized group of people who practice herbalism. The policy requirement of grade 3 school level and at least 25 years of age for those who practice traditional medicine in the rural setting cannot be effectively regulated in South Africa (Grag & Vawda 2018).

Data Analysis of Health Policy Effectiveness

The data used for the analysis of healthcare policy effectiveness were derived from both primary and secondary sources. The research involves the administration of a questionnaire to 1648 respondents such as public sector staff, nongovernmental organizations' employees, traders, academic staff, law enforcement personnel, unemployed citizens, and community and provincial health practitioners. Interviews with 273 respondents, including officials of public and private sectors as well as foreign NGO stakeholders were conducted. The secondary research methods adopted include the review of the National Department of Health in South Africa reports, the World Health Organization white papers, the United Nations Human Development annual report, the Center for Disease Control, and academic as well as professional journal articles. Data were analyzed using SPSS to determine the effectiveness and challenges facing the health policy and quality of the healthcare delivery system in South Africa.

The questionnaire respondents constitute 1252.5 (76%) men and 395.5 (24%) women. Further, 73% of the respondents were single, while 21.2% were married. The remaining 5.35 of the questionnaire respondents were divorced. In addition, 30% of the respondents had completed a high-school diploma, while 67% held a bachelor's degree. Only 2% of the respondents held a master's degree. It was only 1% of the questionnaire respondents that received a doctoral degree. In addition, 58% of the respondents had visited a hospital or clinic to receive treatment at least twice a year before or during the study. Another 26% had also visited a hospital to between 2 and 4 times recently to receive treatment. While 10% of the respondents had visited a clinic or hospital 5–6 times in the previous year to receive some form of treatment, only 6% of them had visited a hospital over 7 times to receive treatment from a physician. Table 2 addresses the first research question.

Research question 1: What are your experiences during the last few times that you have visited a hospital to receive healthcare?

Table 2 questionnaire data reveal that 59.7% of the respondents indicated that hospitals and health centers in South Africa constantly have electricity supply in the country. Further, 58.9% of the respondents stated that they were satisfied with the type of healthcare that they received from either hospitals or health clinics in the country. In addition, 55.3% of the respondents acknowledged that the competencies and skills of medical practitioners "in my town hospital" were very good. Another 55% also confirmed that the hospitals and health centers in the city where they reside were particularly good. On one hand, 74.7% of the respondents indicated that they preferred to receive their healthcare in South Africa, while only 40.8% of the respondents stated that they were not satisfied with the kind of healthcare provided in the country.

There were respondents who expressed some concern about the type of healthcare services that they had received. For example, 59.8% of the respondents indicated that many hospitals and health centers "in their rural town" do not have modern equipment. Another 54% of the respondents also stated that the cost of healthcare in South Africa is not reasonable. A closely related concern expressed by 53.8% of the respondents is that they cannot afford the cost of healthcare and medication in the country without subsidies from the government. It should be noted, that only 47.7% of the respondents confirmed that they could afford the cost of their healthcare in South Africa. It is interesting to note that 52.2% of the respondents acknowledged that most doctors and nurses in their city hospitals are not caring and friendly to their patients. It was also reported by 76.2% of the respondents that many hospitals and health centers "in their country" do not provide emergency services. These experiences of the respondents were observed during the field research in most of the rural health centers. Furthermore, while the average positive experience of the healthcare system in South Africa was 50.5%, the average disagree factor of experiences of the respondents was 49%.

Table 2 confirms that most of the citizens of South Africa have a lot of positive experiences whenever they visit the hospitals and healthcare centers in the country. Thus, the healthcare policies formulated and implemented in South Africa are effective but do not meet the health needs of all the citizens in the country satisfactorily, especially those living the rural areas, and the poor residents of the country.

Table 3 provides a summary of what the respondents think are the major government roles in the provision of affordable healthcare in South Africa. Questionnaire questions 19–28 offer an overview of what the citizens of South Africa think about the role of the government in the provision of affordable healthcare in the country. Table 3 addresses research question 2:

Research question 2: What are the major government roles in affordable healthcare services in South Africa?

Interestingly, only 30.6% of the respondents agreed that the Government of South Africa is providing affordable healthcare to the citizens of the country. While 16.6% of the respondents indicated that the government is performing well in promoting equity in dealing with the healthcare of underserved citizens, another 83.1% disagree with the notion that the government is managing the delivery of healthcare to the citizens effectively.

Questions	Strongly Agree	Agree	Neutral	Strongly Disagree	Disagree	Agree %	Disagree %
1 Hospitals and health centers in my city are particularly good.	423	481	6	350	358	904 55%	738 44.8%
2 The healthcare provided by doctors in my city is highly commendable.	452	456	4	284	452	908 51.1%	736 44.7%
3 I prefer to receive my healthcare in the hospitals in my country.	658	573	3	166	248	1231 74.7%	414 25.1%
4 Competences and skills of medical practitioners in my town hospital are particularly good.	379	532	6	298	433	911 55.3%	731 44.4%
5 Many hospitals and health centers in my rural town have modern equipment.	276	382	5	408	577	658 40%	985 59.8%
6 Many hospitals and health centers in my country do not provide emergency services.	123	267	3	612	643	390 23.7%	1255 76.2%
7 Hospitals and health centers in my city have constant electricity.	388	596	4	307	353	984 59.7%	660 40%
8 Doctors and nurses in my city hospitals are caring and friendly to their patients.	109	675	3	424	437	784 47.6%	861 52.2%
9 The cost of healthcare in my country is reasonable.	213	543	2	343	547	756 45.9%	890 54%
10 I can afford to pay for all my healthcare services.	265	508	4	345	522	773 47.7%	867 52.6%
11 I am satisfied with the type of healthcare services provided in my country.	355	617	4	299	373	972 58.9%	672 40.8%
12 I can afford my Healthcare treatment and medication costs without government subsidies.	251	508	1	375	513	759 46%	888 53.8%
Mean						50.5%	49%

Source: Derived from a Field survey in South Africa in 2019–2023.

Table 3 Government Role in Affordable Healthcare Services in South Africa

	Questions	Strongly Agree	Agree	Neutral	Strongly Disagree	Disagree	Agree %	Disagree %
1	Government effectively supports high-quality healthcare in my country	128	374	5	526	615	502 30.6%	1141 69.2%
2	Government promotes equity in dealing with the healthcare of underserved population	134	139	5	389	273	273 16.6%	1370 83.1%
3	Government policies effectively address why doctors go on strike in my country.	144	510	6	179	809	654 39.7%	988 60%
4	Government effectively addresses medical errors and malpractice by doctors in my country	129	720	6	365	428	849 51.5%	793 48.1%
5	Govt. effectively regulates medical professional licensing and disciplinary boards.	131	513	5	458	672	644 39%	1130 68.6%
6	I get my healthcare from public hospitals in my country.	619	873	4	72	80	1492 90.5%	152 9.2%
7	I get my healthcare from private sector hospitals in my country.	251	262	2	372	761	513 31.1%	1133 68.8%
8	Government pays for my medication in my country	0	112	4	712	821	112 6.7%	1533 93%
9	Government payment of low salaries to doctors and nurses has encouraged their migration to developed nations.	208	811	3	259	367	1019 61.8%	626 38%
10	Most rural government hospitals do not have specialist doctors and nurses	608	577	2	199	262	1185 71.9%	461 28%
	Mean						41.3%	56.6%

Source: Derived from Field survey in South Africa in 2019–2023.

Further, 39.7% of the respondents reported that government policies effectively address why doctors go on strike in my country. Unfortunately, 60% of the respondents disagree. In addition, with respect to the government effectively addressing medical errors and malpractice by doctors in South Africa, 51.5% agree, while 48.1% disagree. On the one hand, the government's ability to effectively regulate medical professional licensing and disciplinary boards received 39% positive votes, while 68.5% of the respondents indicated that the government of South Africa is not doing so well in regulating the practice of medical doctors in the country. Further, only 6.7% of the respondents indicated that the government pays for their medication in the country, while 93% of the respondents stated that they pay for their own medications.

In respect of the government's ability to manage the migration of qualified South African medical doctors to other foreign countries, 38% acknowledge that the government has not been effective in addressing the challenges, while 61.8% of the respondents reported that the government has been effective in managing the issue. In addition, 71.9% of the respondents indicated that most rural government hospitals do not have specialist doctors and nurses.

There is a perception that private hospitals and clinics in South Africa perform better than public medical institutions, as 31.1% of the respondents contend that they obtain their healthcare from the private sector, while 68.8 % confirm that they obtain their treatment from public hospitals. There is a consensus by 69.2% of the respondents that the Government of South Africa is not doing an excellent job in the delivery of high-quality healthcare in the country. Unfortunately, only 30.6% of the respondents indicated that the Government of South Africa is doing well. The average percentage of the respondents who acknowledged that the government is playing a good role in providing affordable healthcare is 41.3%, while those who believed otherwise are 56.6%. Thus, most South Africans confirm that their nation's government is not doing enough to provide affordable healthcare to everyone in the country.

Table 4 provides an analysis of the barriers to high-quality healthcare in the Republic of South Africa. It also provides answers to research question 3.

Research question 3: What are the major barriers to high-quality healthcare in South Africa?

Table 4 provides an overview of the barriers to a high-quality healthcare system in South Africa. According to 89.1% of the respondents, one of the highest barriers to an effective and high-quality healthcare system all over South Africa is the inability of the government to retain qualified doctors in the country due to a high rate of migration. In addition, 73.5% of the respondents indicated that lack of adequate clean water and good sanitation system is a major barrier to good health system especially in the rural and highly populated urban cities in the country. On the one hand, 63.7% of the respondents stated that the low salary of medical doctors, pharmacists, and nurses in the country constitutes barriers to effective healthcare. Other the other hand, 62.4% of the respondents reported that the lack of effective healthcare policy enforcement and implementation is also a major barrier to a high-quality health system in the country. Further, while 61% identified lack of modern technology as a barrier to high-quality healthcare in the country, another 60.7% of the respondents indicated that because

Table 4 Barriers to High-Quality Healthcare System in South Africa

	Questions	Strongly Agree	Agree	Neutral	Strongly Disagree	Disagree	Agree %	Disagree %
1	Political Leaders and rich citizens prefer to seek healthcare services in foreign countries	686	315	4	214	433	**1001** **60.7%**	**647** **39.3%**
2	Lack of trust in the poor healthcare services in the rural districts	213	319	0	437	639	532 **32.3%**	1076 **65.3%**
3	Low payment of salary to doctors, nurses, and pharmacist in the country	487	563	8	234	356	1050 **63.7%**	590 **35.8%**
4	Lack of modern technology and equipment	262	741	5	234	406	1003 **61%**	640 **39%**
5	Very few specialist doctors and hospitals in rural districts	171	822	4	236	415	993 **60.3%**	651 **39.5%**
7	Lack of effective healthcare policy, enforcement, and implementation	374	654	4	268	348	1028 **62.4%**	616 **37.4%**
8	Corruption and unethical behavior of political and administrative leaders.	499	602	0	259	288	547 **33.2%**	1101 **66.8%**
9	Inability to retain qualified doctors in the country due to the high rate of migration.	406	656	4	67	117	1468 **89.1%**	184 **11.2%**
10	Public, private, and community partnership, in healthcare delivery is not strongly encouraged	283	393	2	322	643	676 **41%**	965 **58.6%**
11	Lack of adequate clean water and good Sanitation system.	427	790	4	189	238	1217 **73.5%**	427 **26%**
	Mean						**53%**	**46.7%**

Source: Derived from a Field survey in South Africa in 2019–2023.

political leaders and rich citizens of South Africa prefer to seek healthcare in foreign countries, they are not interested in increasing the budget to provide a better healthcare system that could benefit everyone in the country.

In addition, 66.8% of the respondents stated that corruption and unethical behavior of political and administrative leaders is a major predicament to the high-quality healthcare system in Nigeria. Another 65.3% of the respondents reported that lack of trust in the poor healthcare delivery system constitutes a major barrier to the healthcare system because political leaders and senior public administrators would prefer to engage in medical tourism rather than increase the budget to provide high-quality healthcare in the country. Another major barrier that 58.6% of the respondents indicated is a weak public and private partnership in the delivery of healthcare in the country. Thus, a stronger and more vibrant partnership could galvanize a robust high-quality healthcare system in South Africa. Furthermore, the average agreed barrier factor for high-quality healthcare delivery is 53%, while the average disagree factor is 46.7%. Table 4 confirms that the barriers to high-quality of healthcare delivery are associated with ineffective government leadership in making healthcare delivery in the country a major priority.

Table 5 provides a content analysis of data from the secondary research such as the review of the National Department of Health in South Africa reports, the World Health Organization white papers, and the United Nations Human Development annual report, Center for Disease Control reports. While the World Health Organization recommends that nations around the world should provide an annual budget of at least 15% of their GDP for healthcare, in the past couple of years the Government of South Africa has budgeted an average of just 8.1% of its GDP. Further, the current number of physicians per 1,000 people in South Africa is 91. On the other hand, the ratio of nurses and midwives per 1,000 people is 1.38.

Table 5 Economics and Health Indicators in South Africa

No.	Major Indicators in South Africa	Explanation
1	Population	60.6 million (2022)
2	Gross domestic product (GDP) PPP	US $711 billion (2020)
3	Current health expenditure (% of GDP)	8.1% (2022)
4	Nurses and midwives per 1,000 people	1.31 (2022)
5	Physicians/doctors per 1,000 people	0.91 (2022)
6	Community health workers (per 1,000 people)	0.19 (2022)
7	Birth attended by skilled health personnel	96.7% (2002)
8	Access to basic clean water	92.7% (2020)
9	Population using safely managed drinking water service	44% (2021)
10	Sanitation access to basic toilet	75.8% (2022)
11	Common diseases	HIV/AIDS; ischemic heart disease; stroke; lower respiratory infections; diabetes; tuberculosis; interpersonal violence; neonatal disorders; diarrheal diseases

(Continued)

Table 5 (*Continued*)

No.	Major Indicators in South Africa	Explanation
12	Life expectancy at birth	64.1 years (2022)
13	Life expectancy in 2019 at birth for females	67.7 years (2022)
14	Life expectancy in 2019 at birth for males	60.7 years (2022)
15	Mortality rate for female adults (per 1,000 people)	249 (2022)
16	Mortality rate for infants (per 1,000 people)	28.5 (2022)
17	Mortality rate for male adults (per 1,000 people)	376 (2022)
	Mortality rate of mothers while giving birth per 1,000	119 (2022)
18	Tuberculosis incidence (per 100,000 people)	58% (2022)
19	Population living below income poverty line PPP $1.90 a day	18.9% (2022)
20	Population in multidimensional head count poverty (%)	25.8% (2022)
21	Contribution deprivation in health to multidimensional poverty (%)	39.5% (2022)
22	Infants lacking immunization for measles (5 of one and older)	84% (2022)
23	Malaria incidence (per 1,000 people at risk)	1 (2022)
24	HIV/AIDS prevalence adults (% ages 15–49)	20.4% (2020)

Sources: World Bank Indicators (2023); United Nations Human Development Programme (2020).

The number of community health workers in South Africa was also reported to be 0.19 per 1,000 people. This low ratio of doctors and nurses in the healthcare system in South Africa will confirm the findings of the questionnaire result on the barriers to a high-quality health system. In addition, the population of South Africa using safe managed water services constitutes only 44% of the 60.6 million people in the country. On the other hand, 75.8% of people have access to basic sanitation toilets. The most common diseases in South Africa are diabetes, HIV/AIDS (20.4%), tuberculosis (58%), and Malaria (1.7%). Further, the life expectancy at birth is currently 64.1 years, while the life expectancy in 2019 at birth for females was 67.7 years. On the other, the life expectancy in 2022 at birth for males was 60.7 years. The mortality rate for infants per 1,000 people is 28.5%, while the mortality rate for male adults per 1,000 people is 326. It is also interesting to note that the mortality rate of mothers while giving birth per 1,000 people was 119. The population living below the income poverty line of $1.90 per day is 18,9% of the citizens of South Africa. The number of infants lacking immunization for measles (under five or one year older) is 84%.

According to Asba et al. (2020), Technological predicaments and a lack of up-to-date water management infrastructure have often constituted a challenge to human health in South Africa. In addition, the delay in infrastructure repairs and infrastructure decay, as well as maintenance and improvement, have been serious predicaments in ensuring high-quality safe water and sanitation provision in the country (Asba et al. 2020). The impact of the COVID-19 pandemic in South Africa exposed the systemic weaknesses of both the healthcare system, and the quality-of-service delivery such as water and sanitation services, housing, and infrastructure in various communities across the country (Sekyere et al. 2020). For instance, the healthcare sector experienced a shortage of testing equipment, and intensive care beds as well as ventilators. Other challenges in the health system in Africa include poor water and sanitation facilities in some communities. According to Igamba (2022) and Makaya (2020), some urban and rural communities lack access to clean water and often engage in open defecation. In addition, sanitation facilities are in a deplorable state in many townships, with many households often having to share highly deficient facilities (Chothia 2020; Igamba 2022; Sekyere et al. 2020; Tseole et al. 2022).

Asba et al. (2020) and Igamba (2022) contend that 19% of the rural population lacks access to a reliable water supply and 33% do not have basic sanitation services. While rural citizens suffer the most, over 26% of all schools (urban or rural), and 45% of clinics, have no water access either (Global Data 2022; Igamba 2022). These disparities domestic water resources equation have often resulted in serious negative impacts on domestic hygiene, public health, and the cost of domestic water (Asba et al. 2020; Igamba 2022).

The 273 interview respondents also provided a remarkably interesting perspective on the effectiveness of the health policy in the country. Eighty-two percent of the interview respondents indicated that there is a disparity between Black and White citizens' access to affordable healthcare in the country. Another 77% of the respondents stated that the National Department of Health handled the COVID-19 pandemic crisis better than they did during the crucial HIV/AIDS crisis in the country. Further, 56% reported that there seem to be health system challenges related to poor public health services in the Free State province where they reside. It was interesting to note that 55% of the interview respondents stated that there seems to be a deficiency in antenatal care up to the delivery stage of babies in the country. In addition, 87% of the respondents also indicated that there were medical staff shortages in the hospitals in their province. Furthermore, 67% reported that financial cash flow is a major overall health system challenge resulting in the nonavailability and effectiveness of public health services in their respective provinces. Finally, 93% of the interview respondents indicated that good governance and leadership need to be enhanced in the healthcare system in South Africa as a matter of urgency.

Conclusion

This chapter has examined the effectiveness of the health policies of the Government of South Africa over the past 29 years (1994–2023). It argues that although the government of South Africa has been preparing to adopt universal health coverage that could ensure access to affordable healthcare through the adoption of a new National Health Insurance policy (NHI) and pertinent legislation (Dibie 2022; DPME 2023), the challenges of racial and economic disparities in the country may prevent the attainment of the proposed goal of the policy initiatives. The aftermath of the former apartheid regime in South Africa continues to manifest racial discrimination and segregation in the country. Inequality still exists in rural and urban regions and provinces all over the country (Chikozho et al. 2020; Mafunisa 2003). In addition, the health system in South Africa is currently faced with predicaments such as healthcare worker shortages as well as insufficient budgets to operate at full capacity.

The healthcare analysis conducted reveals that most of the citizens of the country rely on an overburdened, poorly resourced public healthcare system with poor or aging infrastructure. There is also a negative correlation between the challenges of health delivery and physicians and nurses' shortage in the country. Moreover, there is also a negative correlation between public healthcare facilities and inadequate management and corruption. Corruption. This finding also reveals that ethical, good leadership and governance (Mafunisa 2003; Maphunye 2019) should be adopted as a matter of urgency to enhance the high-quality healthcare system in South Africa.

Although the Government of South Africa has enacted impressive health policies since 1994, the health system in the country has not been able to accomplish appropriate governance of its healthcare system. The current governance of the healthcare system has not effectively directed the performance of the healthcare workforce and citizens' values. It is anticipated that a new performance management framework of governance could be adopted in the future that will allow the nation to strive to improve the performance of its health system. There is an urgent need for the Government of South Africa to develop several new indicators as well as monitor medical outcomes, patients' experiences, quality of services, assessment benchmarks surveillance to improve the performance of the country's healthcare system. The introduction of a vibrant information technology system in the country should be considered seriously when moving forward with the country's universal health system goals.

The research findings also reveal that there is a major challenge of shortage of doctors, specialist physicians, and nurses mostly in the rural regions or provinces of the country. Some of the main reasons for experienced health professionals leaving their jobs in South Africa for other countries include unsatisfactory working conditions, concerns about safety and crime, and exceptionally low pay and benefits. These financial and safety issues have also negatively affected their ability to take diligent care of the needs of their immediate family members. Therefore, the Government of South Africa must realize that health workforce planning is very crucial to health system planning and performance (Dibie & Dibie 2021). There is an urgent need to adopt pragmatic strategies that could restore positive benefits and infrastructure of health facilities for doctors and nurses in South Africa (De-Villier 2021; Greer et al. 2016). Enactment of new policies that could help doctors and nurses to leave and perform their duties comfortably in rural communities should also be considered urgent as a strategy to galvanize high-quality performance in both the urban and rural regions of South Africa.

Finally, without effective leadership, cooperation, and collaboration between key stakeholders in the private and public healthcare system of the country, there might never be a vibrant, sustainable, efficient, and effective, health system in South Africa. It is especially important for the Government of South Africa to be mindful that governance shapes markets, and that without appropriate governance, health markets cannot function properly.

References

Asba S. N., Fiko M, Makiwane B., and Mefi N. P. (2020). Water and sanitation challenge the case of a rural South African municipality. Academy of Entrepreneurship Journal (Print ISSN: 1087-9595; Online ISSN: 1528-2686).
Baker C., Lund P., Nyathi R., Taylor J. (2010). The myths surrounding people with albinism in South Africa and Zimbabwe. *Journal of African Cultural Studies*, 22(2): 169–181.
Bloch A. (2010). The right to rights? Undocumented migrants from Zimbabwe living in South Africa. *Sociology*, 44(2), 233–250. DOI:10.1177/0038038509357209.
Britannica (2022). South Africa. https://www.britannica.com/place/South-Africa/Relief. Accessed January 21, 2023.
British Broadcasting Corporation (2022). South Africa country profile. https://www.bbc.com/news/world-africa-14094760. Accessed January 22, 2023.
Britnell M. (2015). South Africa – No more false dawns. *In Search of the Perfect Health System edited by Mark Britnell.* (74–79). New York: Palgrave Macmillian.
Burger R. and Christian C. (2018). Access to healthcare in post-apartheid South Africa: Availability, affordability, acceptability. *Health Economics Policy and Law*, 15(1), 1–13.
Chikozho C., Manaya R., and Dabata T. (2020). Ensuring Access to Water for Food Production by Emerging Farmers in South Africa; What are the Missing Ingredients? Africa Institute of South Africa – HSRC, Pretoria.
Chothia A. (2020). "Lockdown: 87000 cases of gender-based violence reported.
Columbia Public Health (2023). CAPRISA celebrates 20 years of public health progress in southern Africa. https://www.publichealth.columbia.edu/news/caprisa-celebrates-20-years-public-health-progress. Accessed September 15, 2024.
Conmy A. (2018). South African healthcare system analysis. *Public Health Review*, 1(1), 1–8.
Crush J. and Tawodzera G. (2014). Medical Xenophobia and Zimbabwean migrant access to public health services in South Africa. *Journal of Ethnic Migration Studies*, 40(4), 655–670.
Davids I., Theron F., and Maphunye K. J. (2005). *Participatory Development in South Africa: A Development Management Perspective.* Pretoria: Van Schaik Publishers.
Department of Planning, Monitoring and Evaluation (DPME). (2023). http://www.dpme.gov.za/news/Pages/NHI_Update_Sep.aspx. Accessed November 18, 2023.
De-Villier K. (2021). Bridging the health inequality gap: An examination of South Africa's social innovation in health landscape. Infectious Diseases of Poverty. DOI: 10.1186/s40249-021.00804-9. Accessed February 4, 2023.
Dibie R. (2022). Health policy and administartion in Nigeria: A critical analysis, The Journal of African Policy Studies, 28(1): 101–139.
Dibie R. (2018). *Business and Government Relations in Africa.* New York: Routledge Press.
Dibie R., and Dibie J. (2021). Public management and faith-based governance in Nigeria. Journal of the Management Sciences, 57(2), 4–27.
Dovlo D. (2009). The Brain Drain and Retention of Health Professionals in Africa. library. http://library.health.go.ug/sites/default/files/resources/The%20Brain%20drain%20and%20Retention%20of%20health%20Professionals%20in%20Africa.pdf. Accessed September 15, 2024. Accessed February 8, 2023.
Global Data (2022). The five largest gold mines are South Africa. https://www.globaldata.com. Accessed January 23, 2023.

GlobalEdge (2023). South Africa. https://globaledge.msu.edu/countries/south-africa. Accessed January 21, 2023.

GlobalEdge (2022). South Africa. https://globaledge.msu.edu/countries/south-africa/memo. Accessed September 15, 2024.

Government of South Africa (2016). South African Health Review 2016. https://www.hst.org. za/publications/South%20African%20Health%20Reviews/SAHR%202016.pdf. Accessed November 12, 2024.

Greer S. L, Wismar M., and Figueras J. (2016). *Strengthening health system governance: better policies stronger performance.* Berkshire, England: McGraw-Hill.

Grag A., and Vawda Y. (2018). Health policy and legislation. *South Africa Review*, 1(1), 1–17.

Greer S. L, Wismar M., and Figueras J. (2016). *Strengthening Health System Governance: Better Policies Stronger Performance.* Berkshire, England: McGraw-Hill.

How South Africa stumbles on health care for all (2017), July 27. https://www.bloomberg.com/ news/articles/2017-07-27/how-south-africa-stumbles-on-health-care-for-all-quicktake-q-a. Accessed September 16, 2024.

Hlafa B., Sibanda K., Hompashe D. M. (2019). The impact of public health expenditure on health outcomes in South Africa. *International Journal of Environmental Research in Public Health*, 16(16), 2993. DOI: 10.3390/ijerph16162993.

Igamba J. (2022). The water crisis in South Africa: A looming threat. https://www.greenpeace. org/africa/en/blogs/51757/water-crisis-in-south-africa/. Accessed December 23, 2023.

Laitinen A., Annarinna K., Pirkko N., and Honest K. (2019). Healthcare workers' eHealth competences in private health centres in Urban Tanzania. *Journal of Health Informatics in Developing Countries*, 14(1): 1–20.

Life Esidimeni (2021). Life Esidimeni 2021 Report. https://section27.org.za/campaigns/life-esidimeni/. Accessed October 30, 2024.

Mafunisa M. J. (2003). Separation of politics from the South African public service: Rhetoric or reality? *Journal of Public Administration*, 38(2), 85–101.

Makaya E. (2020). Water governance challenges in rural South Africa: Exploring institutional coordination in drought. *Journal of World Water Council*, 22(4), 29–34.

Malakoane B., Heunis J. C., Chikobvu P., Kigozi N. G., Kruger W. H. (2020). Public health system challenges in the free state, South Africa: A situation appraisal to inform health system strengthening. *BMC Health Service Research*, 20–58.

Malema R. N., and Muthelo L. (2018). Strategies for recruitment and retention of skilled healthcare workers in remote rural areas. University of Limpopo, South Africa. EQUINET Discussion paper 115. https://equinetafrica.org/sites/default/files/uploads/documents/EQ%20Diss% 20115%20HR%20ret%20litrev%20Sep%202018.pdf. Accessed February 5, 2023.

Mandela N. (2013). Biography of Nelson Mandela. www.nelsonmandela.org/content/page/ biography.

Maphumulo W. T. and Bhengu B. R. (2019). Challenges of quality improvement in the healthcare of South Africa post-apartheid: A critical review. *Curationis Journal*, 42(1), 1–9.

Maphunye K. J. (2019). Realities facing professional service delivery in South Africa's public sector. *African Administrative Studies*, 84, 35–52. ISSN:2028-6694.

Maphunye K. J. (2006). Towards redressing historical inequities? Gender balancing in the South African civil service. *Public Management Review*, 8(2), 297–311. (ISSN: 14719037).

Malema, R. N., and Muthelo L. (2018). Strategies for recruitment and retention of skilled healthcare workers in remote rural areas. University of Limpopo, South Africa. EQUINET Discussion paper 115. https://equinetafrica.org/sites/default/files/uploads/documents/ EQ%20Diss%20115%20HR%20ret%20litrev%20Sep%202018.pdf. Accessed February 5, 2023.

Meissner R., and Plessis (2022). South Africa's increasing water stress requires urgent informed actions. https://theconversation.com/south-africas-increasing-water-stress-requires-urgent-informed-actions-189659. Accessed February 23.

Mining Technology (2022). Five largest coal mines in South Africa. https://www.mining-technology.com. Accessed January 23, 2023.

Mitchel J., Tediosi F., Egger M., Barnighausen T., McIntyre D., Tanner M. and Evans D. (2020). Universal health coverage financing in South Africa: Wishers vs realty. *Journal of Global Health Reports*, 4, 1–12.

Michel J., Chimbindi N., Mohlakoana N., Orgill M., Bärnighausen T., Obrist B., Tediosi F., Evans D., McIntryre D., Bressers H. T., Tanner M. (2019). How and why policy-practice gaps come about: A South African Universal Health Coverage contex. https://www.joghr.org/article/12185-how-and-why-policy-practice-gaps-come-about-a-south-african-universal-health-coverage-context. Accessed September 15, 2024.

Muller D. (2020). *Addressing the Challenges of Implementing a Health Technology Assessment Policy Framework in South Africa*. Cambridge, England: Cambridge University Press.

National Government of South Africa (2022). South Africa's national government and its related institutions and entities. https://nationalgovernment.co.za/. Accessed January 21, 2023.

National Department of Health (2021). Annual Report 2020/2021. https://www.health.gov.za/wp-content/uploads/2021/11/Annual-Report-2020-2021.pdf. Accessed September 15, 2024.

National Treasury (2021). Budget 2021: Budget review. *Republic of South Africa*. Pretoria, South Africa.

Ned L., Cloete L. & Mji G. (2017). The experiences and challenges faced by rehabilitation community service Therapists within the South African primary healthcare health system, *African Journal of Disability*, 6, 311.

Owolabi O. and Tumbare E. (2022). Four steps toward a stronger African Health workforce in 2030 and beyond. https://www.intrahealth.org/vital/four-steps-toward-stronger-african-health-workforce-2030-and-beyond. Accessed February 5, 2023.

Pauw T. L. (2022). Catching up with the constitution: n analysis of national health insurance in South Africa. *Development South Africa*, 39(6), 921–934.

Republic of South Africa, National Department of Health Annual Report (2021–2022). https://www.health.gov.za/wp-content/uploads/2022/10/2022-Annual-Report-Compressed.pdf Accessed November 18, 2023.

Sekyere E., Narnia Bohler-Muller N., Charles Hongoro C., and Makoae M. (2020). The Impact of Covid-19 in South Africa. https://www.wilsoncenter.org/publication/impact-covid-19-south-africa. Accessed January 24, 2021.

South Africa Government (2023). Let's grow South Africa together. https://www.gov.za/. Accessed January 21, 2023.

South Africa Western Cape Government (2022). The Government of South Africa: overview. South Africa Western Cape Government (2022). https://www.westerncape.gov.za/edat/tags/western-cape-government. Accessed November 12, 2024. Accessed January 22, 2023.

Stewart J. and Wolvaardt G. (2019). Hospital management and health policy: A South African perspective. *Journal of Hospital Management and Health Policy*. DOI: 10.21037jhmhp.2019.06.01.

Tseole N. P., Mindu, T., Kalinda C. and Chimbari M. J. (2022). Barriers and facilitators to Water, Sanitation and Hygiene (WaSH) practices in Southern Africa: A scoping review. *PLoS One*, 17(8), e0271726.

Twala C. (2014). The Causes and Socio-political Impact of the Service Delivery Protests to the South African Citizenry: A Real Public Discourse. *Journal of Social Sciences*, 39(10); 159–167.

United Nations Human Development Programme (2020). Human Development Report 2020. https://hdr.undp.org/content/human-development-report-2020. Accessed November 12, 2024.

University of Minnesota School of Public Health (2018). South African health care system analysis. https://pubs.lib.umn.edu/index.php/phr/article/view/1568. Accessed November 12, 2024.

World Bank Indicators (2023) World Development Indicators. https://databank.worldbank.org/source/world-development-indicators. Accessed November 12, 2024.

Zubane P. (2011). Alternative Service Delivery Models For The South African Public Service For The Year 2020. Research report presented in partial fulfilment of the requirements for the degree of Master of Future Studies at the University of Stellenbosch. Cape Town: Stellenbosch University.

Zwarenstein M. (1994). The structure of South Africa's health service. *African Health Journal*, (3–4), 1–15.

Chapter Sixteen

HEALTH POLICY AND SOCIAL CHALLENGES IN SUDAN

Muawya Hussien, Robert Dibie, and Ayandiji Aina

Introduction

This chapter examines the nature of health policy and implementation in Sudan. It analyzes the challenges of the healthcare delivery system in the country. It argues that despite the previously well-established healthcare system in the country, the challenges of several years of political instability have prevented Sudan's ability to effectively prevent the spread of communicable and noncommunicable diseases. The finding of the research analysis reveals that the ineffective healthcare delivery system has created an aftermath of an increase of chronic and endemic infectious diseases such as malaria, leishmaniasis, and schistosomiasis are incrementally causing substantial morbidity and mortality. Further, antimicrobial resistance has become a major threat throughout the healthcare system, with an emerging impact on maternal, neonatal, and pediatric populations. Communicable and noncommunicable diseases, such as obesity, diabetes, renal disease, and cancer are also increasingly causing high rates of substantial morbidity and mortality. Some recommendations are provided on how to better adapt healthcare delivery strategies that could be more effective in helping Sudan to accomplish its sustainable development and healthcare goals in the future. There is however an urgent need for the nation to focus more on how to meet the healthcare needs of its citizens in both the urban and rural areas by adopting a better economic support system, and health information system, and attracting a better-qualified health and professional workforce. It will also be a sustainable humanitarian service for the Government of Sudan to adopt health laws and social justice policies that support women and girls to make their own decisions about personal sexual and reproductive healthcare.

Brief History of Sudan

The Republic of Sudan is a country in the northeastern part of the African continent. The nation has boundaries with the following African countries. the Arab Republic of Egypt in the north, and the Republic of Ethiopia in the southeast. The Red Sea is located in the northeastern part of Sudan, and the Republic of Eritrea is located in the eastern part of Sudan. Further, the Republic of Sudan has boundaries with the Arab

Republic of Libya in the northwestern part of the country, while the Arab Republic of Chad is located in the western part of the country. The new Republic of South Sudan is located in the southern part of the Republic of Sudan. It should be noted that the nation now called the Republic of South Sudan used to be a region within the Republic of Sudan before it was separated and granted independence in 2011 (Berry 2015).

Some history scholars contend that there were several kingdoms that existed in the present location of the Arab Republic of Sudan between 8 BC and 3300 BC. The major kingdoms were the Nubian Kingdom, Nabatia Kingdom, Mukuria Kingdom, and Alodia Kingdoms of the sixth century, as well as the Kush Kingdom of 1070 BC, and the Shilluk Kingdoms of 1490. These Kingdoms were reported to have practiced the Christian religion (Holt & Daly 2000; Keita 1993; Wikipedia 2023). From the sixth century to the present time, the old Nubian and the Nilo Sharan languages were spoken in the Nile Valley region (Manzo 2017; Najovits 2004). Other archaeologists also indicated that the Nubia and Magadan people of lower and upper Egypt were culturally and ethnically identical to those of the Pharaonic Kingdom of 3300 BC (Fadlalla 2004; Manzo 2017; Najovits 2004; Wikipedia 2023). In addition, between 2500 and 1500 BC, the Kerma Kingdom which was based in the southern region of the Nubia, now part of the central and northern Sudan was defeated in a tribal war and forced to be part of the Egypt Kingdom (Appiah-Mensah 2006).

Although Islam was practiced on the Red Sea coast as far back as the seventh century, the religion did not spread to other parts of the Nile Valley until between the fourteenth and fifteenth centuries as a result of the decline of the Christian kingdoms (Fadlalla 2004; Collins 2008; Holt & Daly 2000; Wikipedia 2023). Between the fifth and seventeenth centuries, cattle herding, fishing on the Nile River, hunting, and graining gathering were the major occupations of the various ethnic groups and kingdoms population along the Red Sea and Nile River. However, a major Sahara Desert drought in the fifth century made the people of the Neolithic culture living in the region start migrating nearer the Nile River Valley (Appiah-Mensah 2006; Holt & Daly 2000; Metz 1991; Wikipedia 2023).

In addition, history scholars indicated that between 1805 and 8010 the Egyptian Kingdom's economic development improved considerably under Muhammad Ali Pasha's leadership. Further, between 1820 and 1821, Muhammad Ali mobilized the Egyptian forces to conquer the northern region of Sudan (British Broadcasting Corporation 2023; Metz 1991; Najovits 2004). During the same period, the Turiyah British missionaries traveled from the current region called Kenya toward Sudan to spread the Christian religion. Furthermore, in 1881, another leader in the region called Muhammad Ahmad declared a war to unify the ethnic groups in central and western Sudan (Chutel 2023; Hassanain et al. 2022; Wikipedia 2023). On January 26, 1885, Muhammad Ahmad (also called Mahdi) called for a nationalist revolt that led to the capture of Khartoum. It is also reported that the British Interim Governor-General of the Sudan, Major-General Charles George Gordon, and over 51,000 people in the city of Khartoum district were killed (Chutel 2023; Holt & Daly 2000; Wikipedia 2023). During the nationalist revolt, the British-appointed governor in Khartoum was killed when the city fell to Muhammad Ahmad (British Broadcasting Corporation 2023). After the death of Muhammad Ahmad in 1885, the United Kingdom sought to re-establish its control over Sudan and change the name of the region to Egyptian Khedive (British Broadcasting Corporation 2023). But in reality, it was a new British colony.

After almost 57 years of control of Sudan as a joint British-Egyptian rule while it was actually a British colony, another crisis emerged in 1952, this time by the Egyptians who advocated Sudanese independence. This revolution triggered Britain to allow both the south and north to vote for independence (Appiah-Mensah 2006; British Broadcasting Corporation 2023; Collins 2008).

On January 1, 1956, Sudan attained its independence from the United Kingdom. The leader of the National Unionist Party Ismail Azhari formed a government as prime minister. However, on July 7, 1956. Abdallah Khalil of the Umma Party defeated Ismail Azhari in a vote of censure in the Constituent Assembly and formed a democratic government for the new nation (Appiah-Mensah 2006; British Broadcasting Corporation 2023; Collins 2008; University of Central Arkansas 2023). Unfortunately, the Republic of Sudan has long been engulfed by civil war and other crises since the nation attained its independence in 1956 (Berry 2015; Hasan 1967). The following is the time frame of the crisis that confronted the Republic of Sudan since its independence: (1) Crisis on November 17, 1958–November 7, 1964; (2) November 8, 1964, to May 24, 1969; (3) Crisis May 25, 1969, to May 15, 1986; (4) Crisis May 16, 1986, to June 29, 1989; (5) Crisis June 30, 1989, to February 25, 2003; (6) Crisis February 26, 2003, to March 18, 2010; (7) Crisis March 19, 2010 to November 10, 2011; (8) November 11, 2011 to October 3, 2020; and (9) Crisis April 15, 2023 to August 15, 2023. The 2023 war in Sudan was between the nation's army and the paramilitary Rapid Support Force which are rival factions of the military government of Sudan in Darfur and Khartoum region (British Broadcasting Corporation 2023; Walsh 2023; Wikipedia 2023). Unfortunately, the various civil wars and political crises in Sudan have had a devastating impact on the health system in the country.

Health Challenges in Sudan

The health system in the Federal Republic of Sudan is considered to be very fragile due to disparities in the delivery of healthcare services between urban and rural regions in the country (Ebrahim et al. 2017; Hassanain et al. 2022; Hemmeda et al. 2023; Kruk et al. 2010). Apart from the lack of investment in the nation's health system has galvanized poor or ineffective curative services, prevention services, low-quality promotion initiatives, fragile rehabilitative roles, and other human rights services to the nation's citizens and residents (Chutel 2023; Ebrahim et al. 2019; Kruk et al. 2010). The Government of Sudan and its related healthcare delivery institutions were originally expected to play a major evidence-based medical social function however the health of communities, the level of democracy, and the degree of freedom of the nation have not been to positively propel the anticipated outcome (Ebrahim et al. 2017; Hemmeda et al. 2023). In most cases whenever the low-income population of the nation visited a hospital or clinic, they were often addressed by nurses and specialist physicians (Chutel 2023; Insecurity Insight 2023). Because of a lack of specialist physicians in some regional health facilities children and women continue to die from preventable or treatable diseases such as malaria, respiratory infections, and diarrhea (Chutel 2023; Hassanain et al. 2022; UNICEF 2022).

Over the past two decades, the Federal Republic of Sudan has been engaging in various civil wars due to the undemocratic transition of power in the country. Each time the nation's political and military leaders engage in civil war, the health system facilities in the country are destroyed (Albarodi 2023; Alfadul et al. 2023; Saied et al. 2021). The unprecedented crisis that occurred on April 15, 2013, between the Sudan Armed Forces and the Rapid Support Forces created a devastating impact on the nation's health infrastructure and workforce (Alfadul et al. 2023; Nashed 2003; World Health Organization 2023). The civil war in Sudan has led to heavy shelling, fires, and direct attacks on healthcare institutions. Currently, over 80% of hospitals in the Republic of Sudan are not functioning. It has also been reported that medical supplies have been looted many health workers killed, and hundreds of patients deliberately obstructed from accessing healthcare services (Doctors Without Border 2023; Insecurity Insight 2023).

Further, the escalation of civil work has galvanized human rights violations, as well as violence against healthcare workers (Buchsee 2023; Schlein 2023). During the devasting war, over a dozen healthcare workers have been reported killed, while many other citizens of Sudan have been reported dead of their illness due to scarcity of basic medical services, and access to hospitals due to the war (Chutel 2023). In addition, many doctors in the country have fled, and it has been reported that the military juntas are kidnaping doctors and nurses and forcing them at gunpoint to treat wounded soldiers (Chutel 2023; Dafallah et al. 2023; Doctors Under Siege in Sudan 2020). Furthermore, the civil war has also led to a shortage of medical supplies, as well as a total breakdown of the supply chain for medical products (Mohammed et al. 2023; Federal Ministry of Health 2017; Noory et al. 2020). Another escalating situation is the inability of doctors and nurses to reach the hospitals as most of the streets in the major cities in Sudan have become battlefields for the two army rivals (Ahmed et al. 2020; Altayb et al. 2020). Moreover, the juntas have been engaging in destroying the supply of electricity and water (Hemmeda et al. 2023). The crisis has also resulted in the blocking of internal trade routes. This pervasive inhuman action of the combatting soldiers has also led to the unavailability of goods, safe water, pharmaceuticals, and fuels (Hemmeda et al. 2023).

These health predicaments include the spread of communicable and noncommunicable diseases, lack of funding for health facilities, poverty, and disparities in both access and affordability of health services to citizens and residents of the country (Charani et al. 2019; Federal Ministry of Health 2020). The health policies that have been enacted in Sudan in the past two decades have not been effectively implemented in the country. This disparity pattern tends to create critical challenges in both the capacity building of healthcare facilities and accessibility to health delivery (Buchsee 2023; Hemmeda et al. 2023). According to Alfadul et al. (2023), Mustafa and Hamed (2018), Yuan et al. (2022), Sudan's fragile health system may soon fail due to poor health governance, lack of transparency, integrity, law and order, regulation, and corruption. The lack of democratic governance in the country has also impeded planning, societal engagement, and system responsiveness (Egere et al. 2021; Schlein 2023). Sudan traditionally has a low score and rank across the six dimensions of governance, indicating overall governance failure. Although the Federal Republic of Sudan has been endowed with natural and human resources, the nation's economy, health system, and social development have performed below expectations (World Health Organization 2023).

The inadequate funding of the Sudan health system is another major challenge in the country. According to the International Trade Administration report (2022), the Government of Sudan spent 6.5% of its gross domestic product (GDP) on healthcare between 2021 and 2022. During the same period, the nation imported US$256 million of medicine. In addition, the Government of Sudan spends about 8.3% of its expenditure on healthcare. It is also reported that out-of-pocket expenses of about 70% or US$84.0 per capita or 22.3% of it constituted the general government expenditure (Ali & Abdalla 2021; Ebrahim et al. 2017). Unfortunately, in 2020, the Federal Government of Sudan only spent 3.02% of its GDP on healthcare (World Bank Indicators 2020). This sudden drop from 6.5% or 8.3% to 3.02% is a major devastating blow to the health system in the country. In the late 1980s, the health services in the country were provided mostly free of charge to the citizens and residents of the country (Noory et al. 2021). The funding challenges of the health system in Sudan could be characterized as incalculable and virtuous in respect of (1) high OOP costs; (2) limited government capacity to collect 27 taxes; (3) state governments unable to generate local revenue; (4) poor coordination between agencies involved in tax collection; (5) inefficient allocation of funds from the Ministry of Finance; and (6) a weak decentralized system (Ebi and Hese 2020; Forsyth 2020; Hassanain et al. 2022). Because of these challenges, the road to universal health coverage is becoming exceedingly difficult to navigate in Sudan (Anib et al. 2022; Habbani et al. 2021).

Furthermore, because of the structural adjustment program (SAP) that was adopted by the country in 1992, a new dimension of financing was adopted, and user fees were reintroduced in Sudan (Hemmeda et al. 2023). Currently, to continue to get access to healthcare most of the low-income population in Sudan often borrow money from their family members who are well off. There has also been a major challenge in medicine distribution in Sudan (Abdeen 2018; Federal Ministry of Health 2017). An alternative way to raise funds for their healthcare is working more hours or reducing expenditure on other vital living expenses (Hassanain et al. 2022; Sharew 2022). Whenever the above options for raising funds to pay for their healthcare, some of the low-income populations in both rural and urban regions in the country often would resort to exploring partially recommended treatments, resulting in further health complications (Ebrahim et al. 2017; Sharew 2022). In addition, other challenges such as the separation of South Sudan, economic sanctions, migration of doctors and nurses to foreign countries drought have also prevented the government of Sudan from accomplishing its health policy goals (Ebrahim et al. 2017; Hemmeda et al. 2023; Republic of Sudan Federal Ministry of Health 2016; World Health Organization 2023).

According to UNICEF (2022), the lack of appropriate funding for Sudan's health system continues to be a major challenge in the nation's healthcare delivery system.

It is also reported that over eight million children under five years old in Sudan are not likely to have access to lifesaving healthcare services in Sudan (Charani et al. 2019; Public Health Institute Federal Ministry of Health 2014; UNICEF 2022). Furthermore, almost 80,000 children under five years of age continue to lose their lives due to a lack of treatment that could have prevented their deaths (Hassanain et al. 2022; International Trade Administration 2022). Further, only 70% of the residents of Sudan have access to hospitals or clinics without traveling at least at least 40 miles (Chutel 2023). Moreover, sick people especially children often arrive at some district health facilities where they could only receive what has been described as insufficient quality treatment (Chutel 2023; UNICEF 2022). A more disturbing predicament is that after traveling a long distance to get to a rural health facility the sick patients are likely to be attended by nonspecialist nurses (UNICEF 2022). Thus, the health services offered to children and mothers in some of the rural health facilities in Sudan are considered exceptionally low compared to those in the urban cities such as Khartoum and are of inferior quality (Hassanain et al. 2022; International Trade Administration 2022; Sharew 2022).

Health workers' shortage challenges in Sudan are getting serious in some states in the country. According to Hassanain et al. (2022) and Sharew (2022), the Federal Republic of Sudan has been struggling to restrain its physicians and nurses in the past few years from migrating to foreign countries to seek a better life and vibrant professional career (Haakenstad et al. 2022; Saleh 2023; Skinner 2023). Many of the nation's health professional staff have been leaving the country for better living standards and working conditions (Ebrahim et al. 2017; Sharew 2022). Unfortunately, the Government of Sudan cannot afford to sustain these efforts in the long term or extend these benefits to all physicians in the country. Sudan currently has a population of over 46.9 million people. However, the nation only has about 27,000 midwives working across the country. In addition, it also reported that 2330 of these midwives work in health facilities in Khanoum the capital city. Further, the midwives address 3–4 births each day (Public Health Institute Federal Ministry of Health 2016; World Health Organization 2023).

Because of the continuous attacks on hospitals, clinics, equipment, and health workers in the country, the combating military personnel are depriving girls and women of life-saving healthcare, with pregnant women seriously affected. According to the World Health Organization Report (2023), over 11 million people urgently need health in Sudan. Among the number that need immediate healthcare in the country 2.64 million women and girls of reproductive age that are considered to need immediate humanitarian and health intervention (World Health Organization 2023). In addition, 262,880 women who are pregnant need immediate access to reproductive health services (Schlein 2023; World Health Organization 2023). It is unfortunate that whenever there is a major improvement in the healthcare delivery system, a few years later another civil war will occur, and the hospitals and clinics will be destroyed again (Saleh et al. 2021; Salim & Hamed 2018). Apart from the deliberate destruction of health facilities and the medicine supply chain crisis, the civil war has also created horrible consequences for citizens and residents of Sudan. Furthermore, the crisis has often created a dire refuge and humanitarian predicaments.

Types of Health Policies

During the past three decades, the Federal Republic of Sudan has enacted several health policies and national health plans. Most of the latest health policies are embedded with a vision to fill the gap in the current health challenges after policy evaluation has been conducted. Below are selected policies of the Government of Sudan.

National Health Policy 2017–2030 enacted in 2017: The goal of this policy is to cover all Sudan's citizens with essential health packages through prepayment arrangements to be financially protected. Sudan is a healthy nation with the highest attainable level of health and health equity for everyone regardless of socioeconomic status through strengthening a multisectoral approach to health and adopting people-centered health systems thereby achieving SDG and universal health coverage and contributing to the overall social and economic development of the country. Other goals of the policy include (1) availing people-centered family health services to all the population across all states and localities; (2) reducing inequities in health; (3) decreasing the burden of Communicable and noncommunicable diseases; and (4) raising life expectancy; and decrease mortality and morbidity of the citizens and residents of Sudan (Sudan Federal Ministry of Health 2017).

Health Finance Policy enacted in 2016: The major goal of this policy is to ensure that all the citizens and residents of the Federal Republic of Sudan are covered by a prepayment arrangement for an essential health package of services and are financially protected. The overall goal is to improve health status and achieve financial risk protection for all population (Sudan Federal Ministry of Health 2016). The health financing policy is providing the direction of the country on how the functions of the health system will be performed to address critical gaps and shape the feature of the system that is to be efficient and equitable resource allocation for health (Sudan Federal Ministry of Health 2016).

The National Health Policy enacted in 2007: The health policy envisages the building of a healthy nation, thereby contributing to the achievement of the targets of the Millennium Development Goals (MDGs) and the overall social and economic development of the country. The National Health Policy is committed to achieving equity and poverty reduction; ensuring investment in health; reaching the targets of the MDGs; maintaining and securing human rights and dignity; preserving the rights of women and children; and fighting disease and ignorance. The National Health Policy envisages building the health system on a comprehensive concept of health which ensures equity, and quality. and accountability which promotes professionalism. The aim is that the health system satisfies both the needs of users and providers, and is based on the principles of citizenship, pluralism, solidarity, and universality (Sudan Federal Ministry of Health 2007).

The Pharmacy, Poisons, Cosmetics, and the Medical Devices Act 2001: The purpose of this policy is to enforce the regulations and increase the frequency of inspection visits to drug companies and retail pharmacies. The act also mandated the state governments to take all steps necessary to ensure compliance with the marketing of registered medicines in licensed premises (Sudan Federal Ministry of Health 2001).

This policy also requires the state regulatory authorities to take advantage of the legal authority granted by the Sudan constitution and the Pharmacy, Poisons, Cosmetics, and the Medical Devices Act 2001 to enforce the regulations and increase the frequency of the inspection visits to drug companies and retail pharmacies (Sudan Federal Ministry of Health 2001; Lucero-Prisno et al. 2020).

Social Health Insurance Policy of 1997: The goal of this policy is to solve the problem of healthcare accessibility in the Federal Republic of Sudan (Public Health Institute Federal Ministry of Health 2014). The social health insurance policy also mandated community engagement through the construction of hospitals and health clinics, as well as top-up of health personnel and the conduction of health education campaigns. Since the formulation of social health insurance in Sudan, Khartoum State has had a very inspiring experience, where health insurance coverage has remarkably increased to between 72.2% and 75.1% (Anib et al. 2022; Habbani et al. 2021). Further, 5.5% of the population in Khartoum State is covered by other health insurance schemes such as police, military, and para-statal organizations (Habbani et al. 2021). In addition, Zakat, which is a form of Islamic charity, and the Ministry of Finance pay premiums annually for the poor (about 350,000 families), but there is still a huge gap as an estimated 2,300,000 poor families are not covered (Public Health Institute Federal Ministry of Health 2014).

Health Administration in Sudan

The health administration system in the Republic of Sudan is divided into three levels. The levels are (1) primary (local), (2) secondary (state), and (3) tertiary (federal) (Federal Ministry of Health 2016). The universities, police, military medical services, and private sector in the country also play a continually active role in the healthcare delivery system in Sudan (Abdullah et al. 2017; African Health Business 2021). The Federal Republic of Sudan has one Federal Ministry of Health and 18 State Ministries of Health (Abdullah et al. 2017; Federal Ministry of Health 2016).

At *the federal or tertiary level*, the Federal Ministry of Health performs the function of formulating national health policies, and strategic health plans. It also manages the mobilization of resources as well as monitoring and engaging in evaluating other health strategies. Furthermore, to enhance the effective implementation of policies that are formulated, the Federal Ministry of Health coordinates, and engages in supervision and training of all the health workforce in the country. It also engages in different forms of external and internal public relations on all issues relating to healthcare, health behavior, and disease prevention activities (Abdullah et al. 2017; Sudan National Health Sector Strategic Plan 2016; Wikipedia 2023). In addition, the federal level is responsible for the provision of nationwide health policies, plans, strategies, overall monitoring and evaluation, coordination, training, and external relations (Abdullah et al. 2017; Federal Ministry of Health 2016; Wikipedia 2023).

The *secondary or state health administration level* mainly focuses on its strategic plan. However, the Department of Health also follows the Federal Ministry of Health guidelines on how to effectively implement health policies that have been formulated by the Federal Ministry of Health (Abdullah et al. 2017; Sudan National Health Sector Strategic Plan 2016; Wikipedia 2023). Further, the state level is concerned with the state's plans, and strategies, and based on federal guidelines funding and implementation of plans (Abdullah et al. 2017; Federal Ministry of Health 2016; Wikipedia 2023).

At *the locality or district level*, the main function is the implementation of policies that have been enacted by both the federal and state Ministry of Health. The district-level health departments are also actively involved in health service delivery (Abdullah et al. 2017; African Health Business 2021).

In addition, the administration of the health system at the federal, state, and district or locality levels is complemented by a continually active private healthcare delivery system in Sudan. According to the African Health Business report (2021), the private healthcare sector is expanding fast from the urban to the rural areas. Most of the organizations that operate in the private health sector constitute not-for-profit and for-profit hospitals and clinics. There are also some not-for-profit health facilities that are operated by religious institutions in Sudan, and foreign own health donors. During the past few decades, the Federal Ministry of Health in Sudan has incrementally adopted a market-based private health service delivery approach for policy regulation (African Health Business 2021; World Bank 2021).

The administration of health facilities especially the curative hospitals is usually within districts, states, and federal levels (Abdullah et al. 2017; Ebrahim et al. 2017). The national health strategic plans have been utilized in tracking the nation's progress toward the sustainable development goals. Another goal of the Federal Ministry of Health is to identify situations of lack of efficiency, and injustice as well as develop strategies that could enable health policies and programs that have galvanized better access to healthcare in the country. However, the challenges of not having sufficient and sustainable funds are aligned with the capacity-building process of the administration of the health system in Sudan.

Data Analysis and Discussion

The goal of this chapter is to examine the nature and impacts of health policies and healthcare services equitably to all the citizens and residents of The Republic of Sudan. The data used for the analysis of healthcare policy effectiveness were derived from secondary research methods. The secondary research methods adopted include content analysis of the Federal Government of Sudan Ministry of Health reports, World Bank indicators, Development Initiatives report, the World Health Organization reports, United Nations Human Development Index annual report, Center for Disease Control, Country Report, and United States Agency for International Development, academic as well as professional journals articles.

Table 1 data were derived from secondary sources. Content analyses were conducted to explore the effectiveness of health policies and healthcare delivery systems in Sudan According to the World Bank Indicators Report (2023) and the United Nations Human Development Index (2022), the Government of Sudan population is estimated to be 46.9 people in 2022. Further, the GDP of Sudan was US$51.66 billion in 2022.

Table 1 Economics and Health Indicators in Sudan

No.	Major Indicators of Sudan	Explanation
1	Population of Sudan	46.9 million (2022)
2	Gross domestic product (GDP)	US$51.66 billion
3	Current health expenditure (% of GDP)	3.02% (2020)
4	Physicians/doctors per 1,000 people	0.3 (2017)
5	Nurses and midwives per 1,000 people	1.1 (2018)
6	Population using at least basic drinking water service (% of population)	65% (2022)
7	People using safely managed sanitation services (% of population)	68% (2017)
8	People practicing open defecation (% of the population)	6% Urban; and 24 Rural (2020)
9	Common disease	Diarrhea, hepatitis A, typhoid fever, malaria, schistosomiasis, rabies, meningococcal meningitis
10	Life expectancy at birth for females	68 years (2021)
11	Life expectancy at birth for males	63 years (2021)
12	Mortality rate for female adults (per 1,000 people)	174 (2021)
13	Mortality rate for infants (per 1,000 people)	39 (2021)
15	Tuberculosis incidence (per 100,000 people)	58 (2021)
16	Population living below income poverty line PPP US$2.150 a day	15.3% (2021)
17	Population in multidimensional handout poverty (%)	49% (2015)
18	Infants lacking immunization for measles (% of one year old)	84% (2021)
19	Malaria incidence (per 1,000 people at risk)	72.8 (2021)
20	HIV/AIDS prevalence adults (% ages 15–49)	0.1% (2021)

Source: World Bank Indicators (2023); United Nations Human Development Program Index (2022); World Health Organization (2023).

In 2020, the Federal Republic of Sudan spent 3.02% of its GDP on healthcare (World Bank 2023). Many scholars contend that apart from the civil wars in the country since the Republic of South Sudan separated from Sudan, the nation has lost about 75% of its oil revenue. Furthermore, the annual percentage of growth rate of domestic product decreased from 7.8% to 3.1% in 2014. The sanctions that the United States imposed have also barred the nation from receiving international funding for healthcare as a result of being included on the terrorism list (Ebrahim et al. 2017; Dafallah et al. 2023; Hassanain et al. 2022). According to Dafallah et al. (2023), the health system in Sudan has been disfranchised due to $700 million of its budget that has been transferred to the military and defense function. Thus, the health budget of Sudan in 2023 has been reduced to just 1.4% of the nation's GDP (Dafallah et al. 2023). Moreover, only 5.4% of the Federal Republic of Sudan's healthcare expenditure are funded with foreign donations (Sharew 2022) The analysis conducted reveals that the funds that the Government of Sudan has been appropriate for its health sector in the past few years are far below the 15% of GDP that all the African Union leaders agreed to at the 2001 Abuja Declaration submit. This shortage of health budget will help to explain the current healthcare challenges in the country.

According to the World Bank Indicators (2023), in 2017, physician/doctor per 1,000 people in Sudan was 0.3, while nurses and midwives per 1,000 people was 1.1 in 2018 (World Bank Indicators 2022; World Health Organization Report 2023). Previously, the physician-to-patient ratio was 0.1 per 1,000 people in 1996, and later it improved to 0.41 doctors per 1,000 people in 2015 (Sharew 2022). In addition, access to safe and basic managed drinking water varies from one state to another. For example, in Khartoum, the rate is 95%, while in North Darfur, the rate of population to basic safe drinking water is reported to be about 30% (Charani et al. 2019).

Furthermore, it is also reported that people using safely managed sanitation services (% of the population in Sudan was 68% in 2017). On the other hand, the people practicing open defecation % of the population constitute 6% in the urban cities and 24% in the rural regions of the country. The analysis conducted revealed that there has been no decrease in the number of people who practice open defecation because, in 2015, 26% of the population were practicing open defecation. It should be noted that people in many parts of Sudan rely on finding water outside their homes because there is no connected piped water distribution. Thus, the water such people depend on could easily become contaminated due to surface water that is not secured (Charani et al. 2019; World Bank Indicators 2023).

According to the Federal Ministry of Health in Sudan Health statistical report, diarrhea, hepatitis A, typhoid fever, malaria, schistosomiasis, rabies, meningococcal meningitis, diseases of the respiratory system, and essential hypertension are among the 10 leading diseases treated in out-patient health facilities as per 1,000 population (Sudan Federal Ministry of Health Statistical Report 2018; World Bank Indicators 2022). Sudan is also susceptible to noncommunicable diseases, and natural and human-caused disasters. Drought, flood, internal conflicts, and outbreaks of violence are quite common which bring about a burden of traumatic disease and demand for high-quality emergency healthcare (Abdullah et al. 2017; Wikipedia 2023). The life expectancy at birth in 2021 was 68 years, for females, while the life expectancy at birth for males in 2021 was 63 years. In addition, the mortality rate for female adults per 1,000 people was 174 in 2021, and 253 per 1,000 for adult males in 2021. The World Bank Indicators (2022) data also show that the mortality rate for infants per 1,000 people was 59 in 2021. Furthermore, the incidence of tuberculosis per 100,000 people has dropped to 58 in 2022 in Sudan. While malaria incidence per 1,000 people at risk was 72.8 in 2021. Sudan has done very well in the area of preventing the spread of HIV/AIDS prevalence among adults ages 15–49. The HIV/AIDS prevalence in the country was 0.1% in 2021. However, due to the civil war, infants lacking immunization for measles percentage of one year was 84% in 2021 (World Bank Indicators 2023). The World Bank Indicators (2022) data also reported that the population living below income poverty line PPP $2.150 a day in the Federal Republic of Sudan was 15.3% in 2022. On the other hand, the population of Sudan in multidimensional handout poverty was 49% in 2015.

Other healthcare challenges that have been identified by many scholars are climate change, geographical barriers, and the distance between some rural communities and healthcare facilities in the urban areas in Sudan. It is postulated that 70% of the healthcare hospitals and clinics are located in Khartoum the capital city while just 20% population reside. Thus, 80% of the population are residents in rural areas where there are few hospitals (Ebi et al. 2021; Egere et al. 2021; Sharew 2022). Although some elements of telemedicine have been adopted in some rural states in the country, challenges associated with software licensing, equipment maintenance, and poor collaboration between scattered telemedicine projects hindered the effective capacity building of the initiative (Hassanain et al. 2022; Sharew 2022). Another challenge is the number of beds available in the health facilities in Sudan. It is reported that the country has 538 hospitals (rate of 1.3/100,000 of the population) with 31,430 beds (rate of 76.4/100,000 of the population), 251 blood banks, 171 X-ray units, and 5,852 primary health centers and units as of 2020. The current political instability in Sudan would continue to be an impediment to resolving this geographical and rate of bed-per-patient predicaments.

Conclusion

This chapter has examined the nature of health policy and implementation in Sudan. It analyzes the challenges of the healthcare delivery system in the country. It argues that despite the previously well-established healthcare system in the country, the challenges of several years of political instability have prevented Sudan's ability to effectively prevent the spread of communicable and noncommunicable diseases. The finding of the research analysis reveals that the ineffective healthcare delivery system has created an aftermath of increased chronic and endemic infectious diseases such as malaria, leishmaniasis, and schistosomiasis are incrementally causing substantial morbidity and mortality. Therefore, improving primary healthcare performance in the Federal Republic of Sudan will require a pressing need to change the culture of constant civil wars, prioritize research efforts, build the field of research around targeted questions, and better understand how to ensure the core service delivery functions of public health coverage in the country.

Apart from the challenges of funding confronting the health system in Sudan, the need to address the shortage of health workers is paramount. This is because physicians, nurses, midwives' pharmacists, and other health workforce personnel are the major drivers of any health system. For the Federal Ministry of Health to be considered a responsive enterprise the hospitals and other health facilities must be embedded with an adequate number of highly qualified health professionals. Further, to retain a highly qualified health workforce, the Government of Sudan must provide comparative salaries, incentives, good working conditions, and modern infrastructure to enable due diligence performance.

One of the reasons why most people in the rural districts in Sudan subscribe to health insurance is a lack of awareness of the benefits of health insurance. In the future, the Government of Sudan should engage in successful community engagement through promotion campaigns in the media such as television, social media, and radio all over the country. A vibrant awareness could propel broader community participation on all issues, including health, ranging from building health facilities, motivating health workers, and conducting health convoys to the 18 states in Sudan.

Furthermore, the Federal Republic of Sudan Government must realize that although healthcare is a human right return of investment in health could be interconnected to several social and economic benefits, notably financial return, social cohesion, and a vibrant motivation for the citizens of Sudan to participate in social and political dialogue that could hence share governance and democracy in the country. In addition, it is paramount for the Government of Sudan to engage in more dialog with the citizens of the country. The autocratic system of governance that has been practiced for more than three decades has not resonated well with the citizens. Thus, engaging dialogue and constant consultation with the different communities and citizens could enhance transparency, capacity building, and well a new brighter vision for the nation.

Finally, moving forward with the establishment of a vibrant health system will require appropriate funding and a stable political system where there is a rule of law, and three equal branches of government such as the executive, legislative, and judicial branches of government. Under such a system nobody should be above the law, and the president is not the boss of the supreme court judges, nor the national assembly members. A check and balance system could propel the nation in the right direction of promoting human rights, social justice, and healthcare for everyone in the Republic of Sudan.

References

Abdeen M. O. (2018). Some aspects of medicine distribution in Sudan. *Archives of Pharmacy and Pharmaceutical Sciences.* DOI: 10.29328/journal.apps.1001009. Accessed October 30, 2023.

Abdullah E. M., Luam G., Tasneem A., Hanafiah J. M. (2017). Health care system in Sudan: Review and analysis of strength, weakness, opportunity, and threats (SWOT analysis). *Sudan Journal of Medical Sciences,* 12(3): 133–147.

African Health Business (2021). Sudan's health sector. https://www.ahb.co.ke/wp-content/uploads/2021/country-overview-Sudan.pdf. Accessed November 7, 2023.

Ahmed A., Dietrich I., Desiree LaBeaud A., Lindsay S. W., Musa A., and Weaver S. C. (2020). Risks and challenges of arboviral diseases in Sudan: The urgent need for actions. *Viruses,* 12(1): 1–16.

Albarodi M. (2023). Sudan conflict leaves health system in total collapse. https://www.gavi.org/vaccineswork/sudan-conflict-leaves-health-system-total-collapse. Accessed October 30, 2023.

Alfadul E. S. A., Abdalmotalib M. M., Alrawa S. S. K., Osman R. O. A., Hassan H. M. A., Albasheir A. T., Hasabo E. A., Mohamed S. O. O., Shaaban K. M. A. (2023). Burnout and its associated factors among healthcare workers in COVID-19 isolation centers in Khartoum, Sudan: A cross-sectional study. *PLoS One.* 21;18(7):e0288638. DOI: 10.1371/journal.pone.0288638.

Ali M. E. M., Abdalla E. M. (2021). Out of Pocket Healthcare Expenditures: Determinants and Impacts on the Livelihoods of Urban Households in Selected Sudanese States. Sudan

Working Paper 2021:01. https://www.cmi.no/publications/7755-out-of-pocket-healthcare-expenditures. Accessed September 19, 2024.

Altayb H. N., Altayeb N. M. E., Hamadalnil Y., Elsayid M., and Mahmoud N. E. (2020). The current situation of COVID-19 in Sudan. *New Microbes and New Infections*. Sep; 37:100746. doi: 10.1016/j.nmni.2020.100746.

Anib V. A., Achiek M. M., Ndenzako F., Olu O. O. (2022). South Sudan's road to universal health coverage: A slow but steady journey. *Pan Africa Medical Journal*, 7(42), (Suppl 1): 1–12.

Appiah-Mensah S. (2006). The African mission in Sudan: Darfur dilemmas. *African Security Review*, 15(1): 1–19.

Bechtold P. K. (2015). Regional disparities in Sudan. In Berry, LaVerle (ed.). *Sudan: A Country Study*. (Fifth Edition). Washington DC: Federal Research Division, Library of Congress. pp. 132–133.

Berry L. (2015). *Sudan a country study*. Washington DC : Unted Staes Library of Congress Publication. Accessed September 20, 2024.

British Broadcasting Corporation (2023). Sudan country profile. https://www.bbc.com/news/world-africa-14094995. Accessed November 11, 2023.

Buchsee D. (2023). The conflict in Sudan is a public health disaster. https://ysph.yale.edu/news-article/the-conflict-in-sudan-is-a-public-disater/. Accessed October 30, 2023.

Charani E., Cunnington A. J., Yousif A. H. A, et al. (2019). In transition: Current health challenges and priorities in Sudan. *BMJ Global Health*, 4: e001723.

Chutel L. (2023). As hospitals close and doctors flee, Sudan's health care system is collapsing. https://www.nytimes.com/2023/04/30/world/africa/sudan-hospitals-doctors-fighting.html. Accessed November 2, 2023.

Collins R. (2008). *A History of Modern Sudan*. (First Edition). London, UK: Cambridge University Press.

Dafallah A., Elmahi O. K. O., Ibrahim M. E., Elsheikh R. E., Blanchet K. (2023). Destruction, disruption and disaster: Sudan's health system amidst armed conflict. *BMC*, 17(42): 1–4.

Doctors under siege in Sudan. The Mail and Guardian (2020). https://mg.co.za/africa/2020-06-26-doctors-under-siege-in-sudan/. Accessed October 30, 2023.

Doctors Without Border (2023). Sudan: MSF condemns looting of medical facilities, harassment of staff. https://www.doctorswithoutborders.org/latest/sudan-msf-condemns-looting-medical-facilities-harassment-staff. Accessed October 30, 2023.

Ebi E. L., Vanos J., Baldwin J. W., Bell J. E., David M., Hondula D. M., et al. (2021). Extreme weather and climate change: Population health and health system implications, *Annual Review of Public Health*, 42(1):293–315.

Ebi K., Hese J. (2020). Health risks due to climate change: Inequity In causes and consequences. *Health Affairs*, 39(12). DOI: 10.1377/hlthaff.2020.01125.

Ebrahim A., Appleby M. V., Axford D., Beale J., Moreno-Chicano T., Sherrell D. A., Strange R. W., Hougha M. A., Robin L. Owenb R. L. (2019). Resolving polymorphs and radiation-driven effects in microcrystals using fixed-target serial synchrotron crystallography. https://journals.iucr.org/d/issues/2019/02/00/ba5292/ba5292.pdf. Accessed November 12, 2024.

Ebrahim M. A. E., Abdalgfar T. G. L, Juni M. H. (2017). Healthcare system in Sudan: Review and analysis of strength, weakness, opportunity, and threats (SWOT analysis). *Sudan Journal of Medical Sciences*, 12(3): 1–18.

Egere U., Shayo E., Ntinginya N., Osman R., Noory B., Mpagama S., Squire S. B. (2021). Management of chronic lung diseases in Sudan and Tanzania: How ready are the country health systems? *BMC Health Services Research*, 21(1): 1–11.

Fadlalla M. (2004). *Short History of Sudan*. Bloomington, IN: iUniverse Press.

Forsyth, A. (2020). What is a healthy place? Models for cities and neighbourhoods. *Journal of Urban Design*, 25(2), 186–202.

Federal Ministry of Health Sudan. (2020). *Sudan Federal Ministry of Health COVID-19 Daily Situation Report 2020*. Khartoum, Sudan: Federal Ministry of Health Publication.

Federal Ministry of Health Sudan Statistical Report (2018). *System of health accounts Report.* Khartoum, Sudan: Federal Ministry of Health Publication.

Federal Ministry of Health Sudan (2017). *Sudan's National Health Policy 2017–2030.* Khartoum, Sudan: Federal Ministry of Health Publication. https://platform.who.int/docs/default-source/mca-documents/policy-documents/policy/SDN-CC-31-01-POLICY-2017-eng-National-Health-Care-Quality.pdf. Accessed November 12, 2024.

Federal Ministry of Health Sudan (2016). *Sudan Maternal Death Surveillance and Response Report 2016.* Khartoum, Sudan: Federal Ministry of Health Publication.

Haakenstad A., Irvine C. M. S., Knight M., Bintz C., Aravkin A. Y., Zheng P., and Lozano R. (2022). Measuring the availability of human resources for health and its relationship to universal health coverage for 204 countries and territories from 1990 to 2019: A systematic analysis for the Global Burden of Disease Study 2019. *The Lancet,* 399(10341): 2129–2154.

Habbani S.Y.I., Karaig E. A. B. A., Al-Fadil S. M., El-Fadul M., Shaheen S. M. A., Gadir N. A. A., Abu Zaid H. A. S., Malik E. M. (2021). Towards universal health coverage: Designing a community-based intervention to scale up coverage with health insurance, in A-Duiem Administrative Unit, Sudan 2018–2019. *Public Health Open Journal,* 6(1): 12–18.

Hasan Y. F. (1967). *The Arabs and the Sudan. From the Seventh to the Early Sixteenth Century.* Edinburgh, United Kingdom: Edinburgh University Press.

Hassanain S. A., Eltahir A., Elbadawi L. I. (2022). Freedom, peace, and justice: A new paradigm for the Sudanese health system after Sudan's 2019 uprising. Economic Research Forum: Working Paper 1555. Dokki, Giza Egypt.

Hemmeda L., Ahmed A. S., Omer M. (2023). Sudan's armed rivalry: A comment on the vulnerable healthcare system catastrophe. *Health Science Report,* 6(8): e1517–e1523.

Holt & Daly (2000). *History of the Sudan: From the Coming of Islam to the Present Day.* New York: Pearson Learning.

Keita S. O. Y. (1993). The subspecies concept in zoology and anthropology: A brief historical review and test of a classification scheme. *Journal of Black Studies,* 23(3): 416–445.

Kruk M. E., Pérignon D., Rockers P. C., Van Lerberghe W. (2010). The contribution of primary care to health and health systems in low- and middle-income countries: A critical review of major primary care initiatives. *Social Science Medicine,* 70(6): 904–711.

Lucero-Prisno D. E., Elhadi Y. A. M., Modber M. A. A., Musa M. B., Mohammed S. E. E., Hassan K. F., and Adebisi Y. A. (2020). Drug shortage crisis in Sudan in times of COVID19. *Public Health in Practice,* 1(November), 100060. DOI: 10.1016/j.puhip.2020.100060. Accessed October 30, 2023.

Insecurity Insight (2023). Sudan violence against healthcare in IN in conflict. /https://insecurity insight.org/wp-content/uploads/2024/05/2023-SHCC-Sudan.pdf. Accessed September 20, 2024.

International Trade Administration (2022). Sudan Country Commercial guide: Healthcare and health technologies. https://www.trade.gov/country-commercial-guides/sudan-health-care-and-health-technologies. Accessed October 30, 2023.

Manzo (2017). Eastern Sudan in its Setting, The archaeology of a region far from the Nile Valley, 33–42 online Archived 2020-01-26 at the Wayback Machine.

Metz K. (1991). Development of explanation: Incremental and fundamental change in children's physics knowledge. *Journal of Research in Science Teaching,* 28(6): 785–797.

Mohammed F. E. A., Viva M. I. F., Awadalla W. A. G., Elmahi O. K. O, Patil D. W. P. (2023). Defending the right to health during Sudan's civil war. *Lancet Global Health.* Sep;11(9): e1327–e1328.

Mustafa S. A. M., Hamed F. H. M. (2018). Exploring health insurance services in Sudan from the perspectives of insurers. *SAGE Open Medical,* 6: 2050312117752298.

Najovits S. R. (2004). *The Consequences: How Egypt Became the Trunk of the Tree.* New York: Algora Publishing Company.

Nashed M. (2023). Sudan doctors targeted with threats and smear campaigns. https://www. aljazeera.com/amp/news/2023/5/9/sudan-doctors-targeted-with-threats-and-smear-campaigns. Accessed October 30, 2023.

Noory B., Hassanain S. A., Lindskog B. V., Elsony A., Bjune G. A. (2020). Exploring the consequences of decentralization: has privatization of health services been the perceived effect of decentralization in Khartoum locality, Sudan? *BMC Health Serv Res.* July 20;20(1): 669–683.

Public Health Institute Federal Ministry of Health. (2016). Health Finance Policy Options for Sudan, (March), 35. https://www.researchgate.net/publication/340263903_Health_Finance_Policy_options_for_Sudan_2016. Accessed September 19, 2024.

Public Health Institute Federal Ministry of Health (2014). *Health System Financing Review Report.* Khartoum: Federal Government of Sudan, Press.

Republic of Sudan National Health Sector Strategic Plan II 2012–2016 (2016). https://extranet. who.int/countryplanningcycles/sites/default/files/planning_cycle_repository/sudan/ sudan_national_health_sector_strategic_plan_nhssp_2012-2016.pdf. Accessed October 30, 2023.

Saleh A. M., Almobarak A. O., Badi S., Siddiq S. B., Tahir H., Suliman M., and Ahmed M. H. (2021). Knowledge, attitudes and practice among primary care physicians in Sudan regarding prediabetes: A cross-sectional survey. *International Journal of Preventive Medicine.* July 5;12:80. doi: 10.4103/ijpvm.IJPVM_164_20. Accessed September 19, 2024.

Saleh D., Hess R., Ahlers-Hesse M., Rischawy F., Wang G., Grosch J., Schwab T., Kluters S., Studts J., Hubbuch J. (2023). A multiscale modeling method for therapeutic antibodies in ion exchange chromatography. *Biotechnology and Bioengineering*, 120(1): 125–138.

Saied E. M, Kabbash I. A, E-Fatah-Abdo S. A. (2021). Vaccine hesitancy: Beliefs and barriers associated with COVID-19 vaccination among Egyptian medical students. Journal of Medical Virology, 93(7): 4280–4291.

Salim A. M. A., Hamed F.H. M., (2018). Exploring health insurance services in Sudan from the perspectives of insurers. *SAGE Open Medicine* Jan 11;6:2050312117752298. doi: 10.1177/2050312117752298. PMID: 29348914; PMCID: PMC5768257. Accessed October 23, 2023.

Schlein I. (2023). UN: Sudan healthcare near collapse due to conflict. https://www.voanew.com/a/ un-suadan-health-care-near-collapse-duetoconflict-/7182156.html. Accessed November 1, 2023.

Security Insight (2023). Sudan Situation Report. https://insecurityinsight.org/wp-content/ uploads/2023/09/Sudan-Situation-Report-Aid-Agencies-Access-and-Security-Management-September-2023.pdf. Accessed November 22, 2023.

Sharew B. (2022). Improving access to healthcare in Sudan. https://borgenproject.org/ healthcare-in-sudan/. Accessed November 1, 2023.

Skinner H. (2023). As Sudan war rages, country's health system nears breaking point. https:// abcnews.go.com/International/sudan-conflict-african-countrys-health-system-nears-breaking/story?id=99564797. Accessed October 30, 2023.

Sudan Federal Ministry of Health (2007). Sudan Antenatal Care and HIV Sentinel Serosurvey. https://ghdx.healthdata.org/record/sudan-antenatal-care-and-hiv-sentinel-serosurvey-2007. Accessed November 12, 2024.

Sudan Federal Ministry of Health (2001). *Sudan National Malaria Control Programme: Short term Malaria Control Strategic Plan 2000–2005.* Federal Ministry of Health, Khartoum: Sudan Publication.

The National Medicine Supply Fund, the Federal Ministry of Health (2017). The National Supply Chain Strategy for Pharmaceuticals and Health Products. June 2017. https://www. nmsf.gov.sdincludes/pdf/UNDP_NCSS.pdf. Accessed October 27, 2023.

UNICEF (2022). Sudan health: Supporting high impact interventions to save lives of mother and babies. https://www.unicef.org/sudan/health. Accessed November 1, 2023.

United Nations (2022). Human Development Data report (2022). https: hdr.undo.org/en/2022-report. Accessed October 30, 2023.

United Nations Human Development Program Index (2022). UNDP human development index 2022: Main components. https://mapstack.io/map/DYs0Dd/undp-human-development-index-2022:-main-components. Accessed September 20, 2024.

University of Central Arkansas (2023). Republic of the Sudan 1956-present. https://uca.edu/politicalscience/home/research-projects/dadm-project/sub-saharan-africa-region/70-republic-of-sudan-1956-present/.

Walsh D. (2023). Gunfire and blasts rock Sudan's capital as factions Vie for Control. https://www.npr.org/2023/04/15/1170249456/gunfire-and-explosions-erupt-across-sudans-capital-as-military-rivals-clash. Accessed September 20, 2024.

Wharton G., Ali O. E., Khalil S., Yagoub H., and Mossialos E. (2020). Rebuilding Sudan's health system: Opportunities and challenges. *The Lancet*, 395(10219): 171–173.

Wikipedia (2023). Health in Sudan. https://en.wikipedia.org/wiki/Health_in_Sudan. Accessed October 30, 2023.

World Bank (2021). Sudan Overview. https://www.wordbank.org/en/country/sudan/overview#1. Accessed November 7, 2023.

World Bank Group (2022a). World Development Indicators. https://databank.worldbank.org/source/world-development-indicators. Accessed November 10, 2024.

World Bank Group (2022b). World Development Indicators. https://databank.worldbank.org/source/world-development-indicators. Accessed November 10, 2024.

World Bank Indicators (2023). Sudan. https://data.worldbank.org/indicator/NY.GDP.MKTP.CD.Locations=CM. Accessed August 16, 2023.

World Health Organization (2023). Sudan Health Emergency. https://www.emro.who.int/images/stories/sudan/WHO-Sudan-conflict-situation-report-15-December_2023.pdf?ua=1. Accessed November 12, 2024.

Yuan Z., Nag R., Cummins E. (2022). Human health concerns regarding microplastics in the aquatic environment – From marine to food systems. *Science of The Total Environment*, 823(1). https://journals.iucr.org/d/issues/2019/02/00/ba5292/ba5292.pdf. Accessed November 12, 2024.

Chapter Seventeen

HEALTH POLICY CHALLENGES IN TANZANIA

Justine Igbokwe-Ibeto

Introduction

This chapter examines the nature of healthcare and the effectiveness of the health policies in Tanzania. It also seeks to explain the factors that led the nation's government to adopt various health strategic plans that could reach all households with essential health and social welfare services. It argues that a strong health system is an essential mechanism for implementing universal health coverage and fulfilling human rights entitlement. The motivation for meeting the healthcare needs of the citizens of Tanzania as much as possible as well as the expectations of the population could yield insights for improvement (Akachi & Kruk 2017; Opuko 2023). Further, adhering to high-quality standards, and applying evidence-informed interventions through efficient channels of the healthcare service delivery system are mechanisms for evaluating success in the health system in Tanzania. The content analysis research method that was used includes analysis of the World Bank's Development Indicator and Tanzania's healthy policy reform United Nations Human Development Report; World Bank Indicators; African Development Bank reports, Walt and Gilson's health policy analysis, academic journals, and World Health reports. The specific objectives include quality improvement of primary healthcare services, delivering a package of essential services in communities and health facilities; equitable access to services in the country by focusing on geographic areas with higher disease burdens and by focusing on vulnerable groups in the population with higher risks; active community partnership through intensified interactions with the population for improvement of health and social wellbeing; a higher rate of return on investment by applying modern management methods and engaging in innovative partnerships and social determinants of health, the health and social welfare sector will collaborate with other sectors, and advocate for the inclusion of health-promoting and health-protecting measures in other sectors' policies and strategies. The findings of the research reveal that for many decades foreign groups have driven health research in Tanzania without creating adequate local capacity in the country. It recommends that investment in information technology systems in the country could propel a positive mechanism for evaluating and refining health policy in Tanzania. This approach could help the Government of Tanzania to attain the right to effectively manage to health delivery system that could benefit citizens and residents of Tanzania.

The African Great Lakes nation of Tanzania was formed out of the union of the much larger mainland territory of Tanganyika and the coastal archipelago of Zanzibar. The former was a colony and part of German East Africa from the 1880s to 1919s when it was under the League of Nations, it became a British mandate. In 1947, Tanganyika became a United Nations Trust Territory under British administration, a status it kept until its independence in 1961. Julius Nyerere, independence leader and *"baba wa taifa"* for Tanganyika (father of the Tanganyika nation), now United Republic of Tanzania, ruled the country for 21 years until his voluntary retirement in 1985 and was succeeded in office by President Ali Hassan Mwinyi 1985–1995, then, Benjamin Mkap 1995–2005, Jakaya Kikwete 2005–2015, John Maguful 2015–2021 before his sudden death in March 2021 which ushered in Samia Suluhu Hassan as the country's first female president and the sixth Tanzanian President.

Successive governments of the United Republic of Tanzania have produced different health policies. As the country strives to reach middle-income status, the health sector has resolved to give more attention to the quality of health services in tandem with the pursuit of universal access. At the same time, better health for the entire population has been promoted through the adoption of health in all policies (National Health Policy 2017; Mikkelsen-Lopez 2014). The country has made impressive gains in reducing under-five and infant mortality, through strengthening immunization services and improved preventive services for malaria and other childhood diseases. The number of new HIV cases has been also decreasing. However, maternal mortality is still high in Tanzania as the Millennium Development Goal (MDG), targets were not attained (NHP 2017; Sprockett 2016).

Health Challenges in Tanzania

The population in Tanzania has increased in the last 10 years. The health system thereby has been adjusting continuously to provide services to an increased number of people. The increase in the population of the country has also galvanized a limited healthcare workforce and inadequate access to healthcare for the citizens and residents of Tanzania. Health services are provided from the grassroots level beginning with community healthcare, dispensaries, and health centers, and proceeding through first-level hospitals, regional referral hospitals, and zonal and national hospitals, all providing increasingly sophisticated and well-defined services. Another challenge is that limitation of access has propelled inadequate improvement in health outcomes in the past two decades (Balogun et al. 2020; Maluka et al. 2018; Sprockett 2016).

There continues to be a major challenge because of the insufficient government spending on the health system in the country. Some scholars contend that the current health system financing is not effectively offering special protection for all the citizens in the country (Kalolo et al. 2022; Kapologwe et al. 2019). Lack of adequate financing has negatively impacted the availability of healthcare equipment that is not equitably distributed to all public hospitals in the country. Furthermore, the state of financing relies too much on out-of-pocket payment (Balogun et al. 2020; Kesale et al. 2022a; Maluka et al. 2018; Opuka 2022). This predicament tends to place a catastrophic financial burden on the low-income population of the country. The World Health Organization recommends a minimum health expenditure of 6% of GDP annually to provide basic health services in each country. On the other hand, the 2001 Abuja Declaration mandates at least 15% of GDP per year for the health system. Unfortunately, the government of Tanzania has not met that trajectory. In 2019, the government only appropriated 1.5% of its GDP for healthcare in the following year (2020) and it budgeted 3.75%. Further in 2021 and 2022, it appropriated 5.6% of its GDP for healthcare. Consequently, Tanzania has not fulfilled both the budget requirements for the Abuja Declaration and the World Health Organization (2011). Maluka et al. (2018) and the United Federal Republic of Tanzania (2022) contend that the nation's health funding comes from two major sources. The sources of financing are (1) central support financing by the national government of Tanzania's general tax revenue, and (2) foreign development partners. The national donors contribute up to 40% of Tanzania's health budget (Kesale et al. 2022b; United Federal Republic of Tanzania 2022).

The shortage of medical workforce such as physicians, nurses, and other healthcare workers in Tanzania has been a major challenge. In 2018, the nation had a physician per 1,000 people to 0.1. While the number of nurses/midwives per 1,000 people was 0.6 World Bank indicators (2023). The total number of health workers required in Tanzania in 2019/2020 was 212,193, and the number that health workers that the nation had was 98,987. This number indicates a 53% shortage of health human resources staff (International Trade Administration 2022). In certain geographical areas, populations still live far away from health services. This has especially been problematic in terms of maternal and newborn care (Balogun et al. 2022; Njaki 2022; Opuka 2022). The referral system does not always function as required, sometimes due to a lack of adequate transport to the next level of care or due to an inability at the referral level to provide adequate services (Maluka et al. 2010; Mujinja & Saronga 2022). Health sector challenges posed by current financing levels and modalities require change to the way financial access to healthcare is organized, greater efforts on resource mobilization, transparency, and social accountability, as well as more determined measures to strengthen the health system as a whole.

Types of Health Policies

The Republic of Tanzania has put in place a conducive environment for the provision of health education and promotion services at all levels. All health sector stakeholders participated in the provision of health education and promotion services. This has been through increasing use of communication media, especially television, internet, mobile phones, and social media such as Facebook, Twitter, blogs, etc. Effective community health education has some positive impact on social welfare (Gilson et al. 1995; Kesale et al. 2022c; Njakoi 2021). There has been an increasing knowledge/awareness toward the protection and promotion of health by the communities in Tanzania. However, Tanzania has no governing principles, acts, regulations, or guidelines established for health education, weak institutional linkages, and community engagement. Below are selected health policies that have been enacted and implemented in the past few decades.

Policy on Reproductive, Maternal, Newborn, Child, and Adolescent Health enacted in 2022: The major objective of the RMNCAH's vision is to have Tanzanian youth and women who are engaged, empowered, and well-informed when making decisions relating to their reproductive health needs, contributing to the country's long-term prosperity, and improving the health outcomes of Tanzanians (United States Agency for International Development 2022). Other goals include (1) Improved access to quality, client-centered RMNCAH services in both health facilities and the surrounding communities; (2) Improved ability of individuals to practice positive health-seeking and self-care behaviors; (3) Enhanced enabling environment for quality RMNCAH service provision. In addition, the policy mandate specific adolescent health services and emergency services during the delivery process has been weak in Tanzania. It also propels or scales up emergency maternal and newborn health services and reduces the rate of maternal and newborn mortality challenges in the country (United Republic of Tanzania 2022).

New National Health Policy enacted in 2017: The objective of this policy was to reach all households with essential health services attaining the needs of the population, adhering to objective quality standards, and applying evidence-informed interventions through resilient systems for health. The other rationale of the policy emanates from the fact that times have changed, there is a new fifth government political regime, increasing health sector challenges, and new demands for drafting processes, format, and contents of national sector policies in Tanzania. The implementation of the National Health Policy—2007 has been in line with implementations of the National Development Vision 2025, the Millennium Development Goals (MDGs), the National Strategies for Growth and Reduction of Poverty (NSGRP I and II) programs, and other development efforts (United Republic of Tanzania 2017).

National Five-Year Development Plan 2016/2017–2020/2021 enacted in 2016: The objective of this policy was to provide quality healthcare ensuring that people are fit to participate in social economic activities. Addressing this depends critically on strengthening of health service delivery system with service delivery geared toward improving the health of mothers and children. It also entails, addressing prevalent illnesses such as malaria, HIV, and AIDS which are major causes of death as well as addressing the human resource crisis, which constrains the provision of adequate healthcare. Specific interventions for the plan include improving the livelihood of Tanzanians; strengthening of referral system; improving the availability of specialized services and strengthening training institutions (United Republic of Tanzania 2016).

Health Sector Strategic Plan 2015–2020 enacted in 2015: The objective of this Health Sector Strategic Plan is to reach all households with essential health and social welfare services, meeting, as much as possible, the expectations of the population, adhering to objective quality standards, and applying evidence-informed interventions through efficient channels of service delivery. The specific objectives include (1) quality improvement of primary healthcare services; (2) delivering a package of essential services in communities and health facilities; (3) equitable access to services in the country by focusing on geographic areas with higher disease burdens and by focusing on vulnerable groups in the population with higher risks; and (4) a higher rate of return on investment by applying modern management methods and engaging in innovative partnerships and social determinants of health (United Republic of Tanzania 2007).

Second National Health Policy enacted in 2007: The goal of the National Health Policy was to facilitate the provision of basic health services that are of excellent quality, equitable, accessible, affordable, sustainable, and gender sensitive. The main objective was to improve the health and well-being of all Tanzanians, with a focus on those most at risk, and encourage the health system to be more responsive to the needs of the people and, thus increase the life expectancy. The NHP 2007 had several specific policy objectives. These included the need to reduce morbidity and mortality and increase life expectancy for all Tanzanians by delivering better health services, which focus on requirements for vulnerable groups such as infants, under-fives, preschool and school children, youths, people with disability, women of reproductive age, and elderly people to access health services (United Republic of Tanzania 2007).

Policy on Traditional and Alternative Medicine enacted in 2002: The policy objective is safety, quality traditional healing, and alternative medicine services. The policy goals also include strengthening basic and scientific research on traditional medicine practices, traditional medicines, and medicinal plants for the improvement of traditional health services, and promoting industrial manufacturing of traditional medicines for malaria. Despite these services being used by the majority, there are concerns about the quality and safety of the practice and products of traditional medicine. Such problems threaten the health of many who are the users of such services (Mujinja & Saronga 2022; United Republic of Tanzania 2002).

Tanzania Vision 1999–2025 enacted in 1999: The goal of this policy was to provide direction and philosophy for the long-term development of the country. The other objectives of this policy include (1) to achieve a quality and good life for all; (2) to achieve good governance and the rule of law; and (3) to build a strong and resilient economy that can effectively withstand global competition. By 2025, Tanzania wants to achieve a high quality of livelihood for its citizens, peace, stability, and unity, good governance, a well-educated society, and a competitive economy capable of producing sustainable growth and shared benefits 2025 (United Republic of Tanzania 1999).

Health Administration in Tanzania

The Ministry of Health in Tanzania is responsible for health matters in collaboration with stakeholders had the responsibility of improving people's health physically, mentally, and socially and their welfare through promotion, prevention, and/or reduction of diseases, disabilities, and deaths. To achieve this objective, the Ministry of Health has the role of developing policies, guidelines, regulations, and laws, which will facilitate the delivery and supervision of promotional, preventive, curative, rehabilitative, and palliative health services. Furthermore, the Ministry of Health has a responsibility to ensure the availability and development of health sector professionals, mobilization and management of funds, equipment, infrastructure, implementable health plans, and provision of quality health services, that are accessible to all people. In addition, the Ministry of Health also has been responsible for strengthening relationships and collaboration with the private sector, and international organizations (United Republic of Tanzania 2022).

The United Federal Republic of Tanzania's health system administration has four levels. The levels are (1) district level; (2) regional level; (3) zonal level; and (4) national level. The structure of the health administration flows from the primary or district level to the secondary or regional level and finally the national or tertiary level. Apart from the public sector health facilities, private that comprise faith-based hospitals also play a major in providing healthcare services to citizens and residents of Tanzania.

The primary- or *district-level* health facilities are closest to the rural communities in the country. The primary-level health facilities consist of dispensaries and healthcare centers. There are currently about 3,250 public dispensaries in Tanzania (Opuko 2023; United Republic of Tanzania 2022). Further, the local government level is divided into 158 districts that consist of urban and rural communities. The primary healthcare hospitals or health centers are located at the district level. The primary-level health facilities are mostly operated by clinical assistants and an enrolled nurse who offers basic outpatient curative care to patients between 6,000 and 10,000 (Maluka et al. 2018). The health facility management team oversees the implementation of health services at the primary district level. The Council Health Management Team is responsible for managing health services at the district level and council level. Further, all district-level health program implementation falls under the authority of the Team. The Team is also responsible for ensuring the implementation of health activities by hospitals, health centers, dispensaries, and communities, as well as monitoring and evaluating the implantation of health activities at the district level (Balogun et al. 2022; Maluka et al. 2018).

At the *regional level*, the Health Management Team manages the health facilities. The regional health system has a decentralized structure. The Regional Health Management Team is responsible for the delivery of health services at the regional level (Maluka et al. 2018; United Federal Republic of Tanzania 2022). It should be noted that multiple districts are merged from regions. Each region has a regional hospital.

The development and administration of the United Federal Tanzania's health system policies are under the control of two ministries. The Ministry of Health is responsible for human resources mobilization and policy formulation and implementation. The Ministry of Health is also responsible for overseeing the delivery of health services at the national hospitals, specialist hospitals, zonal hospitals, and regional feral hospitals (United Republic of Tanzania 2022). The Ministry of Health owns the specialist hospitals. The President's office, Regional Administration, and Local Government are also responsible for managing service delivery at the community level, through mobile and outreach services, dispensaries, health centers, and district hospitals (Balogun et al. 2022; United Republic of Tanzania 2022).

Furthermore, the United Federal Republic of Tanzania tends to have many nonpublic health facilities that are operated by nongovernmental organizations, private for-profit providers, and faith-based organizations. The Government of Tanzania has often signed contracts with nongovernmental health organizations to provide healthcare services to people in some rural districts where there are no public health hospitals or clinics (Maluka et al. 2018; United Federal Republic of Tanzania 2022). The government of Tanzania owns 60% of the health infrastructure in the country while the faith-based health organizations own 23.3%. Furthermore, 41.1% of hospitals are owned by faith-based organizations while the government owns 40% (Maluka et al. 2018).

Data Analysis and Discussion

The objective of this chapter is to analyze the nature and effectiveness of health policies in Rwanda and how the nation's government has been effective in improving mobility, child, and mortality rate over the past two decades after the genocide incident. The research method used for data analysis in this section of the chapter includes content analysis of the United Republic of Tanzania policy documents, United States Center for Diseases Control reports, World Bank indicators and reports, World Health Organization report, Tanzania Ministry of Health reports, United Nations, World Development indicators, and International Trade Administration reports.

The ten major diseases and causes of death in Tanzania are neonatal disorders; lower respiratory infections; HIV/AIDS; stroke; tuberculosis; ischemic heart disease; malaria; diarrheal diseases; congenital birth defects; cirrhosis, and other chronic liver diseases (United States Center for Disease Control and Prevention report 2024). According to the World Bank Indicators report, Tanzania spent 3.75% of its GDP on its health system in 2020. It should be noted that the sources funding the health system in the Tanzania comes from two major groups (1) the central support financed by the United Republic of Tanzania's general tax revenue and (2) the foreign development partners.

Table 1 summarizes the healthcare system profile and indicators. The number of physicians to 1,000 people in Tanzania in 2018 was 0.1, while the ratio of nurses and midwives to 1,000 people was 0.6. The birth of children attended by skilled health personnel in the country in 2016 was 64%. The limited health workers in Tanzania have been argued to negatively reduced access to healthcare for the citizens and residents of the country. This serious predicament is also associated with inadequate improvement in health outcomes in the past two decades in Tanzania. Further, the number of beds per 1,000 people was 1.1 in 2018 (World Economics 2023; World Bank Indicators Report 2023). The United Federal Republic of Tanzania has been reported to provide subsidies to faith-based organizations to provide more beds and staff in districts without a government hospital.

Further, the government also provides operational support to hospitals that are operated by faith-based health facilities (Maluka et al. 2018). The population of Tanzania that had access to electricity in 2021 was 42.7% of the nation's 65.5 million people. The population of Tanzania that is using safe managed drinking water service was 11% in 2022. In addition, the population using at least basic sanitation in the country was 25% in 2022.

Table 1 Economics and Health Indicators in Tanzania

No.	Major Indicators in Rwanda	Explanation
1	Population	65.5 million (2022)
2	Gross domestic product (GDP) PPP	US$1,146 trillion
3	Current health expenditure (% of GDP)	3.75% (2020)
4	Number of physicians/doctors per 1,000 people	0.1 (2018)
5	Number of patients per nurse/midwives per 1,000 people	0.6 (2018)
6	Birth attended by skilled health personnel	64% (2016)
7	Number of bed per 1,000 people	1.1 (2018)
8	Access to electricity	42.7% (2021)
9	Population using safely managed drinking water service	11% (2022)
10	Population using at least basic sanitation	25% (2022)
11	Population practicing open defecation (%)	Urban 0%; rural 10%
12	Common disease in Tanzania	Neonatal disorders; lower respiratory infections; HIV/AIDS; stroke; tuberculosis; ischemic heart disease; malaria; diarrheal diseases; congenital birth defects; cirrhosis and other chronic liver diseases
13	Life expectancy in 2019 at birth for females	68 years (2021)
14	Life expectancy in 2021 at birth for males	64 years (2021)
15	Mortality rate for female adults (per 1,000 people)	192
16	Mortality rate for male adults (per 1,000 people)	253 (2021)
17	Mortality rate for infants (per 1,000 people)	37 (2021)
18	Incidence of malaria per 1,000 people	125.8 (2021)
19	Tuberculosis incidence (per 100,000 people)	192 (2022)
20	HIV/AIDS prevalence adults (% ages 15–49)	0.4 (2022)

Source: World Bank Indicators (2023); United Nations Human Development Programme Human Development Report (2023); United Republic of Tanzania Ministry of Health report (2022–2023).

The gap in the ratio of the health workforce, because of the high turnover and limited career development, is beginning to propel major healthcare challenges in the country. For instance, the mortality rate for female adults in the country per 1,000 people was 192 in 2021, while the mortality rate for men per 1,000 people was 253. The mortality rate for infants per 1,000 people was 37 in 2021. Further, the incidence of malaria per 1,000 people in Tanzania in 2022 was 125.8. While the number of tuberculosis incidence per 100,000 people was 192 in 2022. The HIV/AIDS prevalence for adults' percentage ages 15–49 years old was 0.4% in 2022. This shows significant improvement from what the rate used to be about a decade ago. Another area of improvement in the health system indicators of Tanzania is the life expectancy at birth for females which was reported to be 68 years in 2021. The life expectancy at birth for men was 64 years in 2021. It should be noted that malaria diagnostic treatment services in Tanzania are provided by 6,990 public health facilities, while 872 private hospitals and clinics also provide the same services. Further, 359 faith-based health facilities in the country also provide the same diagnostic services (Severe Malaria Observatory 2023). Moreover, 7,000 pregnant women deliver their babies in reproductive child health facilities annually in Tanzania (Severe Malaria Observatory 2023; Ishungisa et al. 2023).

Although the United Republic of Tanzania has made significant improvements in its health system, there is no doubt that the government needs to increase the development of its healthcare technical and financial capacity, especially in districts where there are no public health facilities. Thus, engaging or awarding contracts to non-state health providers to operate healthcare facilities in some districts is not good enough. This is because this approach creates a disparity between districts that have government hospitals and those that only have faith-based health facilities. Thus, the government should realize the need to equitably distribute public goods to all its citizens. Because over the years, the government tends not to realize the high out-of-pocket cost for its citizens who received their treatment from private providers.

Conclusion

This chapter has examined the effectiveness of the health system and health policy in Tanzania. It argues that despite the efforts that the United Federal Government of Tanzania has made to improve the efficiency of the nation's health system, the recurrent low health system budget has been detrimental to the effectiveness of the healthcare delivery system and poor infrastructure. The chapter also discussed the importance of how well a professionally management health system could be effective between efficient use of human and capital resources, and inefficient waste, which are even more important in a resource-constrained developing country like Tanzania. Because of these healthcare challenges in the United Federal Republic of Tanzania, there is a need to adopt a mechanism of essential healthcare that could meet the expectations of the population.

There is also the need to adhere to the objectives of all the quality standards and evidence-informed interventions that are specified in the health policies that have been enacted by the United Federal Government of Tanzania. As Tanzania strives to reach middle-income status, the health sector has resolved to give more attention to the quality of health services in tandem with the pursuit of universal access. At the same time, better health for the entire population should be promoted through the adoption of universal health coverage policies. It is paramount that the government collaborate with other private sector stakeholders to facilitate the provision of basic health services that are of excellent quality, equitable, accessible, affordable, sustainable, and gender sensitive.

The health policy challenges posed by current health financing levels and modalities require change to the way financial access to healthcare is organized, greater efforts on resource mobilization, transparency, and social accountability, as well as more determined measures to strengthen the health system as a whole. This is needed to achieve a higher rate of return on investment by applying modern management methods and engaging in innovative partnerships.

The findings in this research for this chapter reveal that Tanzania facing major challenges with the timely supply of medicines to all the hospitals and clinics in the nation. Therefore, the government should redesign a vibrant medicine ordering and supply chain system in the country, with greater participation from health workers, and faith-based organizations' senior staff to better understand the challenges, the nation is facing. It is recommended that the United Federal Government of Tanzania various interventions across the health system to strengthen it and improve the availability of medicines. Performance Management mechanism should be adopted to install a better strategic evidence-based approach to solve the problem. It is also recommended that the United Federal Government of Tanzania introduce new methods to galvanize accountability and transparency of the medicines delivery system and force reconciliation between data sources thereby creating information on medicines consumed and the supply chain.

Strengthening the health system will be emphasized in the attainment of better health for the population. The promotion of healthy living and an environment conducive to health protection in households and workplaces will improve the quality of life. Prevention of communicable and noncommunicable diseases, including healthy diets and action against malnutrition, will receive high priority at national, regional, district, community, and household levels. Paid cadres at the community level for social welfare, health promotion, and disease prevention will complement measures to increase access to essential services at facilities and higher levels of the system.

Further, the integration of social welfare and health services and closer collaboration with other ministries, agencies, and nongovernmental organizations will increase accessibility to services for those most in need with a focus on the elderly. This will involve active community partnership through intensified interactions with the population for the improvement of health and social well-being. Gender equity will receive increased attention through concrete measures such as focusing on the prevention of HIV amongst adolescent girls and addressing violence against women. Equal representation of women will be prioritized in committees and boards, and the rights and obligations of duty-bearers and rights-holders will be observed. Tanzania has a successful Sector Wide Approach (SWAp) that will be streamlined to improve joint planning, implementation, monitoring, controlling, and evaluation by all stakeholders.

References

Akachi Y., Kruk M. E. (2017). Quality of care: Measuring a neglected driver of improved health. *Bulletin of the World Health Organization*. 95(6): 46–72.

Balogun A., Bissell P., Saddiq M. (2020). Negotiating access to the Nigerian healthcare system: The experiences of HIV-positive men who have sex with men. *Culture Health Sex*. 22(2): 233–246.

Balogun M., Dada F., Oladimeji A., Gwacham-Anisiobi U., Sekoni A., Banke-Thomas A. (2022). Leading in a time of crisis: a qualitative study capturing experiences of health facility leaders during the early phases of the COVID-19 pandemic in Nigeria's epicenter. https://researchonline. lshtm .ac.uk/id/eprint/4668892/1/Balogun_etal_2022_Leading-in-a-time-of.pdf. Accessed November 12, 2024.

Centers for Disease Control and Prevention (CDC) (2024). CDC in Tanzania. https://www.cdc. gov/globalhealth/countries/tanzania/default.htm. Accessed March 12, 2024.

Gilson L., Magomi M., Mkangaa E. (1995). The structural quality of Tanzanian primary health facilities. *Bulletin of World Health Organization*. 73(1): 105–114.

International Trade Administration (2022). Tanzania Healthcare. https://www.trade.gov/ country-commercial-guides/tanzania-healthcare. Accessed March 11, 2024.

Ishungisa A. M., Mmbaga E. J., Leshabari M. T., Tersbøl B. P., Moen K. (2023). Five different ways of reasoning: Tanzanian healthcare workers' ideas about how to improve HIV prevention among same sex attracted men. *BMC Health Services Research*. 23(1): 807. DOI: 10.1186/s12913-023-09771-3.

Kalolo A., Kapologwe N. A., Samky H., Kibusi S. M. (2022). Acceptability of the Direct Health Facility Financing (DHFF) initiative in Tanzania: A mixed methods process evaluation of the moderating factors. *International Journal of Health Planning Management*. 37: 1381–1401.

Kapologwe N. A., Kalolo A., Kibusi S. M., et al. (2019). Understanding the implementation of direct health facility financing and its effect on health system performance in Tanzania: A non-controlled before and after mixed method study protocol. *Health Research Policy and Systems*. 17: 11.

Kesale A. M., Jiyenze M. K., Katalambula L., et al. (2022a). Perceived performance of health facility governing committees in overseeing healthcare services delivery in primary health care facilities in Tanzania. *International Journal of Health Planning Management*. 38: 239–251.

Kesale A. M., Mahonge C., Muhanga M. (2022b). The quest for accountability of health facility governing committees implementing direct health facility financing in Tanzania: A supply-side experience. *PLoS One*. 17: e0267708.

Kesale A. M., Mwkasangula E., Muhanga M., Mahonge C. (2022c). Leveraging governance strategies adopted by health facility governing committees in response to COVID-19 outbreak at the local level in Tanzania: A qualitative study. *PLOS Glob Public Health*. 2: e0001222.

Maluka S., Chitama D., Dungumaro E., Masawe C., Rao K., Shroff. Z. (2018). Contracting out primary care in Tanzania towards UHC; how policy processes and context influence policy design and implementation. *International Journal for Equity in Health*. 17(1): 118–131.

Maluka S., Kamuzora P., Sebastián M. S., Byskov J., Nadwi B., Karin Hurtig A. (2010). Improving district level health planning and priority setting in Tanzania through implementing accountability for reasonableness framework: Perceptions of stakeholders. *BMC Health Services Research*. 10: 322. http://www.biomedcentral.com/1472-6963/10/322. Accessed March 11, 2024.

Mikkelsen-Lopez K. (2014). Health System Governance in Tanzania: Impact on Service Delivery in the Public Sector. https://core.ac.uk/download/pdf/33298355.pdf. Accessed March 11, 2024.

Mujinja P. G., Saronga H. P. (2022). Traditional and complementary medicine in Tanzania: Regulation awareness, adherence and challenges. *International Journal of Health Policy Management*. 11(8): 1496–1504. DOI: 10.34172/ijhpm.2021.51.

Njakoi G. (2021). Tanzania Health Care System. https://volunteer-africa-blog.org/2021/03/25/ tanzania-health-care-system/. Accessed March 11, 2024.

Opuko B. (2023). Tanzania's Healthcare System. https://issuu.com/foodworldmedia/docs/ healthcare_africa_issue_5_digital/s/23135848. Accessed March 11, 2024.

Severe Malaria Observatory (2023). *Tanzania Health System.* https://www.severemalaria.org/ countries/tanzania/tanzania-health-system. Accessed March 12, 2024.

Sprockett A (2016). Review of quality assessment tools for family planning programmes in low- and middle-income countries. *Health Policy and Planning.* DOI: 10.1093/heapol/czw123. Accessed March 13, 2024.

United Nations Human Development Programme (2023). Human Development Report. https:// hdr.und.or/en/2020-report. Accessed March 12, 2024.

United Republic of Tanzania (1995). National District Health Planning Guidelines. A Paper Presented by the Ministry of Health. Dar es Salaam, Tanzania.

United Republic of Tanzania (1999). *Tanzania Vision 1999–2025.* Dar es Salaam, Tanzania: Government Press.

United Republic of Tanzania (2002). *Policy on Traditional and Alternative Medicine.* Dar es Salaam, Tanzania: Government Press.

United Republic of Tanzania (2003). Second Health Sector Strategic Plan (HSSP) (July 2003– June 2008). Ministry of Health. Dar es Salaam, Tanzania: Government Press.

United Republic of Tanzania (2005). Human Resource for Health Strategic Plan 2008–2013, Ministry of Health and Social Welfare, Retrieved on 20/11/ 2021.

United Republic of Tanzania (2007). *Primary Health Services Development Program – Ministry of Health and Social Welfare.* Tanzania: Dar es Salaam.

United Republic of Tanzania (2007). *Second National Health Policy.* Dar es Salaam, Tanzania: Government Press.

United Republic of Tanzania (2009). Annual Health Statistical Tables and Figures. Ministry of Health and Social Welfare. Dar es Salaam, Tanzania: Government Press.

United Republic of Tanzania (2015). Health Sector Strategic Plan 2015–2020. Dar es Salaam, Tanzania: Government Press.

United Republic of Tanzania (2016). National Five-Year Development Plan 2016/17–2020/2021. Dar es Salaam, Tanzania: Government Press.

United Republic of Tanzania (2017). The National Health Policy 2017, Dares Salam: Ministry of Health, Community Development, Gender, Elderly and Children. Dar es Salaam, Tanzania: Government Press.

United Republic of Tanzania (2022). Policy on Reproductive, Maternal, Newborn, Child, and Adolescent Health. Ministry of Health. Dar es Salaam, Tanzania: Government Press.

United States Agency for International Development (2022). Reproductive, Maternal, Newborn, Child, and Adolescent Health (RMNCAH) 2022–2027. https://www.usaid.gov/sites/default/ files/2022-12/USAID_Afya_Yangu%20RMNCAH_Factsheet.pdf. Accessed March 11, 2024.

World Bank Indicators (2023). Tanzania. https://data.worldbank.org/indicator/NY.GDP. PCAP.CD?locations=NG. Accessed March 11, 2024.

World Economics (2023). Tanzania's Gross Domestic Product (GDP). https://www. worldeconomics.com/Country-Size/Nigeria.aspx. Accessed March 11, 2024.

World Health Organization (2011). Abuja Declaration. https://iris.who.int/bitstream/ handle/10665/341162/WHO-HSS-HSF-2010.01-eng.pdf. Accessed March 12, 2024.

World Health Organization (2022). Tanzania 2022 Annual Report. https://www.afro.who. int/countries/united-republic-of-tanzania/publication/who-tanzania-2022-annual-report#:~:text=The%20Annual%20Report%20summarizes. Accessed November 10, 2024.

World Health Organization (2023). Tanzania 2022–2023 Biennial Report. https://www.afro. who.int/countries/united-republic-of-tanzania/publication/who-tanzania-2022-2023-biennial-report. Accessed November 12, 2024.

Chapter Eighteen

HEALTH POLICY AND CHALLENGES IN UGANDA

Robert Dibie, Jacob Oboreh, and Charles Uchie

Introduction

This chapter investigates the nature of healthcare policy and administration effectiveness in Uganda. It also explores the extent to which the public sector uses healthcare policy and other means to influence the private sector's decision making and practices for the purpose of achieving a lesser burden of communicable and noncommunicable diseases. The chapter provides a detailed description of the key role of the public and private sectors with respect to effectively implementing healthcare policies to address the needs of the citizens and residents of Uganda. It argues that the Government of Uganda and its policies are crucial for the appropriate attainment of effective healthcare delivery services in the country. It uses data derived from primary and secondary sources to analyze the current healthcare system impact in Uganda. The findings indicate that while there have been past weaknesses in the relationship between government and business in the healthcare delivery system in Uganda due to inadequate enforcement of policies, the relationship in both sectors has improved over two decades. In addition, government policies have not been able to effectively address the disparity in healthcare delivery in both urban and rural regions of the nation. The chapter recommends that national and appropriate collaboration with the private sector could effectively impact healthcare administration and life expectancy in Uganda in the future.

Brief History of Uganda

Uganda is a landlocked country located in Eastern Africa. The country has a boundary with the Republic of South Sudan to the north, the Democratic Republic of the Congo to the southwest, Kenya, to the east, Tanzania to the south, and Rwanda to the southwest. The country's southern section is covered by Lake Victoria, which is also shared by the Republic of Tanzania, and Kenya. Uganda has a population of 47.3 million people (World Bank 2023).

The territory now called the Republic of Uganda was previously inhabited by farmers who migrated from central Sudan and the Kuliak-speaking ethnic people who were herders over 3,000 years ago. According to some history scholars, the Bantu ethnic group also migrated from the south to the region, while the Nilotic ethnic group also started migrating to the northeast region about 1,500 AD (Mwakikagile 2009; Schoenbrun 1993). In the fifteenth century, one of the major kingdoms in the region was called Bunyoro-Kitera (Britannica 2023; Mwambutsya 1991). It is also reported that a smaller Buganda kingdom was created offshoot of Bunyoro-Kitara (Britannica 2023; Mwakikagile 2009). However, toward the end of the eighteenth century, the Bunyoro-Kitara kingdom had expanded and extended beyond what the king could not effectively control. This weakness in the kingdom propelled frequent successions of aggressive chiefs (Chrétien 2003; Steinhart 2019; Wikipedia 2023). Furthermore, the name of the country was derived from the Buganda kingdom. The Republic of Uganda has spread over the current territory and beyond Kampala the nation's capital city. The most popular languages spoken in the country are Luganda, and Swahili a Bantu ethnic language (Beachey 1962; Jørgensen 1981; Wikipedia 2023). It should be noted that it was during the period of Buganda's Kingdom that the first group of traders that spoke Swahili visited the east coast of Africa near the current boundary of Uganda in the 1840s (Jørgensen 1981; Lee 1964). Although Swahili was originally regarded as a foreign language spoken only by the Bantu ethnic group, it was later adopted as the Republic of Uganda's second official language due to the nature of its neutrality to the people of the country. Many years later, the Government of Uganda enacted a policy in 2022 to adopt the Swahili language as a subject taught in all the schools in the country (Mwakikagile 2009; Wikipedia 2023).

Furthermore, John Hanning Speke and his British team were the first European explorers, who crossed into the *kabaka*'s territory in 1862. A few years later, in 1875, Henry Morton Stanley, a British-American explorer visited the Buganda Kingdom while Mutesa 1, was the king (Britannica 2023). During Henery Stanley's visit to King Mutesa's palace in 1875, he accepted the proposal presented by the British-American explorer to invite Christian missionaries to Buganda Kingdom (Beachey 1962; Jørgensen 1981). Subsequently between 1877 and 1879, the Church Missionary Society, British Anglican missionaries, and the French Catholic Church priest incrementally started to arrive in Buganda (Jørgensen 1981; Britannica 2023; Wikipedia 2023). According to Pulford (2011), the Imperial British East Company was encouraged to negotiate an agreement in the Uganda region in 1888. In addition, between 1860 and 1878, the Arab trader who traded along East Africa's coastal region, negotiated with the British explorers who were navigating the region to search for the source of the Nile River (Baker 1879; Stanley 1899). Furthermore, between 1886 and 1890, there were several wars in the Buganda region between the Christians and Muslims. On the other hand, there was another set of wars between Christians who were Protestants and the Catholic missionary faction. Because of the British desire to protect the trade route along the Nile River, it decided to annex Buganda (Baker 1879; Pulford 2011; Wikipedia 2023). Subsequently, in 1894, the United Kingdom government established a Uganda Protectorate of the British Empire that was controlled from 1886 to 1962 (Annie 2009; Beachey 1962; Britannica 2023).

Uganda was granted independence by the British Government on October 9, 1962 (Jørgensen 1981). However, as a member of the Commonwealth of Nations, the Queen of England was the Head of State. In addition, the nation changes its title to Republic October 1963. The new nation conducted its first election in 1962, and Milton Obote was elected as the first indigenous Prime Minister. While King Edward Muteesa 11 of the Buganda Kabaka kingdom was appointed as the ceremonial president of the country (Lee 1964; Wikipedia 2023). Because of a power struggle between Prime Minister Obote, and King Musteesa, Milton Obote suspended the nation's constitution and ousted the president and vice president of Uganda in 1967. Further, a new constitution was adopted, and the traditional kingdoms in the country were dissolved. Further, Milton declared himself the president of the Republic of Uganda (Britannica 2023; Jørgensen 1981; Wikipedia 2023).

According to Jørgensen (1981), because of Milton Obote's authoritarian policies and leadership style on January 25, 1971, a military couple led by General Idi Admin overthrew the government, and President Obote was deposed from office as President of Uganda. During General Idi Admin's tenure as Head of State for eight years, he ruled like a dictator. Furthermore, the current president of Uganda, Yoweri Kaguta Museveni ascended to power after what was described as a six-year guerrilla war fair (Britannica 2023; Jørgensen 1981; Wikipedia 2023). Unfortunately, President Museveni continued with the same authoritarian leadership style that Milton Obote and Idi Amin exhibited while they were president of Uganda. One of President Yoweri Museveni's discontents or zealots was the amendment of the nation's constitution, as well as the remover of term limits for president. Because of the remover of the president's term limit his administration has conducted elections a couple of times, and he was elected president in 2011, 2016, and 2021. Museveni has been credited for restoring relative stability and economic prosperity to Uganda following years of civil war and repression under former leaders Milton Obote and Idi Amin (Dibie 2018).

The Republic of Uganda has experienced some economic growth, open markets, and abundant natural resources which includes at least 2.5 billion barrels of recoverable oil. These natural resources provide good opportunities for knowledgeable investors in Uganda (Dibie 2018; US Department of State 2023). According to GlobalEdge (2022), Uganda maintains a liberal trade and foreign exchange regime and adheres to IMF/World Bank programs to fight poverty, maintain macroeconomic stability, and restructure the economy. Despite these positive government initiatives, the country has sluggish bureaucracy, poor infrastructure, insufficient power supply, high energy and production costs, nontariff barriers, and severe corruption problems (Dibie 2018; World Bank 2022). The government has been reported to often interfere in the affairs of the private sector, and this practice constitutes a major challenge to invest in the country (Dibie 2018; US Department of State 2022). In addition, as a result of the multiple levels of government in Uganda, numerous government agencies, and an entrenched bureaucracy, disputes and tensions between these political institutions sometimes lead to conflicting and confusing policies and their implementation (Dibie 2018; U.S. & Foreign Commercial Service and US Department of State 2023).

Health Challenges in Uganda

The Republic of Uganda has a rich health policy framework that has helped the country to make improvements in the health sector. The Government of Uganda has also made major progress toward accomplishing some of the Millennium Development Goals and Sustainable Development Goals. However, the health system in Uganda has been reported to be facing shortage of health workers, underpaid doctors and nurses, inadequate supplies of medicine, insufficient hospital beds, deplorable medical equipment in government health facilities, high out-of-pocket payment, and disparity in the accessibility to healthcare services especially in the rural districts of the country (Africanews 2021; Dowhaniuk 2021; Kakumba 2021; Ministry of Health of Uganda 2020; Nabukeera 2016).

According to the Uganda Bureau of Statistics (2020) and Kakumba (2021) between 2019 and 2020, maternal mortality fell from 505 to 336 deaths per 100,000 live births. Further, infant mortality declines from 87 to 43 deaths per 1,000 live births. On the other hand, under-five mortality also dropped from 156 to 64 deaths per 1,000 live births (Kakumba 2021; Medard et al. 2023; Ministry of Health Uganda 2020; Uganda Bureau of Statistics 2020). Despite these promising improvements in health policies, the healthcare system is still facing substance challenges. In addition, the nation has not been able to fully develop its health infrastructure to meet international and regional standards (Njaye 2022; Mukundane et al. 2016; ThinkMD 2022; United State Department of State 2023). According to many scholars, the major healthcare delivery challenges confronting the Republic of Uganda are inadequate medical supplies of medicine, underpaid health workers, shortage of health workers, insufficient hospital beds, and inadequate supply of essential modern medical equipment. Another major healthcare predicament in the country is the lack of accessibility to healthcare services for citizens and residents of Uganda who reside in the rural regions of the nation (Kakumba 2021; Medard et al. 2023; Ministry of Health of Uganda 2020). Currently, the major healthcare providers in Uganda are the government, nongovernmental organizations' hospitals and clinics, community medicine distributors, drug shops, private clinics, and traditional healers (Koutsoumpa et al. 2020; Medard et al. 2023; Nabukeera 2016).

Furthermore, important medicine health supplies and access to medicine have not been effectively accomplished. Thus, an inadequate supply chain system has increased morbidity and mortality rates in the country. In addition, these challenges have also galvanized avoidable poverty and economic losses to the country's citizens. The shortage of medicine has also spilled over or escalated limited functions and poorly equipped hospitals. According to the United States Department of State Report (2023), most of the regional or district hospitals are only equipped to manage minor healthcare emergencies. This is because most of the district's hospital surgical capabilities are either not available or inadequate. In most cases, blood supply might not be available or is insufficient (United States Department of State Report 2023).

Lugada et al. (2022) contend that a few years ago, there was about 82% of the health facilities in Uganda were stocked out of medicine due to many supply chain calamities such as ineffective supervision, oversight, expired medical commodities, inadequately skilled supply chain system staff, poor storage, ineffective supervision, and poor management drugs to patients (Lugada et al. 2022; Tusubira et al. 2020). The characteristics of hospitals at the district level are that they are only able to provide basic healthcare services. These health predicaments in Uganda have also made most of the citizens and residents in the country lose confidence in the health system (Akello & Beisel 2019; Kakumba 2021; Medard et al. 2023).

The persistent underfunding of the health system in Uganda remains a major challenge. The Ministry of Finance, Planning, and Economic Development (2020) report reveals that the health sector budget has been decreasing in the past two decades from 7.8% in 2010 to 2016 the national budget to 6.1% in 2020–2021. Further, while the total budget in Uganda increased by 47% in 2022/2023, the health system budget was only increased to 7% from 7.7% in the previous year (Amnesty International 2023; Ministry of Health Uganda 2020). The Abuja Declaration that the Government of Uganda is a signatory to mandates African countries to appropriate 15% of the gross domestic product (GDP) funds to their health system (Dibie et al. 2015). Thus, what the government has been budgeting for its healthcare falls short of what it promised to be appropriated each year. Therefore, the nation's failure to implement appropriate financing strategies has constituted a major challenge in priority-setting processes, adequate, quality access unacceptable, and deplorable healthcare conditions in Uganda.

Furthermore, there continues to be overconcentration on macro health policy planning and investment at the expense of micro health policies that have a direct impact on public health facilities (Dibie 2022; Dowhaniuk 2021; Madinah 2016). One other mechanism that the government of Uganda has adopted for its low-income population is to increase access to the remover of use fees in all government-owned hospitals and clinics. In addition, the government of Uganda also provides subsidies to cover 10%–20% of health treatment costs (Dowhaniuk 2021; Medard et al. 2023; Ministry of Health Uganda 2023a).

According to Kim et al. (2022) and Lugada et al. (2022), nonprofit healthcare facilities in Uganda tend to have a 98% higher availability of modern infrastructure and essential medicines for treating patients in government-owned hospitals and clinics. While it has been argued that access to quality health services and safety, as well as affordable critical medicine help to propel higher standards for any health system, the Uganda situation has not done well in this regard (Lugada et al. 2022). Furthermore, there is a considerably elevated level of disparities in the geographic location of hospitals in the country. For example, the five National Referral hospitals are located in Kapala and within one region (Kim et al. 2022; Njaye 2022; Uganda Ministry of Health 2023a). This means that the largest population of the country that resides in the rural districts will have to travel several hundred miles to Kapala to seek specialist healthcare. This major predicament has drastically discouraged the poor rural residents of the country from seeking health or resorting to traditional treatment. Another major health delivery challenge is the lack of ambulance service availability in the Republic of Uganda (Basaza 2020; Dowhaniuk 2021; Uganda Medical Association 2023). In the absence of ambulances and formal emergency services in Uganda, police vehicles and citizens who are bystanders tend to be the only other form of emergency transportation mechanism in the country. There is also a complete absence of emergency services in rural communities and districts due to the nonavailability of police stations and motorable roads.

One other major challenge facing the health system in Uganda is the shortage of physicians and nurses. Although the government has collaborated with foreign health providers the shortage of health workers continues to exist in the country (Koutsoumpa 2020; Medard et al. 2023). While the population of Uganda has grown from 37.8 in 2015 to 47.3 million in 2022, the number of physicians and nurses to 1,000 people is still exceedingly insignificantly low compared to the World Health Standard (World Bank 2022). Some of the factors that have been identified for the health workers shortage include low salary, poor working conditions, brain drain, or migration of doctors and nurses to foreign countries for higher rates of compensation. These major health system challenges are preventing Uganda from moving far away from attaining its vision of universal health coverage (Koutsoumpa et al. 2020). Shortage of health workers in Uganda could be associated with a lack of appropriate funding, and poor management in the recruitment and retention of doctors and nurses (Koutsoumpa et al. 2020; Medard et al. 2023; Njaye 2022).

Other health personnel challenges include the habitual absence of health workers from work due to a lack of motivation and accountability. Some scholars contend that while 80% of the Republic of Uganda's population resides in the rural areas of the country, 70% of all doctors practice in urban areas (Kakumba 2020; Koutsoumpa et al. 2020). Other research findings also revealed that nurses in rural districts in Uganda often argued that there was no need to open their health facility early or go to work regularly because of a lack of medicines or vaccines to treat patients (World Health Organization 2022; ThinkMD 2022). In some cases where health workers are physically present at work, they are not able to fully perform their duties due to a lack of adequate medicine supply, medical equipment, or inadequate managerial specialists (Akello & Beisel 2019; Koutsoumpa et al. 2020; Mukundane et al. 2016). In addition, in some government health facilities, nurses, nursing assistants, midwives, clinical officers, and laboratory assistants are often frustrated because they have to attend to patients under dire circumstances characterized by dilapidated hospitals and health centers, a lack of equipment, and frequent stockouts of vaccines and medicines (Akello & Beisel 2019; Koutsoumpa et al. 2020; Muzyamba et al. 2021). It should be noted, however, that although the Ministry of Health has made considerable progress in improving the health standards in Uganda, the inability to solve the major challenges in the health system such as staffing, drug stocks, hospitals and clinics infrastructure, and inaccessibility of health facilities in hard-to-reach geographical districts among others constitute a major healthcare predicament in Uganda.

Types of Health Policies in Uganda

In the Republic of Uganda, there has been continuous substantial enactment of health policies. This is because the nation's government has been incredibly determined to propel new initiatives either from national or district levels. The resulting health policies are implemented through legislation, public, private, or nongovernmental agencies. Many of these health efforts are disease or capacity-building-specific that are directed toward health problems. Therefore, a variety of national health policies have been formulated to (a) provide or control access to healthcare; (b) enhance quality and reduce the spread of diseases or curtail medical errors in health facilities; and (c) promote change in unhealthy behavior and contain cost. The intent of health policy in Uganda is to enhance the development of the healthcare infrastructure and citizens' access to quality health delivery systems in the country. The dominant social paradigm in the country tends to constitute clusters of values, beliefs, and ideas that influence the nation's citizens' thinking about government effectiveness, shared governance, and individual responsibility in a democratic country. Below are selected health policies that the Republic of Uganda has enacted in the past three decades.

National Alcohol Control Policy enacted in 2019: The objective of this policy is to prevent and resolve alcohol-related harm to individuals, families, communities, and society in Uganda (Republic of Uganda Ministry of Health 2019). Other goals of the policy are (a) to reduce the negative effects, and impact of illicit and informally produced alcohol; (b) to strengthen regulation on production, availability, marketing, and pricing of alcohol in Uganda to protect vulnerable people from mental health, substance abuse; (c) build the capacity of the Government of Uganda and other stakeholders for prevention, treatment and management of alcohol use and related problems; and (d) establish and improve research, monitoring, evaluation, surveillance and dissemination of information use in Uganda (Republic of Uganda Ministry of Health 2019).

National Integrated Early Childhood Development Policy enacted in 2016: The major goal of this policy is to ensure equitable access to quality early child development health services for holistic development of all children in Uganda from conception to at least eight years Republic of Uganda Ministry of Health 2019). Other objectives of the policy include (a) set, improve, and align strategies as well as initiatives within and across public, private, and nongovernmental organizations in Uganda; (b) harmonize existing early childhood development policy-related goals and strategies within and across Uganda; and (c) build and strengthen the capacity of systems and structure to deliver integrated quality and inclusive early childhood development programs (Republic of Uganda Ministry of Health 2019). In addition, the integrated early childhood development policy also includes a variety of strategies and services to provide basic healthcare, adequate nutrition, nurturing, and stimulation with a caring, safe, and clean environment for children and their families (Republic of Uganda Ministry of Health 2019).

Resettlement Policy Framework for Uganda Reproductive, Maternal, Neonatal, and Child Health Improvement Project 2016: The goal of this policy is: (a) to improve birth and death registration services; (b) to improve utilization of essential health services with a focus on reproductive, maternal, newborn, child, and adolescent health services with a focus on reproductive, maternal, newborn, child, and adolescent health services in target districts in Uganda (Republic of Uganda Ministry of Health 2019). Other associated benefits of the policy include enhanced baby delivery and reproductive services, as well as a package of high-impact quality and cost-effective intervention services (Republic of Uganda Ministry of Health 2019).

National Medicine Policy enacted in 2015: The objective of this policy is to galvanize health delivery progress toward universal health coverage in Uganda. The policy also mandates the delivery of essential health and related services needed for the promotion of a healthy and productive life in the country. The 2015 policy is an updated version of similar policies that were formulated in the country in 1993 and 2002 (Republic of Uganda Ministry of Health 2019). It was anticipated that the national medicine policy would compel the Government of Uganda to increase funding for medicines, strengthen partnerships, and collaborate for healthcare delivery; as well as increase the capacity of the nation's Ministry of Health and the district health departments (Republic of Uganda Ministry of Health 2019).

National Oral Health Policy enacted in 2007: The objective of this policy is to provide a framework for the prevention of oral diseases and promotion of health by supporting policies and programs that make a major difference to the health delivery system in the country. The policy also reiterated the importance of equity, integration, community participation, gender empowerment, prevention, and promotion of health research in Uganda. It also prescribes solutions that could help the nation address the inequalities and disparities that affect the population of the country that has the least access to health resources. The oral policy also mandates how to improve the effectiveness and efficiency of the delivery of oral healthcare by adopting safe and effective disease-preventive measures in the country (Republic of Uganda Ministry of Health 2019).

Regardless of the specific health policies or regulations that have been enacted in Uganda in the past few decades, it is paramount that an assessment must be made of the impacts the policies have made on human lives and activities in the country. Further, what is missing in most of the Ministry of Health reports is that there is insufficient inventory risk management assessment. Performance management does not imply growth that tends to continue indefinitely in unchecked health systems. Therefore, sustainable development in the health sector requires economic improvement and efficiencies that are guided by ethical values, shared governance, and democracy, where constant growth only occurs in human health education in the country.

Health Administration in Uganda

According to the Republic of Uganda Ministry of Health Report 2023, the Ministry of Health is mandated to provide guidance leadership, and stewardship to the nation's health system. The Ministry of Health is responsible for the formulation and review of all health policies in the country. In this capacity, the Ministry of Health constantly engages in dialogue with all stakeholders in the nation's health industry in strategic planning, advising other ministries, setting standards and quality assurance, resources mobilization, ensuring quality, health equity, fairness, and the appropriation of funding to the various districts in the country (Ministry of Health of Uganda 2023a). In 2023, there are 6,937 health facilities in Uganda. Government health facilities (hospitals and clinics) constitute 3,133. While the health facilities owned by the private, not-for-profit sector are 1,002. On one hand, the private for-profit sector owns the remaining 2,795 (40.3%). On the other hand, 7 (010%) health facilities are owned by communities in the country (Ministry of Health of Uganda 2023a). It should be noted that the not-for-profit health facilities are operated on a national and local basis and are owned by religious stakeholders (Ministry of Health of Uganda 2023b; World Bank 2010). The major responsibilities of the Ministry of Health are the implementation of the health sector strategic and investment plan. The Ministry of Health is also responsible for the coordination of stakeholders' plans, regulation, policy formulation, and budgeting (Ministry of Health of Uganda 2023b).

Furthermore, the nation's hospitals and clinics are divided into three groups. These three groups are defined based on the type of services that they provide. The Ministry of Health classified the health facilities as (1) health center (HC1), community health workers, (2) health center (HC II), parish level, (3) health center III-sub-county level, (4) referral facility (HCIV)—Hospitals (Ministry of Health of Uganda 2023b). In addition, the District Health Management Team manages the district and sub-districts. These management teams are coordinated by the district's health officer and consist of managers of various health departments in the districts. This group of health officers also engages in the implementation of health services at the specified level, as well as ensuring coherence with national health policies. Further, the Health Unit Management Committee at the district level is composed of health staff, community leaders, and civil society, and their responsibilities include facilitating the link between local hospitals and clinics with community healthcare demands and wellbeing (Tashobya et al. 2006).

The next level of health facilities are classified as *Regional Referral Hospitals*. This level is made up of 17 regional referral hospitals and 62 general hospitals in the country. According to the Uganda Ministry of Health (2023b), the regional referral hospitals (also called Mbale) are considered the district referral facilities for people in Bukwa, Butaleja, Busia, Budaka, Kibuku, Kapchorwa, Manafwa, Mbale, Pallisa, Sironko, and Tororo districts in Uganda (Ministry of Health of Uganda 2023b).

Furthermore, the next health facilities are classified as *National Referral Hospital* (also called Kawempe National Referral Hospital). All the hospitals at this level are located in urban regions of the country. In addition, the National Referral Hospitals include (1) Mulago National Referral Hospital; (2) Kawempe National Referral Hospital; (3) Kiruddu National Referral Hospital; and (4) Butabiika National Referral Hospital (Ministry of Health of Uganda 2023b).

The Republic of Uganda is also reported to have *five specialist hospitals*. The specialist hospitals include (a) Mulago Supper Specialist Hospital; (b) Mulago Women and Neonatal Specialist Hospital; (c) Regional Pediatric Surgical Hospital, Entebbe; (d) Uganda Heart Institute; and (e) Uganda Cancer Institute (Ministry of Health of Uganda 2023b).

Apart from the Ministry of Health, the Uganda Medical Association also plays a crucial role in the administration of the health system in the country. The association provides vibrant programs that help to support social welfare, career development, and interests of physicians in the country. The association also ensures the promotion of universal access to quality healthcare in the country (Buregyeya et al. 2020; Jeppsson 2002; Uganda Medical Association 2022). It is also reported that the government's failure to improve the salary of physicians in the country coupled with its failure to conduct a review of the supply of medicines and other especially important medical equipment consequently led to the Uganda Medical Association strike in 2017 (Kim et al. 2022; Okiror 2017). Analysis of the health administration reveals that although, the Republic of Uganda of formulated new health policies to enhance the healthcare system, it tends not to enhance and better manage hospitals as well as facilitate the coordination and supply chain of essential medicine to treat the sick population of the country. Moving forward would require investment to improve hospital management to enable physicians to better address the administrative challenges of appropriate funding of supply chain coordination in the country.

Data Analysis and Discussion

The goal of this chapter is to investigate the nature of healthcare policy and government regulations in the Republic of Uganda. The data used for the analysis of healthcare policy and regulation effectiveness were derived from secondary research methods. The secondary research methods adopted include content analysis of the Republic of Uganda Ministry of Health reports, World Bank Indicators, United States Department of State reports, World Health Organization reports, United Nations Human Development Index annual report, Center for Disease Control, Country Report, academic as well as professional journals articles.

Table 1 summarizes the nature and effectiveness of health policy in the Republic of Sudan. According to the World Bank Indicators Report (2023) and the United Nations Human Development Index (2022), the Republic of Uganda's population is estimated to be 47.3% people in 2022. Further, the GDP of Uganda was US$45.5 billion in 2022. In 2020, the Republic of Uganda spent 3.8% of its GDP on healthcare (World Bank 2022). This percentage appropriated for the health system is far below the 15% African leader agreed to allocate in their Abuja Declaration of 2001. On one hand, the physicians/doctors per 1,000 people ratio was 0.2 in 2022. On the other hand, nurses, and midwives per 1,000 people was 1.6 in 2020. According to the World Health Organization report (2016), at least 2.5 medical staff (physicians, nurses, and midwives) per 1,000 people are needed to provide adequate coverage with primary care interventions (World Health Organization Report 2016; Ministry of Finance, Planning and Economic Development 2020). Again, Uganda's ratio is far below what is recommended by the World Health Organization.

Furthermore, the common diseases in the Republic of Uganda are hepatitis B, meningitis, yellow fever, typhoid, malaria, HIV, polio, tuberculosis, Marburg hemorrhagic fever, pneumonic plague, and schistosomiasis. The prevalence of HIV/AIDs has dropped to 2.4%, while those of tuberculosis incidence per 100,00 people have also dropped to 82 people in 2021 in the country. The malaria incidence per 1,000 people at risk has also dropped to 284 people in 2021. In addition, the population using safely managed drinking water constituted 19% in 2022. Subsequently, the ratio of people using safe-managed sanitation services is 22% in urban cities and 16% in rural districts in Uganda in 2022. However, people practicing open defecation per percentage of the population was only 4% in 2022. Thus, there seems to be a significant improvement in reducing the unhealthy defecation practice in the country.

In respect of life expectancy at birth for females, the number was 65 years in 2021. Moreover, the life expectancy at birth for male citizens in Uganda was reported to be 60 years in 2021 as well. While the mortality rate for female adults per 1,000 people was 245 in 2020, and the mortality rate for males in 2021 was 345. These data reveal that more men die every year in Uganda than women. In addition, the mortality rate for infants per 1,000 people was 31 in 2021. There has been considerable improvement in the mortality rate of infants in Uganda.

Table 1 Economics and Health Indicators in Uganda

No.	Major Indicators in Uganda	Explanation
1	Population	47.25 million (2022)
2	Gross domestic product (GDP)	US$45.5 billion (2022)
3	Current health expenditure (% of GDP)	3.8% (2020)
4	Physicians/doctors per 1,000 people	0.2 (2020)
5	Nurses and midwives per 1,000 people	1.6 (2020)
6	Population using safe-managed drinking water service	19% (2022)
7	People using safely managed sanitation services (% of population)	18% (2022); urban 22%; rural 16% (2022)
8	People practicing open defecation (% of the population)	4% (2022)
9	Common disease	Hepatitis B, meningitis, yellow fever, typhoid, malaria, HIV, polio, tuberculosis, Marburg hemorrhagic fever, pneumonic plague, and schistosomiasis
10	Life expectancy at birth for females	65 years (2021)
11	Life expectancy at birth for males	60 years (2021)
12	Mortality rate for female adults (per 1,000 people)	245 (2020)
13	Mortality rate for male adults (per 1,000 people)	345 (2021)
14	Mortality rate for infants (per 1,000 people)	31 (2021)
15	Tuberculosis incidence (per 100,000 people	82 people (2021)
16	Population living below income poverty line PPP $2.15 a day	42.2% (2019)
17	Population in multidimensional handout poverty (%)	42.1% (2019)
18	Unemployment total (% of total labor force)	4.3% (2022)
19	Infants lacking immunization for measles (% of one year old)	91% (2021)
20	Malaria incidence (per 1,000 people at risk)	284 people (2021)
21	HIV/AIDS prevalence adults (% ages 15–49)	2.4% (2021)

Source: World Bank Indicators (2022); United Nations Human Development Program Index. Human Development Report (2022); and World Health Organization (2023).

The analysis conducted reveals that the population living below income poverty line PPP \$2.15 a day was 42.2% in 2019. Meanwhile, the population in multidimensional handout poverty (%) was 42.1% in 2019. It is also interesting to note that the unemployment rate was 4.3% in 2022. The analysis of the secondary data reveals that while the Republic of Uganda is facing many challenges in its health system, there are some areas where the government has done very well. As usual, healthcare managerial perception and indicators are especially useful. There are times when it could be incongruous with the actual quality of care that is delivered at any nation's hospitals and clinics. Although the Ministry of Health in Uganda entities are expected to have executive authority over policy formulation and personnel management, there are limitations that they also face due to limited funding.

Conclusion

This chapter has investigated the nature of healthcare policy and government regulations in Uganda. It also explores the extent to which the government of Uganda regulates its healthcare policy for the purpose of achieving a lesser burden of communicable and noncommunicable diseases. The chapter provides a detailed description of the key role of the public and private sectors with respect to effectively implementing healthcare policies to address the needs of the citizens and residents of Uganda. It argues that the Government of Uganda and its policies are crucial for the appropriate attainment of effective healthcare delivery services in the country.

The analysis conducted reveals that although the Republic of Uganda has made substantial improvements in its health system, there are still disparities in both the location of hospitals and clinics around the country, as well as the management performance of health facilities. Further, there is an urgent need for the Ministry of Health to adopt new methods to better manage health facilities all over the country. In addition, investment is urgently needed to improve the management of hospitals so that physicians and health managers can effectively design initiatives by taking strategic mechanisms to improve and elevate a higher-quality healthcare delivery system in the country. One question, the government of Uganda should try and provide an answer to is why the for-profit hospitals in the country have higher essential medicines for treating their patients compared to those of the government? Providing answers to this question could help the government solve most of the current healthcare delivery challenges that Uganda is facing.

Furthermore, the Republic of Uganda should apply due diligence to ensure vibrant governance, policy formulation, and regulation in the country. To accomplish these goals, it will be paramount for the nation's Ministry of Health and other government agencies in the country to take greater responsibility for the effectiveness and implementation of the health supply chain for medicines and medical equipment. There is also the need to strengthen accountability and strategic doing throughout the distribution of medicines to both urban and rural health facilities across all regions in Uganda. In addition, it is especially important that policymakers and public administrators oversee health the budget to prioritize investments and funding toward improving the management of poor-performing government hospitals and clinics in the country.

Because 80% of the Republic of Uganda's population resides in the rural areas of the country there is the need for the government to promote community engagement as an especially important mechanism to enhance the healthcare system in the country. It is paramount to note that the magnitude of healthcare challenges in the country requires a change agent such as community engagement. The new role of the communities in the country could galvanize acceptable intervention, capacities, and resources in the near future. The Government of Uganda needs to build more hospitals in the rural regions of the country.

A cause of disagreement that should be the center of all health issues in the country should be better management could galvanize better outcomes. When government action rises beyond the minimal necessary level, however, it leads inevitably and quickly to the loss of freedom and the support of the business sector. The first freedom affected is often the economic freedom of both the public and private sectors (Dibie 2022; Dibie 2018). It is expected that a new health policy could foster the Government of Uganda's ability to attract multinational corporations to invest in the country as well as increase its levels of foreign direct investment in the healthcare system. A question for future research is whether close relations between business and government have any positive impact on the health system in Uganda.

References

Africanews (2021). Uganda hospitals under pressure amid COVID-19 pandemic second wave. June 10 issue. https://www.africanews.com/2021/06/10/ugandan-hospitals-under-pressure-amid-covid-19-pandemic-second-wave//. Accessed November 28, 2023.

Akello G., Beisel U. (2019). Challenges, distrust, and understanding employing communicative action in improving trust in a public medical sector in Uganda. *SAGE Open*, 1–10. DOI: 10.1177/2158244019893705.

Amnesty International (2023). Building resilience: Public debt management and health financing in Uganda. Accessed November 25, 2023.

Annie K. (2009). Healthcare a major challenge for Uganda. https://www.theguardian.com/katine/2009/apr/01/healthcare-in-uganda. Accessed November 27, 2023.

Baker S. W. (1879). Ismailia: A narrative of the expedition to Central Africa for the suppression of the slave trade, organized by Ismail, Khedive of Egypt. Robarts: University of Toronto. London, Macmillan.

Basaza R., Namyalo P. K., Mayora C., Shepard D. (2020). *The Journey To Universal Health Insurance Coverage: What Are The Lessons For Uganda And The Other Lmic?* New York: Nova Medicine & Health Press.

Beachey R. W. (1962). The rms rade in East Africa in the late nineteenth century. *The Journal of African History*, 3(3): 451–568.

Britannica (2023). History of Uganda. https://www.britannica.com/place/Uganda/additional-info. Accessed November 24, 2023.

Buregyeya E., Atusingwize E., Nsamba P., Musoke D., Naigaga I., Kabasa J. D., Amuguni H., Bazeyo W. (2020). Operationalizing the one health approach in Uganda: Challenges and opportunities. *Journal of Epidemiology and Global Health*, 10(4): 250–257.

Chrétien J. (2003). *The Great Lakes of Africa: Two Thousand Years of History*. New York: Zone Books.

Dibie R. (2022). Healthcare policy and administration in Nigeria: A critical analysis. *The Journal of African Policy Studies*, 28(1): 101–139.

Dibie R. (2018). Business and government relations in Uganda. In *Business and Government Relations in Africa*. Edited by Robert Dibie. New York: Routledge/Taylor and Frances Press.

Dibie R., Edoho F. M., Dibie J. (2015). Analysis of capacity building and economic growth in Sub-Saharan Africa. *International Journal of Business and Science*, 6(12): 1–25.

Dowhaniuk N. (2021). Exploring country-wide equitable government health care facility access in Uganda. *International Journal for Equity in Health*, 2021: 20–28.

GlobalEdge (2022). Doing Business in Uganda. https://globaledge.msu.edu/countries/uganda/statistics. Accessed November 29, 2023.

Jeppsson A. (2002) Defend the human rights of the ebola victims! *Tropical Doctor.* 32(3):181–182. DOI:10.1177/004947550203200330.

Jørgensen J. J. (1981). *Uganda: A Modern History.* New York: St. Martin's Press, 381–403.

Kakumba M. R. (2021). Priority or not? Ugandans continue to cite health as their most important problem, and say access is difficult. Afrobarometer Dispatch No. 465. https://www.afrobarometer.org/publication/ad465-priority-or-not-ugandans-continue-cite-health-their-most-important-problem-say/. Accessed September 22, 2024.

Kakumba M. R. (2020). PP70: Willing to kill: Factors contributing to mob justice in Uganda. https://www.afrobarometer.org/publication/pp70-willing-kill-factors-contributing-mob-justice-uganda/. Accessed October 31, 2024.

Kim J. H., Bell G. A., Bitton A. et al. (2022). Health facility management and primary health care performance in Uganda. *BMC Health Services Research*, 22, 275. DOI: 10.1186/s12913-022-07674-3.

Koutsoumpa M., Odedo R., Banda A., Meurs M., Hinlopen C., Kramer K., Bemelmans M., Omaswa F., Ojoome V., Kiguli-Malwadd E. (2020). Health workforce financing in Uganda: Challenges and opportunities, *European Journal of Public Health*, 30(5): 165.525.

Lee (1964). Uganda's first year of independence. *Political Quarterly*, 35(1): 34–45.

Lugada E., Komakech H., Ochola I., Mwebaze S., Olowo Oteba M., Okidi Ladwar D. (2022). Health supply chain system in Uganda: Current issues, structure, performance, and implications for systems strengthening. *Journal of Pharmaceutical Policy and Practice*, 15(1): 14–25.

Medard T., Yawe B. L., Bosco O. J. (2023). Health care delivery in Uganda; A review. Tanzania. *Journal of Health Resources*, 24(2): 1–7.

Madinah N. (2016). Challenges and barriers to the health service delivery system in Uganda. *Journal of Nursing and Health Sciences*, 5(2): 30–38.

Ministry of Finance, Planning and Economic Development (2020). *National Budget Framework Paper FY 2020–2021.* Kampala, Uganda: Government Press.

Ministry of Health of Uganda (2023a). Hospital. https://www.health.go.ug/hospitals. Accessed November 28, 2023.

Ministry of Health of Uganda (2023b). Uganda Clinical Guidelines 2023 Accessed November 12, 2024. https://library.health.go.ug/sites/default/files/resources/Uganda%20Clinical%20Guidelines%202023.pdf. Accessed October 31, 2024.

Ministry of Health Uganda (2020). *Annual Health Sector Performance Report Fiscal Year 2019–2020.* Kampala, Uganda. Government Press.

Mukundane M., Nannungi A., Dennis Aryaija-Karemani D. B. A., Patrick Ssesanga P., Muhwezi W. W. (2016). *Assessing the Management and Administration in Public Health Facilities of Uganda and the Implications for the Healthcare Service Delivery and Utilization.* Kampala, Uganda: Advocate Coalition for Development and Environment (ACODE) Publication.

Muzyamba C., Makova O. & Mushibi G. S. (2021). Exploring health workers' experiences of mental health challenges during care of patients with COVID-19 in Uganda: A qualitative study. *BMC Research Notes*, 14, 286–297.

Mwakikagile G. (2009). *Ethnicity and National Identity in Uganda: The Land and Its People.* Cape Town, South Africa: New Africa Press.

Mwambutsya N. (1991). Pre-capitalist Social Formation: The case of the Banyankole of Southwestern Uganda. *Eastern Africa Social Science Research Review*, 6(2, 7 no. 1): 78–95.

Nabukeera M. (2016). Challenges and barriers to the health service delivery system in Uganda. *Journal of Nursing and Health Science*, 5(1): 30–38.

Njaye K. S. (2022). Uganda: Is the healthcare system dysfunctional? pulse/Uganda-health-care-system-dysfunctional-kzito-simon-njaye. Accessed November 27, 2023.

Okiror P., Lejju J. B., Bahati J., Kagoro G. R. (2017). Suitability of Kabanyolo Soils for fruit and vegetable production. *Open Journal of Soil Science* 7(2):19–33.

Pulford C. (2011). *Two Kingdoms of Uganda: Snakes and Ladders in the Scramble for Africa*. Daventry: Ituri Publications.

Schoenbrun D. (1993). We are what we eat: Ancient agriculture between the great lakes. *The Journal of African History*, 34(1): 1–31.

Steinhart E. (2019). *Conflict and Collaboration: The Kingdoms of Western Uganda, 1890–1907*. Princeton, NJ: Princeton University Press.

Stanley H. M., (1899). *Through the Dark Continent*. London: United Kingdom: G. Newnes Press.

Tashobya C. K., Ssengooba, F., & Cruz, V. O. (Eds). (2006). *Health Systems Reforms in Uganda: Processes and Outputs*. London: Health Systems Development Programme, London School of Hygiene and Tropical Medicine Publication.

ThinkMD (2022). Addressing healthcare challenges in Uganda. https://thinkmd.org/project/addressing-healthcare-challenges-in-uganda/. Accessed October 30, 2020.

Tusubira A. K., Ssinabulya I., Kalyesubula R., Nalwadda C. K., Akiteng A. R., Ngaruiya C., Rabin T. L., Katahoire A., Armstrong-Hough M., Hsieh E, Hawley N. L., Schwartz J. I. (2023). Self-care and healthcare seeking practices among patients with hypertension and diabetes in rural Uganda. *PLOS Global Public Health*. 3(12):e0001777. DOI: 10.1371/journal.pgph.0001777.

Uganda Bureau of Statistics (2020). *Statistics Abstract*. Kampala, Uganda: Government Press.

Uganda Medical Association (2022). Profile Description. https://research-nexus.net/institution/9002151675/. Accessed October 31, 2024.

Uganda Medical Association (2023). Objectives and what we do. https://www.uma.ug/. Accessed November 30, 2023.

United Nations Human Development Program Index (2022). Human development report. https://hdr.undp.org/data-center/human-development-index#/indicies/HDI. Accessed September 22, 2024.

United States Department of State (2022). 2022 Country Reports on Human Rights Practice: Tanzania. https://www.state.gov/reports/2022-country-reports-on-human-rights-practices/tanzania/. Accessed October 31, 2024.

United States Department of State (2023). Uganda Health System. Accessed November 25, 2023.

Republic of Uganda Ministry of Health (2019). National alcohol control policy. https://www.health.go.ug/wp-content/uploads/2021/07/Uganda-Alcohol-policy-2019.pdf. Accessed September 22, 2024.

Wikipedia (2023). Healthcare in Uganda. https://en.wikipedia.org/wiki/Healthcare_in_Uganda#Antenatal_care,facility_deliveries,and_postnatal_care. Accessed November 25, 2023.

World Bank (2023). Uganda economic update. https://documents1.worldbank.org/curated/en/099020224131540261/pdf/P1798401a450b40361963b12634ab074169.pdf. Accessed September 23, 2024.

World Bank Indicators (2022). Ghana. https://databank.worldbank.org/source/world-development-indicators. Accessed September 22, 2024.

World Bank (2010). Fiscal space for health in Uganda. Africa Human Development Series. 186.

World Health Organization (2022). Annual report: Promotion of health and wellbeing in Uganda. https://www.afro.who.int/sites/default/files/2024-09/WHO%20Uga. Accessed November 12, 2024.

World Health Organization (2023). https://www.who.int/data/gho/data/countries/country-details/GHO/cameroon?countryProfileId=79e4cda0-11b1-4806-9c63-d40904289ced. Accessed November 25, 2023.

World Health Organization (2016). Physician and nurse's ratio per 1,000 people. https://iris.who.int/bitstream/handle/10665/250330/9789241511407-?sequence=. Accessed September 22, 2024.

Chapter Nineteen

HEALTH POLICY AND SOCIAL CRISIS IN ZAMBIA

Robert Dibie and Rayton Sianjina

Introduction

This chapter examines how the nation of Zambia in East Africa has adopted health policies that are modeled along the national health vision of "equity of access to, cost-effective and affordable health services, which is close to the family is possible." The chapter argues that despite Zambia's national health vision rural residents in the country are still faced with major challenges in accessing healthcare services. The aftermath of these challenges is that there is still a higher rate of morbidity and mortality in the rural regions of Zambia. Even though primary health services in Zambia are free, analysis conducted reveals that one other healthcare delivery challenge in the country is the lack of timely access to emergency care for citizens living in rural regions that are more than 50 miles from urban cities. Therefore, most citizens suffer from impaired outcomes such as physical and emotional stress due to difficulties in receiving good and timely access to healthcare. In addition, the nation of Zambia also faces the challenges of a shortage of healthcare professionals as well as financial investment in its health system. Like many other African countries, Zambia also spends less than 10% of its gross domestic product on healthcare. Other challenges discussed in the chapter include inadequate infrastructure and equipment, and weaknesses in the supply of drugs and other medical items. These challenges negatively affect healthcare service delivery in Zambia, particularly in the rural communities, as well as the disadvantaged vulnerable population groups, such as women, children, and those who are disabled. Some policy recommendations are provided that could help the government of Zambia to accomplish more positive healthcare outcomes in the future.

Brief History of Zambia

The Republic of Zambia is a landlocked country located between central Africa, eastern Africa, and southern Africa. It has boundaries with the Democratic Republic of Congo in the northwest, Angola in the east, and the Republic of Botswana in the south. The Republic of Zambia also has boundaries with Zimbabwe in the southeast, Tanzania in the northeast, and the Republic of Mozambique in the east. The origin of the people living in current-day Zambia could be traced to be descendants of those who inhabited in Great Rift

Valley, which runs from the lower Zambezi River in southern Zambia to the headwaters of the Nile in Egypt between the fifth and sixth centuries (Roberts 1976; Lambert 2022; Lewis 1964). Before the fourth century AD, the inhabitants of Zambia were Bushmen, Stone Age hunters and gatherers. Between the fourth and fifth centuries AD, a new wave of Bantu-speaking immigrants arrived from the north (Bjornlund et al. 1992; Lambert 2022). These Bantu ethnic group of immigrants were farmers and they had iron tools and beryl, rubies, sapphires, and other precious or semi-precious stones, which were all mined weapons (British Broadcasting Corporation 2018; Lambert 2022; Lewis 1964).

According to history scholars, the Bantu-speaking ethnic groups migrated to the region formerly known as Northern Rhodesia and now the Republic of Zambia in the sixth century (Henderson 1970; Phiri 2006; Roberts 1976). Further, in the twelfth century, the Shona ethnic groups migrated to the region. It is also reported that the people from the Luba and Lunda empires of Zaire (now the Democratic Republic of Congo) incrementally migrated to the Zambia region to set up kingdoms that were led by kings in the sixteenth century (Henderson 1970; Phiri 2006; Roberts 1976). Furthermore, new kingdoms were established around the fifteenth century. Among the new kingdoms were Bemba and Lunda in the north, Lozi in the west, and Chewa in the east. Other kingdoms include Zulu, Kololo, Lozi, and Ngoni (Bjornlund et al. 1992; Lambert 2022). By the seventeenth and eighteenth centuries, there was competition among the kingdoms, and some overly ambitious kings wanted to expand the kingdom. For example, Shaka, the ruler of Zulu began conquering neighboring villages and people in the early nineteenth century. Historians also contend that by the sixteenth century, some men were buried with gold beads (Henderson 1970; Pettman 1974; Roberts 1976). The kings of these kingdoms in the Zambia region also had glass beads from the Indian Ocean coast (Lambert 2022; Lewis 1964; Van & Jan 1998).

Historians reported that the Portuguese explorers started sailing around the Indian Ocean and near the coast of the eastern part of the African continent in the fifteenth century (Gewald et al. 2008; Henderson 1970). However, the people of Zambia did not have direct contact with the Europeans because of its landlocked location. David Livington was the first European to visit the Zambia land in 1851. Livingstone persuaded the African kingdom to sell cotton and ivory to the Europeans in return for their goods instead of selling slaves, however, his ambition was not successful because of was too difficult to transport goods to the Mozambique sea port (Pettman 1974; Phiri 2006; Roberts 1979). Thirty-five years after David Livingstone's trade ambition failed, Cecil Rhodes another United Kingdom citizen set up the British South African Company to exploit minerals in southern and central Africa (DeRoche & Kaunda 2016; Lambert 2022). Subsequently, Rhode and the British South African Company signed treaties with African ethnic groups and kings in the region to permit his company the right to mine minerals in the Zambia region. Some of the tribes include Tabwa, Lungu, and the Mambe. However, Bemba and the Ngoni refused to negotiate, and they were conquered by force by the British colonial army (Lambert 2022; Lewis 1964). Unfortunately, as soon as the British started mining in the Zambia territory, they went beyond the treaties that they had with the kings of the kingdom and immorally and incrementally took over the governance of the region (Henderson 1970; Roberts 1979; Sardanis 2003). Further, due to competition among British, Belgian, German, and Portuguese interests led to the establishment of Northern Rhodesia's borders in the late nineteenth century (Gordon 2023; Roberts 1976).

British North Rhodesia (Zambia) formerly achieved its independence from Britain and became a member of the *Commonwealth of Nations* (CON) on October 24, 1964. Kenneth Kaunda was elected the first president of the new nation in 1964 (Gewald et al. 2008; University of Central Arkansas 2023). *The election of the National Assembly members* was held on December 19, 1968, and the *United National Independence Party* (UNIP) won 81 out of 105 seats in the National Assembly. The *African National Congress* (ANC) won 23 seats in the National Assembly. President Kaunda was re-elected with 82% of the votes on December 19, 1968 (Gewald et al. 2008; Gordon 2023; University of Central Arkansas 2023). Frederick Chiluba defeated Kaunda and UNIP in the first multiparty elections since 1972.

The current population of Zambia in 2023 was 20.7 million people (World Population Review 2023). The majority of the nation's population resides around Lusaka, the capital city in the northern part of the county, and the Copperbelt province in the northern region. These two regions are regarded as the major economic hubs of the Republic of Zambia (Ihonvbere 1996; Wikipedia 2023). It should be noted that the Republic of Zambia has abundant natural resources, including minerals, wildlife, forestry, freshwater, and arable land. Furthermore, deposits of ironworking in central and western Zambia have been dated to the first five or six centuries (Roberts 1976; Lambert 2022).

The Republic of Zambia is a democratic country. The constitution was changed in 1991 from a one-party system to a multiparty system. According to the 1991 Constitution, the elected president of Zambia serves as the head-of-state and commander-in-chief of the armed forces. The elected president of Zambia can rule not more than two five-year terms (Britannica 2024; Republic of Zambia Constitution 1991). The nation's constitution also allows the president to use his privilege to appoint the vice president, the supreme court chief justice, and members of the high court based on the country's Judiciary Services Commission recommendation (Republic of Zambia Constitution 1991; Republic of Zambia 2016). Further, the Republic of Zambia is also operating as a unitary system of government whereby the Executive, Legislature, and the Judiciary operate as autonomous organs of Government. The Executive is the President who is deputized by a Vice President (Embassy of the Republic of Zambia Washington DC 2023; DeRoche and Kaunda 2016). In addition, President Edgar Chagwa Lungu is the current head-of-state of Zambia.

Health and Social Challenges in Zambia

Zambia was considered one of the world's fastest economically developing lower-middle nations between 2000 and 2009. However, a few years later, the nation's poverty rate increased to about 53% of its population (United States Agency for International Development 2023). In addition, apart from the disparity between the rich and poor in Zambia, the nation's citizens experienced chronic malnutrition that persisted at 35%. This precarious poverty situation eventually hampered the economic development process in the country. Other challenges that the Republic of Zambia has been experiencing include Dutch diseases such as ongoing dependence on copper mining. Zambia has also been struggling with limited economic diversification, poor energy infrastructure, a poor network of roads, a high unemployment rate, and a degradation of natural resources (World Bank Indicators 2020). These challenges also have spillover to low agricultural productivity, high burden of HIV/AIDS, malaria, tuberculosis, COVID-19, and cervical cancer (Geda 2021; United States Agency for International Development 2023).

According to the Center for Global Development (2023), the Republic of Zambia's health system has been struggling to take diligent care of its patients due to inadequate access to drugs, quality healthcare services, and a shortage of health professional workers. Further, a major challenge is that many health facilities in the country do not have enough physicians and nurses (Afriyie et al. 2023). It has also been reported that during the COVID-19 pandemic pick-up period in 2019, several of the medical staff working in the nation's hospitals got infected with COVID-19 (Geda 2021; Zekrya 2022). Additionally, the health personnel working in public hospitals often quit their jobs to seek opportunities in private hospitals that used to offer better salaries (Zekrya 2022).

Although public health systems are expected to function properly in the delivery of services and be adequately financed in order to galvanize quality healthcare for the population of any country, the case in Zambia has limited capacity to accommodate patients, which creates the need for people to seek treatment from expensive private hospitals (Afriyie et al. 2023; Zekrya 2022). Previously in Zambia, the private health system in the country was perceived as a service for the elites, but now, with the implementation of the National Health Insurance Management Authority patients in the country can have access to both public and private hospitals (National Health Insurance Management Authority 2022). In addition, through this scheme, one member of a family that is registered by his/her employer can give access to healthcare services to up to six members of his/her family unit, helping to extend universal health coverage (Republic of Zambia 2022; Zekrya 2022).

Further, Zambia is still experiencing post-COVID-19 challenges. The pandemic underscored the elevated dependency on donors and the lack of emergency preparedness in the country (Center for Global Development 2023). In addition, health insurance is still perceived by the majority of the population in the country as an elite benefit. This perception has propelled, the government of the nation to continue to convince people of the advantages of joining the National Health Management Authority scheme, as private insurance tends to be much more expensive (Zekrya 2022). According to the United States Agency for International Development Report (2023), Zambia has more than 1.2 million people on lifesaving antiretroviral treatment. However, the nation has incrementally overcome the previous high prevalence of HIV/AIDS since the nation adopted the evidence-based approach to prevent the spread of the disease (United States Agency for International Development Report 2023). In addition, the Republic of Zambia has also invested a lot in its citizens to have increased access to maternity and child health, family planning, and nutrition, as well as responding and preventing gender-based violence (Ministry of Health 2017; National Health Strategic Plan 2017–2021). It has previously been reported that 43% of women between the ages of 15 and 49 years old in Zambia have experienced some form of physical violence in their lifetime from their spouse. In addition, 39% of girls between the ages of 13 and 17 years old have experienced physical violence, while 20% of the same age group have also experienced sexual violence (Ministry of Health, National Health Strategic Plan 2017–2021; United States Agency for International Development 2023).

There have been several reports of mismanagement of the health system resources in Zambia (Afriyie et al. 2023; Chansa et al. 2018). One of the most embarrassing of these mismanagement was the 2020 procurement of over US$17 million in defective health kits and medicines. Therefore, with adequate and appropriate capacity in the nation's health system, the standard of health delivery and treatment has been argued to be low in most public hospitals and clinics in the country (Afriyie et al. 2023; Blas & Limbambala 2001). Further, the management of the health delivery system in the country had been compounded by low quality due to long waiting times before sick patients could see physicians or nurses. There are also incidents where patients will have to wait a long time before they can receive their prescribed medicine either because of a lack of medications in the hospital pharmacy or due to an extensive line of people waiting for their drug to be dispensed to them or a shortage of pharmacy staff. Many scholars have also reported that one of the major challenges in the management of the healthcare delivery system in Zambia is the lack of evidence to support effective prioritization by the government of the country (Afriyie et al. 2023; Chansa et al. 2019; Chitah et al. 2018; Geda 2021).

In 2020, the Republic of Zambia introduced a new policy process called Health Benefits Package (HBP). The HBP relies on data evidence and stakeholder consultation. At the time when its HBP was established, the government of Zambia postulated that the HBP process was an ideal mechanism for achieving universal health coverage (UHC) in the country (Center for Global Development 2023). Despite these promises made when the HBP initiatives were introduced in 2022 by the Government of Zambia, the implementation of the HBP roadmap faced multiple leadership, and unresolved funding challenges in its implementation process. Unfortunately, at the time of authoring this book in 2024, only components 1–3 of the HBP roadmap had been accomplished. It is interesting to notice that the Government of Zambia and many other countries in the African continent have formed the habit of enacting policies that they never made efforts to implement (Dibie 2022). The nation has not realized the fact that more health management experts of diverse capacities and experiences are needed to reinvigorate its health system.

According to the Zambia Ministry of Finance (2020) and Paul et al. (2021), there have been financial challenges in the funding of the healthcare system in the past few years. In addition, the allocation of a limited budget for the management of the health system has been detrimental to the quality of health services that are delivered all over the country (Afriyie et al. 2023; Paul 2021). Thus, the decrease in health spending has negatively affected the ability of the various hospitals and clinics in the country to purchase modern medical equipment as well as effectively implement the universal health insurance scheme. Another challenge that is confronting the health system with respect to funding is that there is a major disparity in the way funds are distributed in the country. Unfortunately, a larger proportion of funds are disbursed to the hospitals compared to what is allocated to the primary care facilities in the country (Afriyie et al. 2023; Blas & Limbambala 2001; Chansa et al. 2018).

Another major challenge in the Republic of Zambia is the disparity in the access to basic healthcare between provinces as well as urban and rural regions in the country. According to the Ministry of Health in Zambia report the urban areas have 99% of households that are five kilometers or about three miles from a hospital or clinic (Ministry of Health in Zambia 2024). On the other hand, 50% of the population living in rural regions live about the same distance from health facilities (International Insulin Foundation 2019; Ministry of Health in Zambia 2019). Further, the house expenditure of the population of the country varies from one region to another. For example, some poor households spend about 10% of their income on out-of-pocket payments while the richer population spends less than what the poor people pay each year (Musumali 2020; Prust et al. 2019). In addition, when poor people who live long distances from health facilities add up the cost of transportation, they often wonder if it is worth to such an amount of money to seek healthcare when they have children to care for (Phiri & Phiri 2017; Rudasingwa et al. 2022). Therefore, many of the poor population in Zambia are finding it difficult to pay for the cost associated with the quality medical treatment found in the private hospitals and clinics in the country.

It has been argued that the healthcare provider shortage is more than an inconvenience, it is a public health crisis (Blas & Limbambala 2001; Nyasa et al. 2023). For over two decades, the Republic of Zambia has been experiencing a shortage of health workers in its rural regions. Unfortunately, rural regions in Zambia have the most pressing health needs in the country, yet the population tends to face the highest shortage of healthcare delivery workforce (Manda et al. 2022). This shortage of physicians and nurses in some regions of the country has led to major limitations in the delivery of health services to many of its poor citizens. According to Afriyie et al. (2023) and Zekrya (2022), although the Government of Zambia has made a remarkable investment to improve the number of the health workforce in the country, the nation still lacks about 40% of its estimated health workforce that is needed to galvanize high-quality health system in Zambia (Cosgrave et al. 2019; Phiri & Phiri 2017). While the World Health Organization (2020) recommended 22.8 doctors, nurses, and midwives per 10,000 people, Zambia only has 11.2 doctors, nurses, and midwives per 10,000 people. This threshold of the medical workforce in the country is far below the recommended ratio (Manda et al. 2022; World Bank Indicators 2020). Further, more than 75% of the health workforce in Zambia works in public hospitals and clinics in urban cities as a result, it is the public sector that should be taking the lead in terms of the employment of health workers in the country. However, the country has not recruited enough health workers in the past two decades. Although Zambia trains and graduates about 4,000 health workers from its medical schools each year, the government only recruits around 2,000 to 2,500 new graduates. Thus, the attrition rate is around 2,000–3,000 health workers each year (Afriyie et al. 2023; Sikazwe et al. 2016).

Health Policies

The Republic of Zambia's government has enacted several health policies in the past three decades. The goals of the plans and strategies have been to provide an enabling environment for strengthening the health system in the country. Some of the past strategic plans include the Medical Service Act of 1985; the Governance Action Plan of 2009; the Ministry of Health Action Plan of 2011; the National Malaria Strategic Plan of 2011–2015; the National Child Health Policy of 2011–2016; the National Community Health Worker Strategy 2010; the Human Resources for Health Strategic Plan 2011–2015; the Patriotic Front Manifesto 2011–2016; and The Sixth National Development Plan 2011–2015. The goal of the country has been to incrementally prepare for the formulation of the Universal Health Coverage Policy in the near future. Many of these health policies attempted to address the challenges facing Zambia's health system (Claassen et al. 2021; Phiri & Phiri 2017; Ministry of Health 2021a).

National Health Insurance Scheme enacted in 2018: The goal of this policy has been to ensure that every citizen and resident of Zambia has access to good quality health services without suffering financial hardship, through the provision of a full spectrum of essential, quality health services, from health promotion, treatment, rehabilitation, and palliative care (Chalkidou et al. 2016; Center for Global Development 2023; Government of Zambia 2018). The National Health Insurance Policy also created the National Insurance Management Authority which was mandated to collect a contribution from residence, seeking health services from various hospitals and clinics or post. According to the provisions of the National Health Insurance, employees in the country are mandated to contribute 1% of their monthly salary with employers equally matching contribution (Government of Zambia 2018; Ministry of Health 2019). Further, residents of the country who are self-employed and are working in the private sector are also required to contribute 1% of their declared monthly salary. The citizens of the country who are 65 years or older are exempted from contributing and thus, get their health services free of charge (Government of Zambia 2018; Ministry of Health 2021b).

Pre-exposure Prophylaxis (PrEP) Policy enacted in 2016: The goal of this policy is to adopt measures to prevent the spread of HIV including counseling, family planning, voluntary male medical circumcision, and condom distribution. Between 2014 and 2026, Zambia had an adult HIV prevalence rate of about 11%. This health predicament attracted support from the United States Agency for International Development under the President Emergency Plan for HIV–AIDs Relief (United States Agency for International Development 2023). The PrEP was also established to consolidate guidelines for the treatment and prevention of HIV infection. The PrEP also includes recommending social behavioral change strategies as well as regulation of importation, marketing, and control of PrEP medications (Claassen et al. 2021; Ministry of Health 2020b). The PrEP was also expanded in a 2018 edition. (Claassen et al. 2021; Ministry of Health 2017; Republic of Zambia 2016).

National Health Policy enacted in 2012: The goal of this policy is to set a roadmap for further development of the health sector in Zambia. The policy also mandates the effective provision of equitable access to cost-effective and quality health services as close to the family as possible in a competent, caring, and clean environment for all citizens and residents of Zambia. The policy also envisaged that the Government of Zambia would prioritize primary healthcare services, hospital referral services, human resources development and management, legal framework, medical care financing, medical supplies, and coordination as well as infrastructure development. This health policy also requires action by all stakeholders such as civil society, corporation partners, government, and nongovernmental organizations, to collaborate in working toward the attainment of a better health system in Zambia (Ministry of Health 2012a).

National Health Package enacted in 2012: The major goal of this policy is to provide a wide range of health services across Zambia as well as alleviate the health delivery system in the country. The policy is also mandated to enhance the management of 25 disease control priorities and includes a mixture of infectious and noncommunicable diseases as well as medical specialties (Ministry of Health 2012a). Furthermore, the aim of the Government of Zambia was to implement the National Health Package as a whole rather than adopting a piecemeal approach by funding individual services to its citizens (Ministry of Health 2012b).

Removal of Health User Fees Policy Act of 2006: The goal of this policy was to promote the principles of access to health services to Zambia's citizens as a human right. This is because many people in some rural regions in the country were finding it difficult to have access to healthcare due to long distance, high user fees, and bad road network to hospitals and clinics. There was also the challenge of inadequate and well-trained doctors and nurses who were posted to rural health facilities. According to the Ministry of Health (2012b) and Phiri and Phiri (2017), people in rural districts in Zambia increased their utilization of health facilities after the user fees were abolished.

National Health Service Act of 1995: This policy introduced a meaningful change in the role and structure of the Ministry of Health. The new policy also established an autonomous health service delivery system. This forward led to the establishment of the Central Board of Health (CBH). The role of the CBH was to monitor, integrate, and coordinate the programs of the Health Management Boards (International Insulin Foundation 2019; Ministry of Health 1995).

Health Administration in Zambia

The healthcare system in Zambia has several complex challenges despite the fact the nation has developed well-integrated policies that are fundamental to shaping its pursuit of a high-quality health delivery system. The positive outcome of health policies nevertheless depends on the administration and implementation of formulated strategic health goals. In Zambia, an administrative institution such as the Ministry of Health was created by the government, authorized, and empowered to implement all health policies in the country (Zambia Ministry of Health 2020a; Ministry of Health 2012b). Since the enactment of the National Health Service Act of 1995 in Zambia, the Ministry of Health's role has been primarily the formulation of health policy, and the regulation of all health policies and National Health Strategic Plans, health mobilization, performance audit of the Center Board of Health in Zambia (International Insulin Foundation 2019; Ministry of Health 2017). The health administration and delivery system in the Republic of Zambia is divided into three levels. The health centers or post comprises first level (normally called the district). The second level is also referred to as the provincial health administrative level, while the third level is called the tertiary level.

According to the Zambia Ministry of Health (2012a), the *first or district level* comprises health posts, rural health centers, and district hospitals in Zambia. The health facilities at this level provide mostly preventive healthcare treatments. In most cases, district-level resources are preproperated on a per capita basis considering population density, the prevalence of epidemics, the price of fuel, and availability to commercial banks. In addition, hospitals that are located at the district's levels are based on cost per bed day (International Insulin Foundation 2019; Ministry of Health 2017). The district levels also engage in the prevention of diseases and the promotion of health behavior. The district hospitals in Zambia also provide medical, obstetric, surgical, diagnostic, and clinical services for health center referral in the rural regions of the country (Phiri & Phiri 2017).

The *second or provincial healthcare level* has six main areas of activities: (1) technical support function; (2) monitoring and evaluation; (3) health management information system and health research; (4) logistics supply of drugs, vaccines, and medical equipment supplied from the national level; (5) communication of national health policies and providing other instructions for the districts health boards; and (6) mediation (Phiri & Phiri 2017). The mandates of the National Health Act of 1995 led to the establishment of the Central Board of Health with the mandate to monitor and coordinate the programs of the Health Management Board (International Insulin Foundation 2019). The provincial hospitals also serve as major providers of healthcare services such as internal medicine, dental, internal care, pediatrics, psychiatry, obstetrics, and gynecology. There are about 21 provincial-level hospitals in Zambia (Zambia Ministry of Health 2017; Phiri & Phiri 2017).

The *third or tertiary level* is the highest healthcare system administration in Zambia. The tertiary hospital serves as the referral for all cases deemed too complex for both the districts and provincial hospitals. This is because it is well-equipped and has specialist physicians who can provide state-of-the-art medical treatment and surgery for complicated health cases. The tertiary levels also encompass the National University Teaching Hospitals and the central hospitals. According to the Ministry of Health (2017), these teaching hospitals include Kitwe Central Hospital, Ndola Central Hospital, and other specialist hospitals, that is, Chainama College Hospital, Arthur David Children's Hospitals, and Cancer Diseases Hospital (Zambia Ministry of Health 2017).

Apart from the above three levels under certain circumstances, the Republic of Zambia Government has also indulged in sending patients with critical illnesses that could not be treated in the country's hospitals for specialized treatment abroad since the 1990s (Phiri & Phiri 2017). In most cases, the National University Teaching Hospitals of Zambia refer senior government officials who cannot be treated in the country to the United States, India, South Africa, the United Kingdom, and Zimbabwe for specialist healthcare. Further, the private sector in Zimbabwe also provides healthcare treatment for the population that can afford the expensive cost (Manda et al. 2022).

Data Analysis and Discussion

The objective of this chapter is to analyze the effectiveness of health policy and healthcare delivery system in the Federal Republic of Zambia to determine if the nation has been able to accomplish its vision on equity of access to, cost-effective, and affordable health services. The data used for the analysis of healthcare policy effectiveness were derived from both primary and secondary sources. The primary research involves the administration of a questionnaire to 145 respondents. One hundred and twenty-five or 86.2% of respondents returned their completed questionnaire. The questionnaire respondents constitute 50.4% female and 49.6% male. In addition, 40% of the respondents had visited a hospital or clinic to receive treatment at least twice a year. Another 33% had also visited a hospital or clinic between 3 and 4 times recently to receive treatment. While 21% of the respondents visited 5–6 times a year and 6% also visited the hospital more than 7 times during the same period.

The secondary research methods adopted include the review of the Federal Republic of Zambia Government's Ministry of Health, National Health Plan of Zambia Reports, World Bank Indicators, World Health Organization Reports (2022a) and (2022b), United Nations Human Development Index Annual Report, Center for Disease Control, and United States Agency for International Development, academic as well as professional journals articles. Data were analyzed using SPSS to determine the effectiveness and challenges facing the health policy and quality of the healthcare delivery system in the Federal Republic of Zambia Government.

Table 1 analyzes the nature of healthcare delivery and health policy in the Federal Republic of Zambia Government. The result of the questionnaire reveals that 61.6% of the respondents agree that political leaders and rich citizens of Zambia prefer to seek healthcare services in foreign nations due to lack of trust in Zambia's healthcare system. Furthermore, 74.4% of the respondents agree that the Government of Zambia is effectively regulating medical professional licensing and disciplinary boards. In addition, 70.4% of respondents agree that corruption and unethical behavior of political and administrative leaders in government negatively affect the health system's funding. Furthermore, 68% of the questionnaire respondents stated that the lack of appropriate funding for the healthcare system in my country has negatively affected the quality of healthcare delivery in Zambia.

Further, 72% of the respondents indicated that most rural public hospitals in my country do not have specialist doctors and nurses. On the other hand, 47.2% reported that they can afford to pay for their healthcare treatment and medication costs without government subsidies. While 29.6% of the respondents indicated that they cannot afford to pay for their healthcare.

It was interesting to note that 42% of respondents stated that the healthcare provided by doctors in my city are highly commendable. Further, 38% of respondents indicated that most hospitals in my country do not have modern equipment. In addition, while

	Strongly Agree	Agree	Neutral	Strongly Disagree	Disagree	Agree %	Disagree %
Questions							
1 Healthcare provided by doctors in my city is highly commendable	8	45	37	6	25	53 42%	31 25%
2 Most hospitals in my country do not have modern equipment	9	39	33	12	32	48 38.4%	45 36%
3 I can afford my healthcare treatment and medication costs without government subsidies.	13	46	29	16	21	59 47.2%	37 29.6%
4 Most rural public hospitals in my country do not have specialist doctors and nurses.	53	37	14	15	6	90 72%	21 17%
5 Government pay of low salaries to doctors and nurses has encouraged their migration to foreign countries.	19	39	17	21	27	58 47%	48 38.4%
6 Lack of effective health policy implementation or regulations	6	11	21	45	42	17 13.6%	87 70%
7 Government promotes equity in the delivery of healthcare to underserved citizens in the country.	13	18	19	44	31	31 25%	75 60%
8 Political leaders and rich citizens of my country prefer to seek healthcare services in foreign nations.	33	44	21	16	11	77 61.6%	27 21.6%
9 Government is effectively regulating medical professional licensing and disciplinary boards	59	34	17	7	8	93 74.4%	15 30%
10 Hospitals and health centers in my city have constant electricity.	20	34	32	12	25	54 43.2%	37 30%
11 Lack of appropriate funding for the healthcare system in my country.	35	50	18	8	13	85 68%	21 17%
12 Corruption and unethical behavior of political and administrative leaders in government negatively affect the health system's funding.	51	37	20	10	6	88 70.4%	16 13%
Mean						50.2%	30.8%

Source: Derived from questionnaire administered in Zambia between 2022 and 2024.

47% of the respondents agreed that the government's payment of low salaries to doctors and nurses has encouraged their migration to foreign countries. It was reported by 38.4% of the respondents that they disagreed with the insinuation that low payment of salary is the major course of migration of physicians and nurses from Zambia.

In addition, 60% of the respondents disagree that the Government of Zambia promotes equity in the delivery of healthcare to underserved citizens in the country. Further, 70% of the respondents disagree that the lack of effective health policy implementation or regulations has negatively impacted the health delivery system in their country. Another 36% of the respondents also disagree that most hospitals in Zambia do not have modern equipment. While 30% of the respondents disagree as well that hospitals and health centers in their city have constant electricity. The mean agreement is 50.2%, while the disagreement is 30.8%. The questionnaire data analysis confirms that the health system and policies in Zambia have not been effective.

Table 2 analyzes the state of the health system in the Republic of Zambia economic and health system. Although the Republic of Zambia has appropriated 5.62% of its gross domestic product (GDP) in 2022 for the health system, its health budget is still lower than the 2001 Abuja Declaration of 15% of GDP annual budget that all 52 African nations' Presidents agreed on. Thus, Zambia is experiencing similar health challenges to several other nations on the African continent. The population also has been incrementally increasing in the past decade. The current population of the Republic of Zambia in 2022 is 29.8 million people (World Bank Indicators 2023). The current rate of medical physicians per 1,000 people in Zambia was 0.1 in 2018. Further, the number of nurses and wives per 1,000 people was 1.0, while the hospital beds per 1,000 people were 2.0 in 2022 (World Bank Indicators 2023; World Factbook 2022).

Further, access to safely managed drinking water was 2% in Zambia in 2020. Further, people using safely managed sanitation services (% of the population) was 31% in 2022. On the other hand, people practicing open defecation (% of the population)

Table 2 Economics and Health Indicators of Zambia

No.	Major Indicators in Ghana	Explanation
1	Population	20.02 million (2022)
2	Gross domestic product (GDP)	US$29.8 billion (2022)
3	Current health expenditure (% of GDP)	5.6% (2022)
4	Physicians/doctors per 1,000 people	0.1 (2018)
5	Nurses and midwives per 1,000 people	1.0 (2018)
6	Population using safely managed drinking water service	2% (2020)
7	People using safely managed sanitation services (% of population)	31% (2022)
	People practicing open defecation (% of the population)	6% (2022)

(Continued)

Table 2 *(Continued)*

8	Top ten common diseases in Zambia	1. HIV/AIDS; 2. Neonatal disorders; 3. Stroke; 4. Lower respiratory infections; 5. Diarrheal diseases; 6. Tuberculosis; 7. ischemic heart disease; 8. Malaria; 9. Cirrhosis and other chronic kidney diseases; 10. Hypertensive heart disease
9	Life expectancy at birth for females	64 years (2021)
10	Life expectancy at birth for males	58 years (2021)
11	Mortality rate for female adults (per 1,000 people)	250 (2021)
12	Mortality rate for male adults (per 1,000 people)	369 (2021)
13	Mortality rate for infants (per 1,000 people)	40 (2021)
14	Tuberculosis incidence (per 100,000 people)	307 people (2021)
15	Population living below income poverty line PPP $2.15 a day	60.8% (2015)
16	Poverty head count ratio national poverty line (%)	54.4% (2015)
17	Contribution deprivation in health to multidimensional poverty	Not available
18	Infants lacking immunization for measles (% of one year old)	91% (2021)
19	Malaria incidence (per 1,000 people at risk)	187.7 people (2021)
20	HIV/AIDS prevalence of adults (% ages 15–49)	10.8% (2022)

Source: World Bank Indicators (2022); United Nations Human Development Program Index. (2022). United Nations Human Development Report (2022); and World Health Organization (2022a; 2022b; & 2023).

constitute 6% in Zambia in 2022 (World Bank Indicators 2023). Only 46.7% of the population of Zambia has access to electricity.

Furthermore, HIV/AIDS, neonatal disorders, stroke, lower respiratory infections, diarrheal diseases, tuberculosis, ischemic heart disease, malaria, cirrhosis, other chronic kidney diseases, and hypertensive heart diseases continue to be the major causes of mortality in Zambia (World Health Organization 2022a). Life expectancy has improved in the country. While life at birth is currently 64 years for females in 2021. The life expectancy in 2021 for males has increased to 58 years. On one hand, the mortality rate for females per 1,000 people is 250 in 2021. On the other hand, the mortality rate for male adults per 1,000 people is 369 in 2021 (World Bank Indicators 2023). Unfortunately, the mortality rate for infants per 1,000 people has dropped to 40 in 2021.

The incidence of tuberculosis per 100,000 people was 307 people in 2021 (World Bank Indicators 2023). The population living below income poverty line PPP $2.15 a day was 60.8% in 2015. Further, the poverty head count ratio national poverty line (%) was 54.4% in 2015. The sad news was that the number of infants lacking immunization measles % of one year old in 2021 in Zambia was 91% (World Bank Indicators 2023). While the malaria incidence per 1,000 people at risk was 187.7 people in Zambia in 2021, the HIV/AIDS prevalence of adults % aged 15–49 has dropped to 10.8% in Zambia in 2022 (World Bank Indicators 2023; World Health Organization 2022b).

Conclusion

This chapter has examined the Republic of Zambia's health policies that were modeled along the provisions of the national health vision of "equity of access to, cost-effective and affordable health services, which is close to the family is possible." It argues that despite Zambia's national health vision rural residents in the country are still faced with major challenges in accessing healthcare services. The aftermath of these challenges is that there is still a higher rate of morbidity and mortality in the rural regions and urban cities due to the lack of access to affordable healthcare by the citizens of Zambia. Analysis conducted reveals that over 61% of the population of the people in Zambia live in rural districts in the country, however, this group of poor people lack access to needed primary healthcare services. This predicament of the low-income people in Zambia confirms that the healthcare system and policies have not been effective over the past three decades.

Analysis conducted reveals that the Republic of Zambia's health system has improved considerably since the nation enacted its Medical Service Act of 1985, and the National Health Service Act of 1995. In addition, over the past three decades, more than a dozen health policies and National Health Strategic Plans have been formulated and implemented. The policies introduced have propelled significant changes in the role and structure of the Ministry of Health as well as progress toward the adoption of Universal Health Coverage in the country. The ambition of the government of Zambia to accomplish universal health coverage through the initial formulation of universal health insurance has been extremely high.

Furthermore, despite the strategic health plans and health policies enacted, the transformation of the ambition into the accomplishment of universal health coverage has been faced with very many challenges. Some of the major obstacles that are preventing the Republic of Zambia from accomplishing its healthcare delivery vision include lack of enough healthcare budget, health workers shortage, poor healthcare infrastructure, and inability to motivate and retain healthcare staff. Other challenges include the lack of appropriate medical equipment, lack of effective essential drugs supply chain, the disparity in the location of health facilities in rural regions in the country, and the lack of access to health facilities by poor people living in rural regions of the country.

Moving forward to solve these challenges will require investment and setting major priorities for performance management. Furthermore, the solution to the shortage of health workers, that is, physicians and nurses in the country calls for the urgent need for new strategies to improve the rural health workforce by providing incentives and higher pay to attract and retain them in rural communities in Zambia (Manda et al. 2022;

Prust et al. 2019). Furthermore, to solve the problem of disparity at higher levels of care previously discussed in this chapter, there is an urgent need for the Republic of Zambia government to put in place measures to facilitate access to public hospitals by the poor citizens of the country (Rudasingwa et al. 2022).

It is especially important for the Republic of Zambia's government to redefine the administration of the healthcare system in the country as well as identify the most important variables and interrelationships that will affect future decisions and the health workforce. Because of a weak control system, the healthcare system lacks direction causing difficulty in accomplishing its strategic vision goals. Moving forward would require setting direction and empowering people to make their own decisions on how best to accomplish the healthcare vision for Zambia. The healthcare system at the district and provincial levels should be regarded as an integrated system with each part of the subsystem proving a unique interdependent contribution. The above approach should be considered to increase healthcare workers in the country. The government of Zambia should also provide more incentives in addition to good housing and transportation systems for doctors and nurses deplore to work in rural regions of the country. Scholarships should be awarded to students who are studying to become doctors, and nurses. One of the conditions for giving the award should mandate the recipients to work at least five years after graduation from medical or nursing schools, at the district or provincial health facilities.

Finally, the medication and medical supply chain system in Zambia needs to be reinvigorated. To sustain the supply of drugs to medical facilities and pharmacies in the country the Zambia, medicines and medical supplies agency should be enhanced to better coordinate and ensure the timely supply of essential medicines in the country. The medicine and medical supplies agency needs to be better financed with an adequate budget, and highly qualified staff that are trained in supply chain management. There is also the need to purchase more vehicles for the agency to ensure the timely distribution of medicines and medical equipment to districts and provincial hospitals and clinics to save lives.

References

Afriyie D. O., Masiye F., Tediosi F., Fink G. (2023). Purchasing for high-quality care using national health insurance evidence from Zambia. *Health Policy and Planning*, 38(1): 681–688.

Bjornlund E., Bratton M., Gibson C. (1992). Observing multiparty elections in Africa: Lessons from Zambia. *African Affairs*, 91: 405–431.

Blas E., Limbambala M. (2001). The challenge of hospitals in health sector reform; The case of Zambia. *Health Policy and Planning*, 16(2): 29–43.

Britannica (2023). History of Tanzania. https://www.britannica.com/topic/history-of-Tanzania. Accessed November 13, 2024.

Britannica (2024). The Editors of Encyclopaedia. "Zambia summary". *Encyclopedia Britannica*, 29 Apr. 2021. https://www.britannica.com/summary/Zambia. Accessed 6 October 2024.

British Broadcasting Corporation (2018). Zambia profile—Timeline. news/world-africa-14113084. Accessed October 8, 2023.

Center for Global Development (2023). *Towards Universal Health Coverage: Zambia's Experience Developing a Roadmap to Support Health Benefit Package Reform*. Washington DC: Center for Global Development Publication.

Chalkidou K., Glassman A., Marten R., Vega J., Teerawattananon Y., Tritasavit N., Gyansa-Lutterodt M., Selter A., Kieny M. P., Hofman K., Culyer A. J. (2016). Priority-setting for achieving universal health coverage. *Bulletin of the World Health Organization*, 94(6): 462. Accessed October 14, 2023.

Chansa C., Mastebula T., Piatti M. et al. (2019). *Zambia Health Sector Public Expenditure Tracking and Quantitative Services Delivery Survey*. Washington DC: World Bank.

Chansa C., Workie N. W., Piatti M., Mastebula T., Yoo K. J. (2018). *Zambia Health Sector Public Expenditure Review*. Washington DC: World Bank.

Chitah B. M., Chansa C., Kaonga O., Workie N. W. (2018). Myriad of healthcare financing reforms in Zambia: Have the poor benefited? *Health System & Reform*, 4(1): 313–323.

Claassen C. W.; Mumba D., Njelesani M., Nyimbili D., Mwango L. K., Mwitumwa M., Mubanga E., Mulenga L., Chisenga T., Nichols B., Hendrickson C., Chtembo L., Okuku J., O'Bra H. (2021). Initial implementation of PrEP in Zambia: Health policy development and service delivery scale-up. *BMJ Open*, 11(1). Accessed October 16, 2023.

Cosgrave C., Malatzky C., Gillespie J. (2019). Social determinants of rural health workforce retention: A scoping review. *International Journal of Environment Resources Public Health*, 16(3): 314–325.

DeRoche A., Kaunda K. (2016). *The United States, and Southern Africa*. London, United Kingdom: Bloomsbury Press.

Dibie R. (2022). Healthcare policy and administration in Nigeria: A critical analysis. *The Journal of African Policy Studies*, 28(1): 101–139.

Embassy of the Republic of Zambia Washington DC (2023). Government of Zambia. https://www.zambiaembassy.org/. Accessed October 8, 2023.

Ferguson J. (1999). Expectations of Modernity: Myths and Meanings of Urban Life in the Zambian Copperbelt. Berkeley: University of California Press.

Geda A. (2021). *The Economic and Social Impacts of COVID-19 in Zambia*. Geneva, Switzerland: United Nations Conference on Trade and Development.

Gewald J. B., Hinfelaar M., Macola G. (2008). *One Zambia, Many Histories: Towards a History of Post-Colonial Zambia*. Boston, MA: Brill Press.

Gordon D. (2023). Zambia: Oxford bibliographies. Accessed October 6, 2024.

Government of Zambia (2018). The National Health Insurance Act (No. 2 of 2018). Lusaka, Government Republic of Zambia.

Henderson I. (1970). *The Journal of African History*, 11(4): 591–603.

Ihonvbere J. (1996). *Economic Crisis, Civil Society and Democratization: The Case of Zambia*. Trenton, NJ: Africa World Press.

International Insulin Foundation (2019). Zambia health system. Accessed October 16, 2023.

Lambert T. (2022). A short history of Zambia. Accessed October 9, 2023.

Lewis G. H. (1964). *A History of Northern Rhodesia: Early Days to 1953*. London: Chatto and Windus Press.

Manda K., Silumbwe A., Kombe M. M., Hongoma P. (2022). Motivation and retention of primary healthcare workers in rural facilities: An exploratory qualitative study of Chipata and Chadiza districts, Zambia.

Ministry of Health (2021a). *Agenda for Review of National Health Care Package Roadmap*. Lusaka: Government Republic of Zambia.

Ministry of Health (2021b). *National Health Care Package Rroadmap Stakeholder Validation Workshop-Presentation by the Director, Planning & Budget*. Lusaka: Government Republic of Zambia.

Ministry of Finance and National Planning (2020). 2020 Annual Economic Report. Accessed October 6, 2024.

Ministry of Health (2020a). *Health Care Priority Setting in Zambia: A Scoping Review*. Lusaka: Government Republic of Zambia.

Ministry of Health (2020b). *Terms of References for Health Benefits Package Technical Workshop-Presentation by the Director, Planning & Budgeting*. Lusaka: Government Republic of Zambia.

Ministry of Health (2019). *National Health Insurance Scheme Tariff and Benefit Package Operation Manual*. Lusaka: Government Republic of Zambia.

Ministry of Health (2017). *National Health Strategic Plan 2017–2021*. Lusaka: Government Republic of Zambia. Accessed October 14, 2023.

Ministry of Health (2012a). *National healthcare package*. Lusaka: Government Republic of Zambia.

Ministry of Health (2012b). *National Health Policy*. Lusaka: Government Republic of Zambia.

Ministry of Health (1995). Zambia National Health Accounts 1995-1998. Accessed October 6. 2024.

Ministry of Health in Zambia (2024). Zambia experiencing high resistance to antibiotics and other antimicrobial. https://www.moh.gov.zm/?p=3951. Accessed November 14, 2024.

Ministry of Health Zambia (1995). National Health Services Act, 1995. https://zambialii.org/akn/zm/act/1995/22/eng@1996-12-31. Accessed November 14, 2024.

Musumali C. (2020). Zambia's deepening crisis in COVID era: a shortage of health workers. Accessed December 15, 2023.

Musumali M., Qutieshat A. (2022). A brief review of literature on issues and challenges of business continuity management for small and medium-sized enterprises in developing countries. *International Journal of Business Continuity and Risk Management*, 12(4), 362–382.

National Health Insurance Management Authority (2022). Zambia: National Health Insurance Authority Strategic Plan (2023–2026). Accessed November 25, 2023.

National Health Strategic Plan (2017–2021). Zambia: Building robust and resilient health systems. Accessed January 29, 2024.

Nyasa M., Chipungu J., Ngandu M., Chilambe C., Nyirenda H., Musukuma K., Lundamo M., Simuyandi M., Chilengi R., and Sharma A. (2023). Health care workers' reactions to the newly introduced hepatitis B vaccine in Kalulushi, Zambia: Explained using the 5A taxonomy. *Vaccine* X;13:100274. DOI: 10.1016/j.jvacx.2023.100274.

Paul V. B., Finn A., Chaudhary S., Mayer Gukovas R., Sundaram R. (2021). COVID-19, Poverty, and Social Safety Net Response in Zambia. *Policy Research Working Paper; No. 9571*. Washington, DC: World Bank.

Pettman, J. 1974. Zambia's second republic – The establishment of a one-party state. *The Journal of Modern African Studies*, 12(2): 231–244.

Phiri F., Phiri M. (2017). The health system in Zambia, merits, opportunities, and challenges. *IOSR Journal of Humanities and Social Sciences*, 22(11):56–63.

Phiri B. J. (2006). *A Political History of Zambia: From the Colonial Period to the 3rd Republic*. Trenton, NJ: Africa World Press.

Prust M. L, Kamanga A, Ngosa L, McKay C, Muzongwe C. M, Mukubani M. T, Chihinga R, Misapa R, van den Broek J. W, Wilmink N. (2019). Assessment of interventions to attract and retain health workers in rural Zambia: a discrete choice experiment. *Human Resource Health Journal*. 3;17(1):26. doi: 10.1186/s12960-019-0359-3. Accessed September 30, 2024.

Republic of Zambia (2016). *Constitution of Zambia Amendment no. 2 of 2016*. Lusaka, Zambia: Government Press.

Republic of Zambia (1991). *Constitution of the Republic of Zambia*. Lusaka, Zambia: Government Press.

Republic of Zambia (2017). National Health Strategic Plan 2017–2021. https://faolex.fao.org/docs/pdf/zam191199.pdf. Accessed November 13, 2024.

Republic of Zambia (2022). National Health Insurance Management Authority (2022). https://p4h.world/en/news/the-national-health-insurance-management-authority-provides-an-update-on-the-performance-and-status-of-the-zambia-national-health-insurance-scheme/. Accessed October 31, 2024.

Republic of Zambia Ministry of Finance and National Planning (2020). Advert for call for proposals-public-private partnership projects. https://www.mofnp.gov.zm/?p=7979. Accessed November 13, 2024.

Roberts A. (1976). *A History of Zambia*. Portsmouth, NH, USA: Heinemann Press.

Roberts H. (1979). Women and medicine. *Sociology*, 13(3), 557–558.

Rudasingwa M., Allegri M., Mphuka C., Chansa C., Yeboah E., Bonnet E., Ridde V., Chitah B. M. (2022). Universal health coverage and the poor; to what extent are health financing policies making a difference? Evidence from a benefit incidence analysis in Zambia. *BMC Public Health*, 22(1): 1546–1557.

Sardanis A. (2003). *Africa: Another Side of the Coin: Northern Rhodesia's Final Years and Zambia's Nationhood*. London, United Kingdom: B. Tauris Press.

Sikazwe A., Musumali M., Siboonde M., Chabala R., Mufunda J. and Chime J. K. (2016). Improved financial probity in the health Sector following the WHO reforms in Zambia. *Medical Journal of Zambia*, 43(1). https://library.adhl.africa/handle/123456789/11428. Accessed November 13, 2024.

Simfukwe P., Edward S. M., Alfred D. (2022). Accessing future mixed beans yield in Zambia under a changing climate scenario. DOI:10.26502/ijpaes.4490144.

The World Fact book (2022). Zambia hospital bed numbers to 1000 people. https://www.cia.gov/the-world-factbook/countries/zambia/. Accessed October 22, 2023.

United Nations Human Development Report (2022). Changing the world: Working with the people of Zambia to build a resilient and diversified economy. Accessed October 6, 2024.

United Nations Human Development Program Index (2022). Human development report. https:hdr.undo.org/en/2022-report. Accessed October 18, 2023.

United States Agency for International Development. (2023a). Tanzania Project Briefer. https://www.usaid.gov/sites/default/files/2023-10/USAID_Tanzania_Project_Briefer_July_2023.pdf. Accessed November 10, 2024.

United States Agency for International Development. (2023b). USAID Tanzania Strategy 2020–2025. Accessed October 31, 2024.

United States Agency for International Development (2023c). Zambia: Country overview. Accessed September 25, 2024.

University of Central Arkansas (2023). Zambia: 1964–present. Accessded Septmeber 30, 2024.

Van D., Jan K. 1998. Reflections on donors, opposition and popular will in the 1996 Zambian general elections. *Journal of Modern African Studies*, 36 (1): 71–99.

Wikipedia (2023). History of Zambia. https://en.wikipedia.org/wiki/2023_in_Zambia. Accessed October 8, 2023.

World Bank Indicators (2023). Zambia. Accessed October 6, 2024.

World Bank indicators (2022). Zambia. https://data.worldbank.org/country/zambia. Accessed October 18, 2023.

World Bank Indicators (2023) World Development Indicators. https://databank.worldbank.org/source/world-development-indicators. Accessed November 12, 2024.

World Bank (2020). World development indicators. World Bank Group. https://www.worldbank.org/en/country/zambia/overview. Accessed October 14, 2023.

World Health Organization (2023). Zambia. https://data.who.int/countries/894. Accessed October 18, 2023.

World Health Organization (2022a). Annual report WHO Zambia. default/files/2023-09/WHO%20Zambia%20Ann. Accessed October 6, 2024.

World Health Organization (2022b). Zambia: For a safer, healthier and fairer world. Accessed October 6, 2024.

World Health Organization (2020c). Mental Health Atlas 2020 Country Profile: Zambia. https://www.who.int/publications/m/item/mental-health-atlas-zmb-2020-country-profile. Accessed November 13, 2024.

World Population Review (2023). Zambia population. https://worldpopulationreview.com/countries/zambia. Accessed October 8, 2023.

Zekrya, H. (2022). How is Zambia improving universal health coverage? We asked a local parliamentarian. Accessed October 14, 2023.

Chapter Twenty

HEALTH POLICY AND SOCIAL CRISIS IN ZIMBABWE

Robert Dibie and Halima Khunoethe

Introduction

This chapter examines the challenges facing health policy implementation and the health delivery system in Zimbabwe. It argues that the present health system in Zimbabwe tends not to effectively preserve the health of the citizens of the country. This is because the nation's healthcare system and funding mechanism do not recognize the citizens' rights to affordable health and other protected interests. The chapter uses a value-based health service conceptual framework to explain how the nation could adopt high-quality health services to improve its citizens' health safety and cost efficiency. The findings of the research conducted reveal that citizen of Zimbabwe suffers from a high rate of communicable and noncommunicable diseases. The nation's citizens also suffer from severe clean water and sanitation crises. Despite these health challenges, the nation's health system also faces a shortage of healthcare staff, limited access to healthcare facilities by citizens, high out-of-pocket expenses, exceptionally low funding for healthcare delivery, high congestion at healthcare facilities, and poor-quality healthcare services. In addition, citizens and residents of Zimbabwe especially those living in the rural regions do not have good access to any medical insurance. This is because access to medical insurance differs by area of residence and level of wealth. The chapter recommends that the deteriorating health challenges in Zimbabwe require an immediate review of the nation's health insurance system, as well as appropriate reinvigoration of the healthcare system. The Government of Zimbabwe must ensure that universal health coverage policies are adopted to improve the healthcare of all its citizens. The nation's government must also consider taking steps to better equip the hospitals with state-of-the-art equipment and other health infrastructure, as well as make more pragmatic efforts to retain highly qualified health practitioners as well as discourage the flight of nurses and physicians from the country.

Brief History of Zimbabwe

Zimbabwe is a country located in Southeast Africa. The country was formally called Southern Rhodesia before it became an independent country in 1980 (Makumbe 2006) The nation has no direct access to the Indian Ocean hence it is often referred to as a landlocked nation. It has a border with the Republic of Mozambique on the eastern and northeast, and the Republic of Zambia on the northwest. The country also shares a boundary with the Republic of Botswana and South Africa in the south. The geography of Zimbabwe is mostly high plateau and mountains in the east. The current population of Zimbabwe is about 16.4 million people (World Population Review 2023). The government system is a parliamentary democracy (Government of Zimbabwe 2017). History scholars contend that the Bantu-speaking ethnic group was one of the first people to settle in the current land now called Zimbabwe around 400 AD (Britannica 2024; Guthrie 1971; Huffman 2007; Phillipson 1989; Rexová et al. 2006). The Bantu were farmers and established farms and villages along rivers in central Zimbabwe. Other precolonial ethnic groups that settled in the land called Zimbabwe include the Matebele people (Bastin et al. 1999; Gray 1956; Victoriafalls 2020; Wikipedia 2018). A few centuries later 1830, the Ndebele people came to Zimbabwe from the south, and their chief, Mzilikazi established the capital at Bulawayo between 1810 and 1830 (Britannica 2024; South African History Online 2020). In addition, the Matebele people were led by Mzilikazi, their King and commander in several wars in the region. After the death of Mzilikazi in 1968, his son Lobengula became the King of the Matebele people. Like his father Mzilikazi, King Lobengula fought vehemently to extend his Kingdom until the white settlers from the south under the pretest of the British South Africa Company pushed northwards toward the Zimbabwe River valley (Beach 1979; Bret 2005; South African History Online 2020).

According to Parsons Neil (1993), Palley Claire (1966), and South African History Online (2020), Cecil Rhodes a director of British South Africa connived to arrange a trade contract with King Lobengula for the mineral rights of the country in exchange for ammunitions, guns, and money. As a result of a dispute that arose due to the misunderstanding in the implementation of the contract between the two parties' tensions escalated to become a major war (Neil 1993; Pakenham 1992; South African History Online 2020). Despite the joint effort of the Matebele and Mashona to prevent the British South Africa Company's colonization, they were unsuccessful. At the end of the crisis, the British South Company captured the territory and changed its name to Southern Rhodesia. Further, in 1890, the British African Company was chartered (Britannica 2024; South African History Online 2020; Wikipedia 2024; Wikipedia 2018). The intention of spreading their control made the British African Company proclaim Southern Rhodesia as a British colony in 1923.

After four decades, the Matebele and Mashona ethnic people requested the decolonization of their land, however, the British colonial regime resisted, and the outcome led to a brutal civil war between the white colonial government and the majority African people that advocated for their independence (Cuneo et al. 2017; History World 2007). Between the early 1950s and 1970s, the majority of black African people in Rhodesia formed two political parties namely (a) the Zimbabwe African National Union (ZANU) and (b) the Zimbabwe African People's Union (ZAPU) (History World 2007; Wikipedia 2018). In an attempt to prevent the activities of the two political parties, the Rhodesia white colonial government banned the activities of the political parties, and their leader was thrown in jail. This action of the white Rhodesia colonial administration further escalated the Chimurenga bloody bush war staged by black African freedom fighters in the country (History World 2007; Wikipedia 2024). The positive outcome of the brutal war led to several negotiations between the British Government and the freedom fighters (Leoewenson et al. 1991).

In 1980, Rhodesia became an independent country. The name of the new nation was changed from Rhodesia to Zimbabwe. Further, Robert Mugabe was elected the first Prime Minister of the new country called Zimbabwe from 1980 to 1987 (History World 2007; South African History Online 2020; Wikipedia 2018). Robert Mugabe also served as president of Zimbabwe from 1987 to 2017.

In addition, after becoming an independent nation in 1980, Zimbabwe had a diversified economy, well-developed infrastructure, and an advanced financial sector. In the first few years of President Mugabe's administration, Zimbabwe was an economic success story (Bret 2005; Britannica 2024; Dibie 2018; Kuye & Ogundele 2013). However, the nation was plunged into economic crisis when Zimbabwe adopted the structural adjustment policy (SAP) in the mid-1980s. The GDP recording is far much lower compared to that before the adoption of the SAPs (Britannica 2024; Kidia 2018). Therefore, some scholars have argued that the problems of Africa are directly linked to ventures of Western exploitation of Africa, corruption, and bad leadership of political leaders (Dibie 2018; Drezner 2011; Mamdani 2008; Moyo 2009). The Zimbabwe elite during President Mugabe's administration did not promote true community participation and engagement that could have provided civil society leaders to explore the needed sustainable development goals of the country. Instead, the Zimbabwe elites pragmatically alienated the majority who have sunk into further impoverishment due to the strings attached to the Economic Structural Adjustment Policy formulated in the 1980s by the nation (Britannica 2024; Dibie 2018; Mhazo & Maponga 2022).

Zimbabwe is now one of Africa's poorest countries (Dibie 2018). The economy of Zimbabwe started moving in the wrong direction when the administration of President Mugabe formulated a radical land redistribution policy in the early 2000s. The land redistribution policy mandated taking land that originally belonged to the black citizens of Zimbabwe that was vehemently taken by the white colonial settlers (Mhazo & Maponga 2022; Kidia 2018). Immediately after the land redistribution policy was adopted by President Mugabe, many Western industrialized countries responded by imposing various forms of sanction on Zimbabwe (Freeman 2014; Mhazo & Maponga 2022; Sylvester 1985). The Western countries that imposed sanctions on Zimbabwe include the United Kingdom, many member nations of the European Union, and the United States. The sanctions that were imposed made it difficult for foreign aid organizations to deliver food, healthcare aid, and many other forms of humanitarian services to Zimbabwe (Drezner 2011; Government of Zimbabwe 1997; Kidia 2018; Mamdani 2008).

In addition, the sanctions imposed on Zimbabwe also discourage foreign direct investment in the country. On one hand, the European Union nation's members adopted a policy to terminate development assistance to Zimbabwe. On the other hand, the United States formulated a Zimbabwe Democracy and Economic Recovery Act of 2001 (Jaeger 2016; Mhazo & Maponga 2022). This policy restricted the United States from voting in support of any form of development assistance to Zimbabwe from international financial institutions (Mhazo & Maponga 2022). During these economic predicaments, few donors and nongovernmental organizations started funding Zimbabwe citizens by bypassing the government and dealing directly with non-state institutions (Freeman 2014; Kawewe & Dibie 2000; Mhazo & Maponga 2022). Unfortunately, President Mugabe died on September 6, 2017, at the age in Singapore due to cancer. A few months before President Mugabe's death, he was forced to resign after a military coup in November 2017. While he was the president, he used to secretly travel to Singapore to seek healthcare (Mhazo & Maponga 2022; Mnangagwa 2018).

The current president of Zimbabwe is Emmerson Dambudzo Mnangagwa. He resumed office of the Presidency on November 24, 2017. The new administration of the new Republic of Zimbabwe was structured like a democratic nation. The chief of state is the Executive President, and the head of government is the Prime Minister. Zimbabwe has a mixed economy in which there is limited private freedom, but the economy remains highly controlled by the government (OECD 2014). Zimbabwe is a member of the African Union (AU), the African Economic Community (AEC), and the Common Market for Eastern and Southern Africa (COMESA) (Dibie 2018; United Nations Human Development Report 2014).

In 2017, Emmerson Dambudzo Mnangagwa, the new President of Zimbabwe asked the international community to lift the sanctions that were imposed on his country. President Mnangagwa contends that the sanction has not only destroyed the economy of his nation but also punished most of the poor and vulnerable black citizens of Zimbabwe as well as galvanizing human rights abuses in all ramifications (Mnangagwa 2018). Since 2017, President Emmerson Mnangawa's administration has proposed several economic and health policies that are directed toward health financing. There is also evidence of new political and redistributive processes that could help the nation to revitalize its healthcare systems. Therefore, President Mnangawa's adoption of economic policy reforms could be considered compatible with the contemporary style for achieving sustainable national economic development. The Republic of Zimbabwe has now established a vibrant partnership with local and international health partners to reinvigorate the healthcare system for all its citizens.

Healthcare Challenges in Zimbabwe

Zimbabwe as previously discussed used to be a vibrant, productive, resilient, and productive country in Southeast Africa (United Nations Human Development Index 2023; USAID 2023). Historically, the nation had an outstanding teaching hospital system and highly trained healthcare practitioners such as doctors and nurses (Kidia 2018; UNICEF 2020 & 2022). However, a challenging or deplorable economic condition over the past two decades has led to a high cost of living, insufficient healthcare workers, and a lack of advanced medical care for the citizens of Zimbabwe (USAID 2023). In addition, ineffective leadership, political crisis, ineffective health policies; corruption by elites, wrong economic policies, and the control of its economy by minority white own corporations. have led to a major disaster in education, public health, and infrastructure (Mkandawire 2020; Razvi et al. 2020; USAID 2022).

Mhazo, Maponga, and Mossialos (2023) argued that market failure and weak public policy as well as regulations or inadequate implementation have contributed to healthcare disaster in Zimbabwe. Over the past two decades, the economy has been in crisis. To compound the health challenges, the gross national product has dropped by more than 50%. On the other hand, inflation is running at more than 100, 000% (Mhazo et al. 2023). More than 80% of the country's 12 out of 14 million citizens of the country are living below the government's own poverty line. Further, there is also a widespread shortage of food, and more than 4.5 million people need food aid from foreign nongovernmental organizations in the country (Government of Zimbabwe 2017; Masuku & Macheka 2020; Nhapi 2019).

Makoni (2020) contends that because of the neglect of the health sector in Zimbabwe by the Government of Zimbabwe, the citizens and healthcare workers have lost confidence in the system. This major perception of the above group has resulted in a brain-drain of qualified and skilled healthcare workers in the country (Makoni 2022). Another level of the escalating challenge is the fact that healthcare clinics and hospitals in some regions of the country are now operated by junior doctors, student nurses as well as staff that are still under training. Over the past decade, the deplorable healthcare delivery system in Zimbabwe has led to high mortality and morbidity levels (Makoni 2022). Furthermore, most of the pharmacies in the rural regions of the country are empty with no drugs to administer to sick people or for patients to purchase (Government of Zimbabwe 2020; Makoni 2022; Meldrum 2008; Nhapi 2019).

One of the critical beginnings of the collapse of a once vibrant health system in Zimbabwe is the authoritarian system of governance and sanctions that was imposed on the nation by the European Union and the United States. According to the USAID (2023) report because of the implementation of the United States' President's Emergency Plan for AIDS Relief (PEPFAR) in 2006, there continues to be an incremental decrease in the death of people due to HIV/AIDS by 81%. Further, deaths related to HIV/AIDS have also dropped from 121,000 in 2005 to 24,100 in 2017. Despite the decrease in the number of death rate due to AIDs, there is great concern that the HIV/AIDS pandemic is still a major health challenge in Zimbabwe (Cuneo et al. 2017; USAID 2023; World Health Organization Report 2022).

While malaria remains one of the major health challenges in Zimbabwe. It has been reported that women and children in the country are highly vulnerable to disease. This is because more than 50% of the citizens of Zimbabwe live in rural areas where there are lots of mosquito insects. Pragmatic malaria control programs established by foreign organizations such as Global Fund, USAID, and the Ministry of Health in Zimbabwe have helped to reduce malaria cases from 1.2 million reported cases in 2008 to 264,278 in 2018 (USAID 2023). This 78% reduction rate of malaria continues to encourage the Zimbabwe Ministry of Health to form more collaborations to effectively address its health challenges.

In the mid-1980s, some scholars contend that President Mugabe incited infliction against his political opponents. He also constantly harassed doctors and nurses who provided healthcare for his political victims (Kidia 2018; Todd et al. 2010). President Mugabe also denied the existence of an outrageous cholera pandemic in the country that led to the death of over 4500 citizens (Cuneo et al. 2017; Mason 2009). In addition, due to the sanction that was imposed on Zimbabwe, the economy including the health system also most completely collapsed. Most of the healthcare clinics and hospitals' infrastructure became delipidated and in some instances, some hospitals and clinics neither have running water nor electricity. Further, the Ministry of Health found it difficult to pay health workers on time, and when they were paid the rate of pay was very low compared to what it used to be. These low pay challenges and working conditions galvanized about 23% of the doctors and nurses who migrated to practice medicine in other foreign countries (Todd et al. 2010). Rather than encouraging Zimbabwe's citizens who are doctors and nurses to remain or continue to stay in the country by paying them better pay and providing higher living standards for them, the Mugabe administration preferred to invite Cuba's government to send many of their physicians to Zimbabwe (Chikanda 2006; Mhazo & Maponga 2022). It is interesting to observe that rather than encouraging the retention of Zimbabwean citizens who are nurses and doctors, the focus of the government was to have the foreign doctors train the national citizens who later travel abroad after graduation to seek better standards and pay (Willis-Sattuck et al. 2008). It was also reported that during the same period, the financing of the healthcare system in the country was reduced from 7% in 2000 to 4% in 2007 (Green 2018; Kidia 2018).

It is also reported that 9.5 million of the population in Zimbabwe live in rural areas where there are very few clinics and hospitals. Thus, the black citizens of the country barely have access to good healthcare services, while their white counterparts living in the urban cities could afford the best healthcare system (Kidia 2018; World Bank 2015). In addition, with the sanction that was lifted or ended in the country and the changes that took place in the country, there seems to be a disparity in building a national healthcare system for the Black African majority in the country compared to their White minority. This is because a large European White minority tends to propel the private practice health sector in Zimbabwe to serve their own privilege. This disparity practice among Black and White citizens is not new. The nation tends to have inherited a racially divided healthcare system. On one hand, white citizens who are a minority group enjoy the most vibrant and sophisticated healthcare system. On the other hand, most of the poor Black citizens of Zimbabwe mainly depend on poorly dilapidated public hospitals and clinics (Mhazo et al. 2023; Mhazo & Maponga 2022).

In low-resource settings such as Zimbabwe, the accessibility of healthcare services is usually determined by the considerable distances and time required to reach healthcare facilities, the financial means to cover transportation expenses and healthcare costs, and the presence of essential medications and skilled healthcare professionals (Kazel 2020; Manenji et al. 2020). Thus, people living in rural communities of Zimbabwe normally find themselves having to cover distances ranging from 10 to 50 miles to reach the closest healthcare facility (Mhazo & Maponga 2022). Furthermore, inadequate infrastructure, including poorly maintained, unpaved roads, and the presence of road hazards such as potholes, can worsen the challenge of access to healthcare (Manenji et al. 2020).

The hospitals in the rural regions of Zimbabwe do not operate with modern medical imaging technology to enhance patients' records, communicate to seek the best medical practice, or evidence-based treatment (Masuku & Macheka 2020). Further, most hospitals in the country do not have state-of-the-art advanced medical imaging. There is also a major challenge that some health workers in public hospitals do not know how to operate computer tomography (CT) scan machines. This lack of CT scan machines and MR technology scanners has often led to inadequate clinical decision making and a high mortality rate that could have been avoided (Green 2018; Mhazo et al. 2023). Poor network and lack of electricity in some rural regions also makes it difficult for the effective use of modern medical technology in the country.

The trends in the healthcare financing system in the country have also varied tremendously over the past two decades. Healthcare expenditure and financing methods in Zimbabwe are also facing a lot of challenges. The budget is financed by the public and private sectors. Unfortunately, most of the money derived from these sources is directed toward the payment of employee-related costs and salaries. The practice of spending about 30% on employee-related costs and 4% on low capital investment tends to negatively affect the availability of a better health system in the country. Because there is no publicly funded healthcare system in the country, life has been hard for poor citizens who are sick (Zimbabwe Ministry of Health and Childcare 2010; Mhazo et al. 2023). This is because healthcare is mainly financed by individual out-of-pocket payments. As a result of these major health finance challenges, access to good healthcare and financial protection could be considered biased toward the wealthier urban-based citizens of Zimbabwe (Masuku & Macheka 2020; Mhazo et al. 2023). Further, because of the way the current public health insurance enrollment is structured, the system tends to favor mostly the privileged and rich people in the country (Mhazo et al. 2023). The Public Health Insurance efficiency has somewhat reduced due to supplier-induced demand, abuse, waste, and fraud (Mhazo et al. 2023; Mufudza & Naidoo 2018).

Types of Health Policies

The Republic of Zimbabwe has so many health policies. However, the ineffectiveness of implementing the nation's health policies is a major problem. In addition, the implementation strategies adopted are also limited because of unavailable financial and physical resources in the past two decades (Mabaso 2022). In the past four years, the administration of President Emmerson Dambudzo Mnangagwa has adopted planning instruments to propel the healthcare system in the country to improve the situation. The nation's Ministry of Health and Childcare has also been mandated to supervise and ensure a better health delivery system in the country (Government of Zimbabwe Ministry of Health and Childcare 2023).

The 2013 Constitution of the Republic of Zimbabwe specified that all citizens and permanent residents of the nation have the right to basic healthcare including health reproductive health. Further, people with chronic illnesses in the country have the right to access basic healthcare and health services. In addition, permanent residents in the country cannot be refused emergency medical treatment in any healthcare institution.

The Constitution also mandates the Government of Zimbabwe to take reasonable legislative measures to achieve the progressive realization of the rights set in Section 76 subsections 1–4 of the constitution (Republic of Zimbabwe Constitution 2013).

Based on the mandates of the constitution, the Government of Zimbabwe has enacted many health policies as well as formulated three or four National Health Strategies. The goal of 2009–2013 is to provide a framework for the immediate resuscitation of the health sector as well as put Zimbabwe back on track toward achieving the millennium development goals (Zimbabwe National Heath Strategy 2009). The outcome of the various surveys, which were conducted by the Zimbabwe Ministry of Health and Childcare before 2009 revealed the nation had severe predicaments. The challenges include a lack of adequate health financing, poor health information technology system, inadequate medical doctors, and nurses; a high shortage of medical products, dismal health service delivery, and poor health administration and leadership (Zimbabwe National Heath Strategy 2009). Thus, the main goal of the Zimbabwe National Heath Strategy 2009 was to find the best solutions to the health problems listed above. Table 1 shows some of the health policies that have been formulated and implemented in the past three decades.

Table 1 Some Health Policies Enacted by the Government of Zimbabwe

	Type of Health Policy	Year Adopted	Purpose
1	Planning for Equity in Health Policy	1980	This health policy was in response to the disparity between black and white as well as social economic challenges that existed in the country before it gained its independence.
2	The Food and Food Standard Act	2001	This policy provides healthy food standards and regulates the sales as well as the importation of manufacturing food commodities.
3	The Health Professional Act	2001	This policy was established by the Medical and Dental Practitioner Council of Zimbabwe. The goal of the policy is to provide registration for health professionals after verifying their academic credentials. The Council also provides the registration of persons in the health profession and the issue of practicing licenses to practice in the country.
4	Public Health Act	2002	This policy provides the legal framework of the health sector in Zimbabwe.
5	The Health Service Act	2002	The goal of this policy is to provide guidelines for the administration of the health system in Zimbabwe.

(Continued)

Table 1 (*Continued*)

6	The Environmental Management Act	2002	This policy regulates and ensures sustainable management of natural resources and the environment in the country.
7	The Water Act	2002	This policy regulates the planning and development of healthy water resources in Zimbabwe
8	The Food and Nutrition Security Policy	2011	The goal of this policy is to strengthen the national structures, mechanisms, and capacity to effectively resolve the food and nutrition security in the country.
9	Public Health Act	2018	This act was enacted with the purpose of providing guidelines in preventing disease, injury, and disability as well as promoting health and well-being and preparing the nation against health threats tracking the spread of any pandemic in Zimbabwe.
10	National Health Strategy of Zimbabwe	1997–2007	The goal of this national strategic plan is to improve the quality of life in Zimbabwe by working for quality and equity.
11	National Health Strategy of Zimbabwe	2016–2020	The goal of this health strategy was not only to sustain the gain that was achieved previously but also to improve the health delivery system in the country.
12	National Health Strategy of Zimbabwe	2021–2025	The purpose of this policy is to improve the health and well-being of the population and eventually ensure universal health coverage.
13	Drought Risk Management Strategy and Action Plan	2017–2025	This strategic action plan was enacted to effectively support the implementation of suitable drought mitigation practices and interventions in the country.
14	Start Network Policy	2022	The policy was formulated to protect more than 800,000 people in Zimbabwe from drought risk during the 2021/2022 agricultural season.

Source: Government of Zimbabwe Ministry of Health and Childcare 2023; National Health Strategies 2009–2013; 2016–2020; and 2021–2025.

The devasting state of health emergency that had occurred in Zimbabwe before 2021 made the Government of the nation to start researching for new policy solutions. According to the Zimbabwe Ministry of Health and Childcare (2021), the health sector is regarded to be a major pillar of national development in the country. To galvanize the national development process, in 2021, the Government of Zimbabwe adopted a strategic plan to facilitate the enhancement of the health and well-being of the entire citizens of Zimbabwe (Public Health Act 2018). Although the National Health Strategy of Zimbabwe 2021–2025 was adopted to improve the health of the citizens as well as to ensure universal access to health services by the population in the country these goals have not been accomplished. The national strategy also advocated efficiencies in the utilization of resources in the country by the Ministry of Health and Childcare (Zimbabwe National Health Strategy 2025). Despite, these great health policy initiatives to improve the healthcare system in Zimbabwe, the government has not appropriated enough funding to galvanize the health system in the country. Unfortunately, the Government of Zimbabwe has only appropriated an average of 3.4% of its GDP for the health sector annually for the past few years.

Nature of Health Administration in Zimbabwe

The administration of healthcare in Zimbabwe is divided into five major levels: (a) the primary or rural level; (b) the secondary or district level; (c) the tertiary or provincial level; (d) central or national level; and (e) the quinary level (Ministry of Health and Childcare 2021; Zimbabwe National Health Strategy 2021–2025).

The *primary level* is basically located in the rural regions and provides community health services as well as minor treatment of health issues. There are also private clinics on farms and commercial organizations such as industrial sites (Zimbabwe National Health Strategy 2021–2025).

The secondary or district-level hospitals offer ambulatory and inpatient services. It should be noted that there is only one hospital in each district in Zimbabwe. The provincial hospitals are mandated to offer specialist, ambulatory, and specialist services to the citizens of Zimbabwe. Hospital at the national level offers specialist inpatient services. The medical institutions at the national level constitute University teaching hospitals and medical schools.

The quinary level oversees conducting medical research and developing collaboration with manufacturing organizations as well as the Ministry of Health and Childcare. This highest level of health administration institutions in Zimbabwe is also mandated to liaison with the new divisions of biomedical engineering science, pharmaceutical, and biopharmaceutical production in the country (Mabaso 2022; Zimbabwe National Health Strategy 2021–2025).

The delivery of healthcare is typically based on the seriousness of the sickness and complications of medical care. According to the Government of Zimbabwe (2021) report, the primary healthcare centers provide basic services to patients. In the case of a medical complicated issue, a patient could be transferred to a higher level such as the district, provincial, or national levels. Furthermore, most provincial and national hospitals in Zimbabwe are in the urban cities.

Depending on the complication of the medical issue the hospitals or clinics in the country will use government ambulances to transfer intensive care patients from the lower level to a higher-level hospital at the either provincial or national level. According to the Zimbabwe National Health Strategy (2021–2025) report, the provincial hospital provides treatment at the ratio of 0.2 and 0.4 hospitals per 10,000 patients. However, the national average is 2 hospitals for 10,000 patients. Further, the lack of sufficient highly qualified healthcare workers in the country as well as inadequate medicines and health equipment has not only limited the capacity of these levels of hospitals to provide good healthcare services. The outcome of these limited human and capital resources is the unnecessary referral of patients to both private and public hospitals all over the country, depending on the patient's ability to pay for the cost of treatment (Mabaso 2022).

Data Analysis and Discussion

The goal of this chapter is to examine the effectiveness of health policy and the health delivery system in Zimbabwe. The research for this chapter involves content analysis of more than 52 sources, The sources include the Government of Zimbabwe National Health Strategy (1997–2007, 2009–2013, 2016–2020, and 2021–2025), World Health Organization report on Zimbabwe (2021–2023), United Nation Human Development Program Human Development Report (2020–2023), Global Sustainable Development Goal Indicators Database, Zimbabwe Ministry of Health and Child Care Reports (1985–2022), Centers for Disease Control and Prevention (CDC) reports, and many academic journal articles on health performance in Zimbabwe. Table 2 summarizes the health indicators and performance effectiveness in the past few decades.

Table 2 shows that the estimated current population of Zimbabwe is 16.4 in 2023 (World Bank Indicators). The gross domestic product (GDP) dropped from US$42 billion in 2019 to US$20.68 billion in 2022. The Government of Zimbabwe also spent 3.43% of its 2020 GDP on healthcare in 2020, previously it spent 6.6% in 2019 (United Nations Human Development Program 2021). As indicated above health budget per capita in the past few years was far below the World Health Organization benchmark of US$86 per capita and lower than the regional counterpart whose average was US$146 (Mabaso 2022; Nkala 2021). There is no doubt that an inadequate health budget makes it very difficult for the healthcare delivery system in Zimbabwe to strive for more high-quality practices. Further, it is also reported that the healthcare system currently faces challenges such as massive migration of doctors and nurses; quantity, size, absorption of health workers, geographic and health facility level distribution of health workers, as well as skill mix and health workforce management capacity (Mugarisi 2022; USAID 2022).

There are 1,848 health facilities in Zimbabwe. The number of hospitals is 214. Out of this, there are 32 private hospitals, and 69 private clinics, as well as 25 mission clinics. The total number of clinics is 1,122. There are also 62 hospitals that are in the rural regions all over the country. In addition, there are 6 central hospitals, 8

Table 2 Economics and Health Indicators in Zimbabwe

No.	Major Indicators in Zimbabwe	Explanation
1	Population	16.4 million (2023)
2	Gross domestic product (GDP)	US $20.6 billion (2022)
3	Current health expenditure (% of GDP)	3.46% (2020)
4	Nurses and midwives per 1,000 people	1.93 (2021)
5	Physicians/doctors per 1,000 people	0.21 (2021)
6	Birth attended by skilled health personnel	86.1% (2022)
8	Access to safe and clean water	64% Urban cities; rural regions 36% (2021)
9	Population in rural regions without access to safely drinking water service	67% (2021)
10	People with basic sanitation	36.2% (2021)
11	Sanitation—no toilet and practice open defecation	34.7% (2021)
12	Common diseases	Respiratory infections: tuberculosis, enteric (intestines) diseases, neglected tropical diseases and malaria; maternal and neonatal; nutritional deficiencies; neoplasms (cancers); cardiovascular (heart) diseases; chronic respiratory diseases
13	Life expectancy at birth	61.5 years (2021)
14	Life expectancy at birth for females	63 years (2021)
15	Life expectancy at birth for males	56 years (2021)
16	Mortality rate for female adults (per 1,000 people)	326 (2022)
17	Mortality rate for infants (per 1,000 people)	35.79 (2022)
18	Mortality rate for male adults (per 1,000 people)	456 (2022)
19	Tuberculosis incidence (per 100,000 people)	190 (2021)
20	Population living below income poverty line PPP $2.15 a day	33,9% (2021)
21	Population in multidimensional head count poverty (%)	25.8% (2022)
22	Contribution deprivation in health to multidimensional poverty index	23.6% (2022)
23	Infants lacking immunization for measles (% of one and older)	27.2% (2021)
24	Malaria incidence (per 1,000 people at risk)	51% (2022)
25	HIV/AIDS prevalence adults (% ages 15–49)	12.7% (2021)
26	COVID-19 vaccination rate (per 1,000 people)	74.89 (2022)

Sources: World Bank Indicators (2023); United Nations Human Development Programme Human Development Report (2022).

provincial hospitals, and 44 district hospitals (DataReportal 2023; Zimbabwe Ministry of Health and Childcare 2021). The data show that most healthcare institutions are at the primary care level. The primary-level clinics basically refer complicated health cases to the districts or provincial-level hospitals (Government of Zimbabwe 2021; Chivhenge et al. 2022).

Communicable diseases are reported to lead to high mortality and illness rates because of an under-resourced health delivery system in Zimbabwe (Zimbabwe National Health Strategy 2021–2025; Ministry of Health and Childcare Report 2021). The nation's healthcare system continues to be overstretched by the high burden of HIV/AIDS prevalence in Zimbabwe.

The residents of Zimbabwe also have a high rate of respiratory infections such as tuberculosis (TB) incidence at the rate of 190 per 100,000 people (United Nations Human Development Program Index 2021, USAID 2022). Further, the Zimbabwe Ministry of Health and Childcare reported that the TB incidence in 2018 was 210 per 100,000 residents of the country (Global TB Report 2019). Unfortunately, it was the male residents of the country between the age of 25 and 44 who suffered the burden of TB due to their tobacco smoking behavior and working environment that exposed them to industrial smoke pollution (Mabaso 2022). It should be noted that Zimbabwe does not have an effective occupational health and safety policy.

Another communicable disease that continues to kill residents of Zimbabwe is malaria (Center for Disease Control 2022; USAID 2022). The malaria incidence per 1,000 people at risk constitutes about 51% in 2021 (United Nations Human Development Program Index 2021). In addition, the case of malaria incidence per 1,000 residents in Zimbabwe has decreased from 153 in 2004 to 19 in 2018 (Zimbabwe Ministry of Health and Childcare 2021). The number of malaria cases has also decreased from 1.2 million in 2008 to less than 265,000 in 2018. This decrease constitutes a 78% reduction rate (USAID 2022).

The life expectancy at birth in the country in 2020 was 61.5 years. While the life expectancy at birth for females was 63 years. During the same period, the life expectancy for male residents of Zimbabwe was 56 years (World Bank Indicators 2021; United Nations Human Development Program Index 2021). The data show a major improvement from what the indicators were in 2015. This is because in 2015, the life expectancy for women was 61.3, while that for men was 56.2 (United Nation Human Development Program Human Development Report 2023–2024; World Health Organization Indicators 2015; Zimbabwe Ministry of Health and Childcare 2016).

Another health indicator that has not changed that much over the past decade is the maternal and child mortality rate. The child mortality for infants under five years rates has incrementally declined in Zimbabwe. However, between 2014 and 2019, maternal newborn intervention has improved from 71.4% to 82% for mothers, while newborn rate has also improved from 82% to 91% (Zimbabwe Ministry of Health and Childcare 2021). In addition, the mother's mortality rate dropped from 651 maternal deaths per 100,000 live births in 2014 to 462 per 100,000 live births in 2019 (Zimbabwe Ministry of Health and Childcare 2021). The mortality rate for female adults per 1,000 people was 326 in 2021, while that of men adults was 456 per 1,000. Despite these differences in female and men adult indicators, the mortality rate for infants per 1,000 people was 35.7 (United Nations Human Development Program Index 2022).

As a result of the high-rate turnover of healthcare workers in Zimbabwe, the ratio of physicians per 1,000 people is 0.21, while the ratio of 1 nurse to 1,000 people is between 1.9 and 2.0 (World Bank Indicators 2023; United Nation Human Development Program 2022; Global Sustainable Development Indicators Database 2022). In addition, health professionals working in the country are reported to be less than 23 per 10,000 patients. This low number of health professionals could be classified as below the required health workers' specified rate for the delivery of good health service in any country (Mugarisi 2022; World Health Organization 2022).

Retaining health workers such as doctors, pharmacists, and nurses continues to be a major predicament for the Government of Zimbabwe. In the mix of the aging infrastructure and equipment, supply of medicine, poor working conditions, very low salaries for health workers, and massive migration to foreign countries, the government seems to know the best approach to address the needs of health practitioners in the country. In early January 2023, the health workers who have been frustrated with their deplorable working conditions in the hospitals and clinics in the country publicly protested about the predicament that they have been facing for many years. Rather than negotiating with the health workers, the Government of Zimbabwe passed a new law banning health professionals from striking for more than three days (Chingono 2023). Those found guilty of violating the new law could be imprisoned for six months or face a major fine (Chingono 2023).

Although the medical workers shortage has been and continues to be a major and devastating challenge to the healthcare delivery system in Zimbabwe for more than two decades, the government still does not know how to professionally provide solutions to the problem (Chirwa et al. 2014; Mabaso 2022). Despite the many National Health Strategies and policies that have been enacted between 1997 and 2023, the health workers shortage predicament continues to prevail (Mhazo et al. 2023; Nhapi 2019). Further, the implementation of all the formulated National Health Strategies has been ineffective due to inadequate funding, and physical and human resources (Chingono 2023; Deve 2020; Mhazo et al. 2023; Mobaso 2022; Nhapi 2019).

Conclusion

This chapter has examined the nature of health policy in Zimbabwe. It argues that the present health system in Zimbabwe tends not to effectively preserve the health of the citizens of the country. This is because the nation's healthcare system and funding mechanism do not recognize the citizens' rights to affordable health and other protected interests. The chapter also argued that achieving a high-quality healthcare system dependent on equitable distribution and a well-performing medical professional workforce. The challenges of healthcare delivery and health policies identified in our research reveal that Zimbabwe's public health insurance has not been effective in providing fiscal relief to both the citizens and the government of the country. This is because access to healthcare and financial protection continue to favor the richer and urban population of the country. Unfortunately, Zimbabwe's citizens are dismally covered by private health insurance. The current pattern of healthcare insurance tends to cover a minority and relatively richer population of the country. In addition, the political will to address the nation's citizens' health needs is not forthcoming.

The Government of Zimbabwe should consider establishing a new Public Health Insurance that could be used to address the poor stakeholders' healthcare in the country. The administration of the healthcare system as well as policy implementation in Zimbabwe still involve command and control in line with provisions of the nation's obsolete Civil Protection Act of 1989. Further, political patronage rather better strategy to resolve health challenges and vulnerabilities in the country is still a common practice. Democracy and shared governance cannot take place in Zimbabwe if the poor citizens, women, youths, and people with black skin are deliberately marginalized by a government that is made up of a majority of black politicians and administrators.

Although, Zimbabwe's Constitution and National Health Strategy 2016–2020 and 2021–2025 acknowledge the right to health for its citizens. This mandate has not been fully fulfilled by the government. Moving forward, the Government of Zimbabwe should make every effort to take more direct control and ownership of its healthcare delivery system and financing. Depending on the rest of the world to contribute almost 27% of Zimbabwe's healthcare financing could be very problematic if this funding stops flowing into the country soon. Precautionary measures need to be taken to avoid a dependency trap like what happened when sanctions were placed on Zimbabwe.

For any country to develop a sustainable health system it must hire more doctors, nurses, and other health professionals. Zimbabwe suffers from the brain drain of citizens who are trained within the country due to low wages and poor working conditions. The current doctor-to-people ratio in Zimbabwe is 0.21 physician to 1,000 (Nhapi 2019; World Bank 2020; World Health Organization. 2022). This overpopulated doctor to patients' ratio in Zimbabwe is against the World Health Organization rules of one doctor to 600 patients. Continuing with this outrageous ratio could put the citizens of the country at a major health risk. In addition, funding of the healthcare system in Zimbabwe remains one of the major challenges for achieving all the National Health Strategies that have been adopted between 1997 and the current 2021–2025.

There is no doubt that the health system in Zimbabwe has been incrementally improving since 2019 (Deve 2020). According to the World Health Organization (2022) and the Zimbabwe National Health Strategic (2021–2025) report, maternal mortality and infant mortality rates have improved from what they used to be about a decade ago. There is also the need for equitable collaboration among multi-sectoral partnerships, that is, private, public, and nongovernmental organizations, in research and development (Dibie 2022). Finally, the Republic of Zimbabwe should ensure that setting funding priority for the health delivery system in the country should be a major priority.

References

Bastin Y., Coupez A., Mann M. (1999). Continuity and divergence in the Bantu languages: Perspectives from a lexicostatistic study. *Annales Sciences Humanities.* 162: 315–317.

Beach D. N. (1979). Chimurenga: The Shona rising of 1896–97. *The Journal of African History.* Cambridge University Press. 20(3): 395–420.

Bret E. A. (2005). From corporatism to liberalization in Zimbabwe: Economic policy regimes and political crisis, 1980–97. *International Political Science Review.* 26(1): 91–106.

Britannica (2024). History of Zimbabwe. https://www.britannica.com/place/Zimbabwe. Accessed September 27, 2024.

Centers for Disease Control and Prevention (CDC) report (2022). CDC in Zimbabwe. https://www.cdc.gov/globalhealth/countries/zimbabwe/. Accessed July 12, 2023.

Chikanda A. (2006). Skilled health professionals' migration and its impact on health delivery in Zimbabwe. *Journal of Ethnic Migration Studies.* 32(1): 667–680.

Chingono N. (2023). Health workers in Zimbabwe dismayed as law curbing strikes is passed. https://www.theguardian.com/global-development/2023/jan/12/health-workers-in-zimbabwe-dismayed-as-law-curbing-strikes-is-passed. Accessed July 2023.

Chirwa Y., Mashange W., Chadiwa P., Buzuzi S., Munyati S., Chandiwana B., Witter S. (2014). Policies to attract & retain health workers in rural areas in Zimbabwe. https://assets.publishing.service.gov.uk/media/57a0899140f0b64974000150/rebuild_report_16_zimbabwe_hw_kii.pdf. Accessed September 27, 2024.

Chivhenge E., Mabaso A., Museva T., Zingi G. (2022). *Zimbabwe's Roadmap for Decarbonization and Resilience: An Evaluation of Policy (In) Consistency.* DOI:10.2139/ssrn.4029469.

Cuneo C. N., Sollom R., Beyrer C. (2017). The cholera epidemic in Zimbabwe, 2008–2009: A review and critique of the evidence. *Health Huan Rights.* 19(1): 249–253.

DataReportal (2023). Digital 2023: Zimbabwe. https://datareportal.com/reports/digital-2023-zimbabwe#:~:text=Zimbabwe's%20population%20in%202023,of%20the%20population%20is%20male. Accessed July 12, 2023.

Deve C. R. (2020). Perception of health professionals on the changes brought about by health system reform in Zimbabwe. https://uir.unisa.ac.za/handle/10500/27018. Accessed September 27, 2024.

Dibie R. (2022). Health administration in Nigeria. *Journal African Policy Studies.* 28(1): 101–139.

Dibie R. (2018). *Business and Government Relations in Africa.* New York, N.Y.: Routledge Press.

Drezner D. W. (2011). Sanctions sometimes smart: Targeted sanctions in theory and practice. *International Studies Review.* 13(1): 96–108.

Freeman L. (2014). A parallel universe - competing interpretations of Zimbabwe's crisis. *Journal of Contemporary African Studies.* 32(3): 349–366.

Global Sustainable Development Indicators Database (2022). https://unstats.un.org/sdgs/iindicators/database. Accessed August 18, 2022.

Government of Zimbabwe (2021). *Zimbabwe National Heath Strategy 2021–2025.* Harare: Government Press.

Government of Zimbabwe Ministry of Health and Childcare (2020). *Zimbabwe Population-Based HIV Impact Assessment Survey.* Harare, Zimbabwe: Government Press

Government of Zimbabwe (2017). *Capacity Assessment of the Disaster Risk Management System in Zimbabwe.* Harare, Zimbabwe: Government of Zimbabwe Press.

Government of Zimbabwe (2016). *Zimbabwe National Heath Strategy 2016–2020.* Harare: Government Press.

Government of Zimbabwe (2009). *National Health Strategy for Zimbabwe 2009–2013.* Harare, Zimbabwe: Government of Zimbabwe Press.

Government of Zimbabwe (2009). *Zimbabwe National Heath Strategy 2009–2013.* Harare: Government Press.

Government of Zimbabwe (1997). *Zimbabwe National Heath Strategy 1997–2007*. Harare: Government Press.

Government of Zimbabwe Ministry of Health and Childcare. (2023). Health parastatal signed performance contract. https://www.herald.co.zw/health-parastatals-sign-performance-contracts/. Accessed October 31, 2024.

Government of Zimbabwe Ministry of Health and Childcare. (2023). National Health Strategy 2021–2015. https://faolex.fao.org/docs/pdf/zim225019.pdf. Accessed November 14, 2024.

Gray J. A. (1956). A country in search of a name. *The Northern Rhodesia Journal*. III(1): 78. Accessed June 5, 2023.

Green A. (2018). Zimbabwe post-Mugabe era: Restructuring a health system. *Lancet*, 391: 17–18.

Guthrie M. (1967–71). *Comparative Bantu: An Introduction to the Comparative Linguistics and Prehistory of the Bantu Languages*. Gregg International.

History of Zimbabwe (2022). https://www.goway.com/travel-information/africa-middle-east/zimbabwe/history/. Assessed July 31, 2023.

History World (2007). History of Zimbabwe. http://www.historyworld.net/wrldhis/plaintexthistories.asp?historyid=ad28#ixzz86FGW2xm2. Assessed June 19, 2023.

Huffman T. N. (2007). *Handbook to the Iron Age*. University of KwaZulu-Natal Press. p. 123.

Jaeger M. D. (2016). Constructing sanctions: Rallying around the target in Zimbabwe. *Cambridge Review of International Affairs*. 29(3): 952–969.

Kawewe S. M. & Dibie R. (2000). The impact of economic structural adjustment programs (ESAPs) on women and children: Implications for social welfare in Zimbabwe. *The Journal of Sociology and Social Welfare*. 27(6):79–107.

Kazel M. (2020). Improving access to clean water and sanitation in Zimbabwe. https://borgenproject.org/clean-water-in-zimbabwe/. Accessed July 10, 2021.

Kidia K. K. (2018). The future of health in Zimbabwe. *Global Health Action*. 18(110): 1–4.

Kuye O., Ogundele O., Alaneme G.C. (2013). Strategic roles of business, government and society: the Nigerian situation. *International Journal of Business and Social Science*, 4(12): 223–243.

Leoewenson R., Sanders D., Davis R. (1991). Challenges to equity in health and healthcare: A Zimbabwean case study. *Social Science Medicine*. 32(10): 1079–1088.

Mabaso E. (2022). Disaster Risk Management system and policies in Zimababwe: opportunities and constraints for national development. In Zhou G. and Zvoushe H. *The Public Policy Question in Zimbabwe's Evolving Development Agenda*. Soshanguve, South Africa: SAPAAM Publishing.

Makoni M. (2020). Covid-19 worsens Zimbabwe's health crisis. *Lancet*. 396(10249): 457–463.

Makoni T., Kadziyanhike G., Mademutsa C., Mlambo M., Malama K. (2022). Community-led monitoring: a voice for key populations in Zimbabwe. *Journal of the International Aids Society*, 25(S1): https://doi.org/10.1002/jia2.25925.

Makumbe J. (2006). Electoral politics in Zimbabwe: Authoritarianism versus the people. *Africa Development*. 31(3): 45–61.

Mamdani M. (2008). Lessons of Zimbabwe. *London Review of Books*. 17–21.

Manenji M., Roet L., Van-Rensberg E.J. (2020). Accessibility of healthcare in rural Zimbabwe: The perspective of nurses and healthcare users. *African Journal of Primary Health Care & Family Medicine*, 12(1). DOI:10.4102/phcfm.v12i1.2245.

Mason P. R. (2009). Zimbabwe experience the worst epidemic of cholera in Africa. *Journal of Infection in Developing Countries*. 3(1): 148–151.

Masuku S., Macheka T. (2020). Policy making and governance structures in Zimbabwe: examining their efficacy as a conduit to equitable participation (inclusion) and social justice for rural youths. *Congent Social Sciences*. 7(1): 1–18.

Mavhinga D. & Nyamande F. (2018). 100 days of Mnangagwa in the health sector. Newsday. https://www.newsday.co.zw/opinion-amp-analysis/article/69636/100-days-of-mnangagwa-in-the-health-sector. Accessed September 27, 2024.

Meldrum A. (2008). Zimbabwe's healthcare system struggles on. *World Report*. 371(9618): 1059–2060.

Mhazo A. T., Maponga C. C., Mossiatos E. (2023). Inequality and private health insurance in Zimbabwe: history, politics, and performance. *International Journal for Equity in Health*. 22(54) 1–13.

Mhazo A. T., and Maponga C. C. (2022). The political economy of health financing reform in Zimbabwe: A scoping review. *International Journal for Equity in Health*. 21(42) 1–14.

Ministry of Health and Childcare (2021). *Capacity Assessment of the Disaster Risk Management System in Zimbabwe*. Harare, Zimbabwe: Government of Zimbabwe Press.

Mkandawire T. (2020). Zimbabwe's transition overload: An interpretation. *Journal of Contemporary African Studies*. 38(1): 18–38.

Mnangagwa E. (2018). We are beginning about the new Zimbabwe. New York Times (March 11). https://www.nytimes.com/2018/03/11/opinion/zimbabwe-emmerson-mnangagwa. html. Accessed September 27, 2024.

Moyo D. (2009). *Dead aid: Why Aid is Not Working and How There Is a Better Way for Africa*. New York: Macmillan Press.

Mufudza T., Naidoo V. (2018). Customer perceptions and expectations of medical insurance service quality rendered by companies in Zimbabwe. *Journal of Contemporary Management*. 15(1): 48–77.

Mugarisi V. (2022). Zimbabwe conducts health labour market analysis. https://reliefweb.int/ report/zimbabwe/zimbabwe-conducts-health-labour-market-analysis. Accessed September 9, 2023.

Neil P. (1993). *A New History of Southern Africa*, Second Edition, 1993. London: Macmillan. pp. 178–181.

Nhapi T. G. (2019). Socioeconomic barriers to universal health coverage in Zimbabwe: Present issues and pathways toward progress. *Journal of Developing Societies*. 35(1): 153–174.

Nkala B., Mudimu C., Mbengwa A.M. (2021). Human resources for health talent management contribution: A case for health systems strengthening in the public health sector. *World Journal of Advanced Research and Reviews*, 9(2): 192–201.

Organization for Economic Corporation and Development (OCED). (2014). Zimbabwe Report. https://www.oecd-ilibrary.org/zimbabwe_5jz44fdt4j31.pdf?itemId=2Fcontent %2Fcomponent%2Faeo-2014-66-en&mimeType=pdf. Accessed November 14, 2024.

Pakenham T. (1992). *Scramble for Africa: White Man's Conquest of the Dark Continent from 1876 to 1912*. New York: Avon Books. pp. 503–669.

Palley C. (1966). *The Constitutional History and Law of Southern Rhodesia, 1888–1965: With Special Reference to Imperial Control*. London: Oxford University Press.

Phillipson, D. W. (1989). *Bantu-Speaking People in Southern Africa' in Obenga* (ed), Les Peuples Bantu. Paris. p. 156.

Public Health Act (2018). Allied health practitioners' council of Zimbabwe. http://www.cfuzim. com/wp-content/uploads/2018/09/healthact18.pdf. Accessed July 13, 2023.

Razvi S. S., Douglas R., Williams O. D., Hill P. S. (2020). The political economy of universal health coverage: A systematic narrative review. *Health Policy Plan*. 35(3) 364–372.

Republic of Zimbabwe (2013). *The Constitution of Zimbabwe Amendment Act of 2013*. Harare, Zimbabwe: Government Press.

Rexová K., Bastin Y., Frynta D. (2006). Cladistic analysis of Bantu languages. *Naturwissenschaften*. 93(4): 189–194.

South African History Online (2020). The role of Cecil John Rhodes' British South African Company in the conquest of Matabeleland. https://www.sahistory.org.za/article/role-cecil-john-rhodes-british-south-african-company-conquest-matabeleland#:~:text=Cecil%20 John%20Rhodes%20who%20was,declared%20war%20on%20the%20King.   Accessed September 27, 2024.

Sylvester C. (1985). Continuity in Zimbabwe's development history. *African Studies Review*, 28(1): 9–27.

Todd C., Ray S., Madzimbamuto F. (2010). What is the way forward for the health in Zimbabwe? *Lancet*, 375: 606–609.

United Nations Human Development Index (HDI). (2023). https://hdr.undp.org/data-center/human-development-index#/indicies/HDI. Accessed November 13, 2024.

United Nations Human Development Program Index (2023–2024). https://hdr.undp.org/content/human-development-report-2023-24. Accessed September 27, 2024.

United Nations Human Development Program Index (2020–2023). https://www.google.com/search?sca_esv=8536d3cccb765549&sca_upv=1&rlz=1C1GCEA_enUS1031US1031&sxsrf=ADLYWIKYYp8hzicuG4lSwn3mva3-wOwm8w:1727475002793&q=United+nations+human+development+program+index+2020+2023. Accessed September 27, 2024.

United Nations Human Development Program Index (2022). https://hdr.undp.org/content/human-development-report-2021-22.

United Nations Human Development Program (2021). Human development report. https;//hdr.undp.org/en/2020-report. Accessed May 10, 2023.

United Nations Human Development Program Report (2014). https://hdr.undp.org/content/human-development-report-2014. Accessed September 27, 2024.

UNICEF (2020). Zimbabwe: Water, sanitation, and hygiene (WASH). https://www.unicef.org/zimbabwe/water-sanitation-and-hygiene-wash. Accessed May 10, 2021.

United States Agency for International Development (USAID). (2022). Zimbabwe: Country development cooperation strategy. https://www.usaid.gov/sites/default/files/2022-12/Zimbabwe%20CDCS%202022-2027%20External%20Version%20%281%29_1.pdf. Accessed November 13, 2024.

Victoriafalls (2020). History of Zimbabwe. https://www.victoriafalls-guide.net/history-of-zimbabwe.html. Assessed July 1, 2023.

Wikipedia (2024). History of Zimbabwe. https://en.wikipedia.org/wiki/History_of_Zimbabwe. Accessed September 27, 2024.

Wikipedia (2018). History of Zimbabwe. https://en.wikipedia.org/wiki/Historyof Zimbabwe#:~:text=Until%20roughly%202%2C000%20years%20ago,Mapungubwe%20and%20Kingdom%20of%20Zimbabwe. Assessed July 1, 2023.

Willis-Shattuck M., Bidwell P., Thomas S., et al. (2008). Motivation and retention of health workers in developing countries: A systematic review. *BMC Health Service Research*. 8(1): 247–249.

World Bank (2023). Zimbabwe population: World development indicators. https://databank.worldbank.org/reports.aspx?source=2&series=SP.POP.TOTL&country=ZWE. Assessed July 25, 2023.

World Bank (2020). World Development Report 2020 Chapters and Data. https://www.worldbank.org/en/publication/wdr2020/brief/world-development-report-2020-data. Accessed September 27, 2024.

World Bank (2015). *Health Public Expenditure Review: Zimbabwe*. Washington DC: World Bank Publication.

World Health Organization Indicators (2015). https://iris.who.int/bitstream/handle/10665/173589/WHO_HIS_HSI_2015.3_eng.pdf. Accessed November 13, 2024.

World Bank Indicators. (2021). https://databank.worldbank.org/source/world-development-indicators. Accessed November 12, 2024.

World Bank Indicator (2023). https://data.worldbank.org/indicator/SH.XPD.CHEX.GD.ZS?locations=ZW. Accessed July 14, 2023.

World Health Organization (2019). Global Tuberculosis Report. chrome-extension://efaidnbmnnnibpcajpcglclefindmkaj/https://iris.who.int/bitstream/handle/10665/329368/9789241565714-eng.pdf. Accessed November 14, 2024.

World Health Organization report on Zimbabwe (2021–2023). Zimbabwe Annual Report 2023. https://www.afro.who.int/sites/default/files/2024-08/WCO%20 Zimbabwe%20 Annual%20Report%202023_pdf. Accessed November 13, 2024.

World Health Organization (2022). Environmental Health Zimbabwe 2022 country profile https://www.who.int/publications/m/item/environmental-health-zimbabwe-2022-country-profile. Accessed September 27, 2024.

World Population Review (2023). Zimbabwe population. https://worldpopulationreview.com/countries/Zimbabwe-population. Accessed July 12, 2023.

Zimbabwe Ministry of Health and Childcare (2025). *Zimbabwe National Health Strategy 2025*. Harare Zimbabwe: Government Press.

Zimbabwe Ministry of Health and Childcare (2021). National Health Strategy 2021–2025. https://faolex.fao.org/docs/pdf/zim225019.pdf. Accessed September 27, 2024.

Zimbabwe Ministry of Health and Childcare (2018). *Zimbabwe National Health Account*. Harare Zimbabwe: Government Press.

Zimbabwe Ministry of Health and Childcare (2016). *National Health Strategy for Zimbabwe 2016–2020*. Harare, Zimbabwe. Government Press.

Zimbabwe Ministry of Health and Childcare (2010). *Zimbabwe National Health Account*. Harare Zimbabwe: Government Press.

Zimbabwe Ministry of Health and Childcare (2009). *National Health Strategy 2009–2013*. Harare, Zimbabwe. Government Press.

Chapter Twenty-One

CHALLENGES OF MEDICAL TOURISM IN AFRICA

Robert Dibie

Introduction

This chapter examines why African leaders, senior public administrators, and rich citizens prefer to seek their healthcare in England, France, Spain, Portugal, Canada, the United States, India, Singapore, and so on. It also discusses challenges such as poor funding and infrastructure, adequate regulation and poor standards, lack of highly qualified medical staff, as well as negative perceptions that could be major reasons for a mass exodus of Africans seeking healthcare in countries outside their continent. The chapter also argues that although there are a couple of well-established private hospitals, health centers, and clinics in some African countries, there are still convoluted perceptions of poor healthcare services. The fact that patients admitted to such hospitals may not get the value for their money is also a major challenge. Therefore, to prevent gambling with their life, political leaders and rich African elites prefer to travel outside their respective nations to countries outside the continent to seek healthcare. The research conducted reveals that because of the huge gap in the healthcare sector in the African continent, many entrepreneurs from outside the continent, especially India are beginning to explore opportunities in the African continent by investing heavily in providing state-of-the-art medical facilities. Even then many rich African leaders especially those who have stolen public funds prefer to travel abroad to seek medical care. Some recommendations are provided on how African nations could start to change the poor nature of their health infrastructure, and negative perception of their healthcare delivery system.

Medical tourism is defined as a situation that galvanizes a sick person to travel to a foreign country to seek medical care, or wellness treatment (Stolley & Watson 2012). Medical tourism also occurs when consumers elect to travel across international borders to receive some form of medical treatment (Organization for Economic Cooperation and Development (OECD) Report 2007). The sick people who travel to foreign countries to seek healthcare are called medical tourists (Dalen & Alpert 2018). According to Beland and Zarzeczny (2018) and Kim and Hyun (2022), the idea of seeking treatment outside the boundaries of a person's country of residence or nation of origin has led to a new type of health industry. It has also been reported that the medical tourism industry has expanded systematically over the past two decades (Kim & Hyun 2022).

Some scholars have also argued that the increase in medical tourism and cooperation in the health, and. medical sector may be a path to improving relationships between countries (Balaban & Marano 2010; Kim & Hyun 2022). Health policies and health delivery have traditionally been bounded by the nation state. However, because of the desire to engage in outsourcing of healthcare services, there has been a need for quality healthcare to continue to grow beyond boundaries of nations (Stolley & Watson 2012).

A new development in the medical tourism industry is that developed countries such as the United States and some Western European countries no longer have monopoly of superior health systems that meet the needs, of the citizens of the world (Glinos et al. 2010; OECD 2009). This is because some developing nations notably India, Singapore, Japan, Philippines, and South Africa to mention a few have now adopted top-notch medical facilities that are equally outstanding with state-of-the-art technology, and highly trained medical doctors and nurses. Further, the competition for medical tourism patients between developed and developing countries has also escalated because the developing countries could provide superb modern healthcare services far cheaper than what the treatment costs could be in the developed countries. Murphy (2023) contends that many people in the United States now prefer to travel to other countries for medical care that is either not available in America or costs a lot less in developing countries such as Mexico. In most cases, the majority of the United States citizens seeking medical tourism tend to explore cheaper treatment for dental procedures, plastic surgery, cancer treatments, and prescription drugs, experts (Murphy 2023). Apart from Mexico, other common destinations that United States citizens travel to seek healthcare treatment include Canada, India, and Thailand (Murphy 2023).

According to the Patients Beyond Borders report (2024), the 2019 medical tourism market size is about US\$74–92 billion, based on 21–26 million cross-border patients worldwide spending an average of US\$3,550 per visit, including medically related costs, cross-border and local transportation, inpatient stay, and accommodations. It is also estimated that some 2.1 million United States citizens traveled outside the country to seek cheaper medical care in 2019 (Patients Beyond Board Report 2024). Therefore, the magnitude of income from medical tourism often propels seven nations and cities to actively spend a lot of money on advertisements to attract medical tourism patients (Patients Beyond Borders 2024; United States International Trade Commission 2021). One of the reasons for seeking treatment abroad is to save 50%–80% of the cost they would have paid in the United States for heart bypass, facelift, dental care, cosmetic surgery, elective surgery, and fertility treatment. These medical tourists often seek treatment overseas from doctors who were previously trained in North America (Obuh et al. 2020). In the past two decades, Dubai, India, Malaysia, and Singapore have been reported to vigorously contest medical tourism patients from both developed and developing countries. According to Hotelier (2020), Dubai has maintained its position as the Arab region's top medical tourism destination for the past few years.

Patients without Boarders (2024) and Hotelier (2020) contend that the Dubai Health Authority has also continued to embark on initiatives that could strengthen the medical tourism sector in the Emirates as well as enhance its economic diversification. Hotelier (2020) also reported that Dubai issued 3.397 licenses to health facilities in Dubai, while

45 new health facilities, a hospital, and 10 general and specialized medical clinics were inaugurated during the period. Moreover, Dubai has 20 licensed centers specializing in complementary, and alternative medicine (TCAM). These centers currently offer eight TCAM services and employ 234 professionals (Hotelier 2020). In addition, more than 20 dedicated medical centers are being managed by licensed health professionals that are operating in the emirate toward accomplishing its medical tourism goals (Hotelier 2020).

According to the World Health Organization Report (2022), the incremental growth in the medical tourism industry is due to the decreasing costs of travel and the increase in advertising by companies that wish to attract patients, as well as the improved availability of health technology (World Health Organization 2022). In addition, the global growth in the flow of patients and health professionals as well as medical technology capital funding and regulatory regimes across national borders has given rise to new patterns of consumption and production of healthcare services over recent decades (Stolley & Watson 2012; Wilensky & Teitelbaum 2020; World Bank 2015a). Some scholars also contend that a new vibrant mechanism of a growing trade in healthcare continues to involve the movement of patients across borders in the pursuit of medical treatment and health; a phenomenon commonly termed medical tourism (Glinos et al. 2010; Holsinger 2017; OECD 2009; Suess et al. 2018).

Africa and the Nature of Medical Tourism

In the past seven decades, after African nations started gaining independence from the European countries that colonized them, political leaders, senior military officers, public administrators, and some African elites often tended to engage in medical tourism (Dibie 2022; Obuh et al. 2020). Unfortunately, one of the common immoral practices of the African leader mentioned above is that they use public funds that could have been used to build state-of-the-art health facilities in their own country to travel to developed nations that had effectively utilized their nation's funds with due diligent to build outstanding health infrastructures (Africanglobe 2012: Dibie 2022; Mogaka et al. 2017). Some scholars contend that while African leaders want to preserve their lives or enhance their physical appearance if they cannot get such treatment in their respective nations, they would rather use public funds to travel to foreign countries to seek better healthcare at the expense of the common people in their respective African nations (Abdebayo 2020; Mogaka et al. 2017; Oleribe et al. 2019).

It has been argued that the value of importance that a nation's leaders and citizens place on the health of their citizens is categorically reflected in the amount of funding, policies, infrastructure, and resources devoted to the pursuit of a vibrant healthcare system in the country (Dibie 2022; Kraft & Furlong 2021; Longest 2016 2018). In addition, the objective of any healthcare system is to improve the health of all citizens in a country. A good leader or president of any health system is expected to promote strong ethical and social justice values (Dibie 2018; Van de Walle 2001). The moral and social justice values that must be promoted as well as practiced by leaders should involve the integration of the principles of freedom, social and ethnic equality, and the worth and dignity of all the people in the continent of Africa. The practice of collaborative governance that promotes the principles of brotherhood and sisterhood of all human beings could ensure a good life for everyone (Dibie 2018, Ferrel et al. 2019; Gatwiri et al. 2020).

Research reveals that the value or importance that a nation's leaders and citizens place on the health of their citizens is categorically reflected in the amount of funding, policies, infrastructure, and resources devoted to the pursuit of a vibrant healthcare system in the country (Dibie 2022; Kraft & Furlong 2021; Longest 2016; Marks et al. 2018). Further, it should be emphasized in many African countries that the determinants of healthcare in the country includes people's behavior physical environment in which they work, their biology, family history, physical and mental health problems. There are also social factors such as socioeconomic position, and income distribution, as well as other economic circumstances (Dibie 2022; Frimpong-Ansah 1992). Therefore, the major goal of the country is how to determine what factors could propel a "healthy people." There is also no doubt that the existence of multiple determinants could galvanize the government to engage in strategic doing with a larger option to explore in the pursuit of vibrant healthcare system that could lead to a society of healthy people in the country. A good steward leader or moral president of any country should work diligently to cater for the wellbeing of all citizens by focusing on the healthcare needs of everyone in the nation. It is also especially important to. improve the quality of healthcare delivery system in his/her country. The current healthcare challenges in the country requires a systematic promotion of a vibrant ethical and social justice values (Dibie 2018; Froeb et al. 2018). The moral and social justice values that must be promoted as well as practiced by leaders should involve the integration of the principles of freedom, social and ethnic equality, and the worth and dignity of all the people in the African continent (Dibie 2022; Johnson & Stoskopf 2010; Longest 2016).

The practice of shared governance that promotes the principles of brotherhood and sisterhood of all human beings could ensure a good life for everyone (Dibie 2018; Ferrell et al. 2019; Gatwiri et al. 2020). Unfortunately, the health systems in many African countries are in deplorable conditions, rather than the presidents and political elites to solve the dilapidated state of their healthcare system they frequently travel outside their respective countries to seek better treatment in foreign countries (Anna et al. 2020; Zana 2017).

Abdebayo (2020) and African Development Bank Report (2012) contend that unethical presidents and their political elite are busy amassing fortunes in European and North American countries while the majority of their citizens are living in abject poverty. It is also mind-boggling that these poor African people do not have access to basic public goods or social services such as good health system, elementary schools, sanitation, safely managed drinking water, and electricity, yet their presidents own majestic buildings and palaces in foreign countries and in their home countries (African Development Bank 2012; Zana 2017). It is unfortunate that while their citizens are dying of diseases, and sick patients sleeping on the floor of hospitals due to the availability of beds, political leaders travel to receive better healthcare in western developed countries (Bachrach & Daley 2017; Jchiwanza 2018). It is also incredibly sad that African countries do not demand certified records of the health condition of candidates who are contesting for the presidency of their respective, nations. If they do it would have been possible for them to eliminate candidates that do not have the cognitive capacity, and intellectual acumen to withstand the rigors of the position of the presidency. The debilitating and degenerative illnesses that affected elderly presidents of developing countries presidents and elites are starting to create a culture of medical tourism. In most cases, during the period when various presidents of African countries are receiving treatment in foreign countries, there tends to be poor or no coordination between the government and administration because the leader of the nation is not available for consultation on how to manage the affairs. The bewilderment of governance is also galvanized when such a president refuses to hand over power to the vice president to act in his absence (Dibie 2022; Gatwiri et al. 2020; Martin 2017).

The World Economic Forum Report (2014) reveals that about 30,000 Nigerians spend US$1 billion annually on medical tourism to IM8f: countries like Canada, England, France, India, Indonesia, Spain, and Dubai. In addition, Nigerian elites spent 60% of their foreign health payment on four major disease areas: cardiology, orthopedics, renal dialysis issues, and cancer (International Trade Organization 2023). According to Anna (2020) and Zana (2017), African presidents who engage in medical tourism do so because they lack confidence in the health system that they are expected to fund, provide modern equipment, and employ high-quality doctors and nurses. This is the obvious reason that African leaders are the culprits who have created the unbelievably bad healthcare systems that exist in their respective countries (Anna 2020; Chiwanza 2018). Rather than buying modern equipment, they refer to using taxpayers' money to travel to seek better healthcare in foreign countries while their fellow citizens die (Zana 2017). In addition, to the above deplorable situation, doctors and nurses migrate to North America and Europe to seek better pay and working conditions (Bachrach & Daley 2017). The lack of political will by some African political leaders to increase the funding appropriated for their health system has negatively affected the projected progress in the achievement of health goals for the African continent which each president has agreed to accomplish for their respective countries (Jchiwanza 2018; WHO 2020).

Reasons for Medical Tourism by People Living in African Countries

The challenge of poor health delivery systems in many African countries is the cause of disagreement while both rich and middle-income residents of the African continent tend to explore alternative sources of better treatment in foreign countries (Adeoye 2023; Biz Community 2019). Research reveals that the function of current governments regardless of the systems used, is the creation and implementation of health policies which reflects the immediate and future needs of the people. Healthcare, security, political stability, and development projects are all affected by poor governance (Patients Beyond Borders 2024). Many scholars have identified the reasons why African elite travel to foreign countries to seek medical treatment. Research also reveals that the common reasons why the elites in Africa engage in medical tourism are the following:

1. Poor domestic healthcare infrastructure, and poor standards of health professionals;
2. Long waiting times for approval of medical procedures.
3. Low or inadequate funding.
4. Lack of confidence in several African countries healthcare systems.
5. Ineffective regulation and implementation of healthcare policies.
6. Poor healthcare standards.
7. No specific medical and cosmetic treatments are available or are illegal;
8. Dilapidated hospital buildings, lack of modern medical equipment, and lack of constant electrical supply.
9. Shortage of specialist physicians and nurses especially in rural medical facilities;
10. Negative perception of citizens about healthcare delivery in the country;
11. Lack of effective collaboration or partnership with public and private health sectors.
12. Disparities in the health delivery system in the urban and rural regions.
13. Poor governance of the health sector; and
14. Corruption of political leaders and senior public administrators (Abdebayo 2020; Biz Community 2019; Liepaja 2017; Martin 2017; Obuh et al. 2020; Olanrewaju 2017).

The above list of reasons for the poor health system reveals why most African leaders and elite travel to the United States, France, United Kingdom, Canada, India, Thailand, Singapore, Turkey, Dubai, and many other foreign countries to seek healthcare. Some scholars have also argued that African leaders and governments have not specified healthcare as a priority (Abdebayo 2020; Anna 2020; Dixit et al. 2019; Mmotia 2019; Zana 2017). It is also mind-boggling that African government leaders cannot comprehend the fact that the effectiveness of healthcare system in the foreign countries that they go to seek treatment is functioning well because they were appropriately funded, maintained, and staffed with visionary health experts (Abdebayo 2020; Anna et al. 2020). Among the list of treatments that are sought by Africans that engage foreign medical procedures include the following. Cardiovascular health, cosmetic surgery, dermatology, eye surgery, in vitro fertilization, liver and kidney transplants, neuro-surgical surgery, spinal surgery, and weight loss (Adeoye 2023; Deb 2024, Dixit et al. 2019; Health Tourism 2024).

Furthermore, the presidents of 52 African countries attended a health conference in Abuja, the capital city of Nigeria, and signed a document called the Abuja Declaration in 2001. The 2001 Abuja Declaration constituted a commitment by the 52 African Presidents who attended the health conference to appropriate 15% of their gross domestic product (GDP) each year for healthcare. Rather than appropriating the committed funds each year, they would prefer to use most of such funds for their family members and themselves to seek better treatment in foreign countries. Thus, self-aggrandizement is preventing them from investing in their respective nation's health system so that all their citizens can benefit from a vibrant state-of-the-art health delivery (Dibie 2022).

In the past five years, the Republic of Nigeria has also experienced a dramatic decrease in the specialist health workforce in the country. It is estimated that the ratio of doctors to patients is 1:3,500. The rate of brain-drain is also reported to be getting worse incrementally every year (Pollard et al. 2023). Moreover, the Federal Government of Nigeria has also acknowledged that the nation spends between US$1.2 and US$1.6 billion every year. The former president of Nigeria Muhammadu Buhari's 237 days state paid medical treatment in the United Kingdom was unprecedented. This is because Buhari operated and landed parking cost airplane trips cost between US$2.43 and US$9.5 million (Pollard et al. 2023). The cost of former President Buhari's medical tourism expenses in London, England, was estimated to be equivalent to 0.07% of Nigeria's health budget (Abdebayo 2020; Anna 2020; Martin 2011). Pollard et al. (2023) contend that President Buhari's government budgeted US$2.97 million (N297 million Naira) for the Nigerian Health Insurance Scheme. However, he planned to spend US$25 million (N2.5 billion Naira) on his presidential foreign medical tourism trip, and local travels within his country in 2023. Furthermore, Nigeria loses at least $2 billion every year to medical tourism, according to the Nigerian Medical Association (International Trade Organization 2023). The current president of Nigeria Bola Ahmed Tinubu has also embarked on a couple of medical tourism trips to France since he became president of Nigeria in 2023. Late President Mugabe used to snub his nation's hospitals and flew to Singapore to seek medical treatment because he did not provide enough funding. While he was the president, the hospitals in Zimbabwe were reported not to have basic medicines like painkillers and antibiotics (Mmotia 2019; Zana 2017). Unfortunately, former President Mugabe died in Singapore on September 6, 2019.

Over the past few years, the current president of Zimbabwe Emmerson Mnangagwa has secretly traveled to China to seek treatment. Some scholars have argued that African leaders from the Republic of Benin, Malawi, Ethiopia, Zambia, Ghana, Cameroon, and many more have engaged in medical tourism to receive treatment from foreign countries while their poorly funded hospitals and clinics limp in with underfunded and understaffed hospitals in their respective nations. Unfortunately, many presidents of African countries such as former presidents of Nigeria, Malawi, Zambia, and Zimbabwe have all died in foreign countries and their bodies flown back to their home country for burial (Buchanan 2016; Oluwasanmi 2020). While these African presidents have massive resources at their disposal, their greed, power, and wickedness have influenced their lack of social justice virtue. At the end of their life greedy style, they died in foreign countries lonely and humiliated (Oluwasanmi 2020). What a legacy they have really accomplished.

According to Martin (2017) and Pollard et al. (2016), African nations spent over US$1 billion on medical tourism in 2015. Furthermore, Galal (2024) contends that despite the challenges of medical tourism in some African countries, it is estimated that in 2012, travel and tourism contributed 5.9% to Africa's GDP, up from 4.4% in the previous year. In addition, in 2023, travel tourism has been estimated to contribute to 6.5% of the African continent's GDP. The year 2019 provided the highest contribution of travel tourism with 6.5% of the continent's GDP (Galal 2024).

Corruption is not only a major pandemic in many African countries but also regarded as a way of life (Dibie 2022; Martin 2017). The unethical challenges of corruption have permeated all life facets from simple things like access to healthcare, schools, and jobs in public and private sectors in all Sub-Saharan African nations. It ranges from public servants demanding bribes, before providing what is supposed to be free to citizens. Corruption also facilitates the unfair awarding of government contracts to favor business associates, relatives, and friends of government officials (World Bank 2020). Sometimes senior political leaders secretly award government contracts to their private companies (Dibie 2018; Obuh et al. 2020).

Another commonly used form of corruption in many African countries is the deliberate action of senior government leaders, such as presidents, vice presidents, or prime ministers to capture and distort how government institutions work and select who should control them in such a way that the outcomes may benefit them (Froeb et al. 2018; Transparency International 2016; World Bank 2020). The problems associated with corruption in many African countries have elevated the level of unfair inequalities both in access to healthcare services from government offices as well as opportunities for investment with many local and foreign firms that are discouraged and forced to close business (Gaspar et al. 2019; World Bank 2020). Misappropriation of public funds and bias in the awarding of contracts often comprise the quality of service available to the citizens of the country (Dibie 2022; Ejifoma 2021; Oleribe et al. 2019).

The incidence discussed above confirms that many African nations' presidents lack the steward leadership principles and understanding of how the modern world operates. Unfortunately, if they realize that technology and modernization are increasing horrendously in the foreign countries that they have been visiting, they could have put their self-aggrandizement, greed, ambition, and differences aside and rethink a better strategy to confront these change dynamics in the healthcare system in their respective countries, ignorance, greed, and the mechanism that has propel their foolishness and blindness to act nobly in addressing the social and economic needs that could benefit everyone in their nations.

There is no doubt that the hospitals where some African presidents seek healthcare are better than what might be available in their respective nations. The question, we wish to ask is: why can an African country government build at least two or three similar advanced hospitals? Why can African nations producing gold diamond, crude petroleum, and other natural resources not able to form partnerships with private foreign partners to build modern hospitals in Africa that are better equipped? The injustice in governance, and democracy that prevail in many African countries, as well as the mentality of the winner, takes all without investing in public goods has made nations in the continent to be poor and lack modern infrastructure.

According to Keck et al. (2012) and Rowitz (2009), hospitals and healthcare systems are where leadership skills are embedded and must be strengthened by utilizing the core functions of public health and its essential services as a guide to the changes that should occur to benefit all citizens. Therefore, to provide a high-quality health system for everyone as a human rights service, leaders must evaluate the health status of the population. African political leaders must also conduct a critical analysis of the capacity of the region, state, community, and nation to effectively address its health priorities, as well as implement preventive measures to reduce the impact of or even avoid health crises in the country. One other especially important function of health system leaders is to help restructure the policies and laws that govern health and public health in the country.

Despite this lack of social justice values and political will to enhance the health system by leaders of some African countries, the money made available for health services is shrinking annually in many countries on the continent. This challenge has often prevented healthcare practitioners not to being better prepared to treat all the citizens who need care. Further, lack of adequate funding tends to prevent practitioners from seeking the best and modern equipment for most of the answers for the healthcare needs of their citizens and patients. According to the World Health Organization Report (2022), insufficient investment by many African countries' governments in the health sector or in actions to tackle the environment and social determinants of health is a serious obstacle to improving health outcomes in Africa (Dibie 2022; Olinos et al. 2010; Piper 2023). Table 1 shows a list of current and former African presidents who sought health treatment in foreign countries such as in Europe, North America, and Asia.

Table 1 List of Some African Presidents Who Sought Health Treatment in Foreign Nations

Name of Country	Name of President	Country where they received their treatment
Algeria	Abdelaziz Bouteflia	France
Angola	Jose Eduarado dos Santos	Spain
Benin	Patrice Talon	France
Botswana	Mokgweetsi Masisi	Namibia
Cameroon	Paul Biya	France
Chad	Pascal Yoadimnadi	France: Died overseas
Ethiopia	Meles Zenawi	Belgium
Gabon	Omar Bongo Ondimba	Spain
Ghana	John Atta Mills	United States
Guinea	Lansana Conte	Switzerland and Morocco
Guinea	Ahmed Sekou Toure	France
Guinea Bissau	Bacai Samha	France
Nigeria	Bola Ahmed Tinubu	France
Nigeria	Mohammed Buhari	England
Nigeria	Umaru Musa Yar'Adua	Saudi Arabia: Died overseas
Malawi	BinQUwa Mutharika	South Africa: Died overseas
Zambia	Levy Mwanawasa	France: Died overseas
Zambia	Michael Sata	England
Zimbabwe	Robert Mugabe	Singapore: Died overseas
Zimbabwe	Constantino Jchiwenga	China

Source: Anna (2020) and Jchiwanza (2018).

This human-caused predicament bears the bulk of the global morbidity and mortality burden for maternal and infant death, Ebola, COVID-19, and HIV/AIDS (Dibie 2022; Kim & Hyun 2022; Piper 2023). Some scholars have previously argued that the majority of the countries in Africa are confronted with the challenges of lack of collaborative governance and leadership (Adedeji 1979; Ajei 2018; Ake 1996; Ayittey 2005; Dibie 2018). According to Dibie (2018) and Olanrewaju (2017), the prosperity of a nation is an indication of the kind of decisions that its political leaders make. These scholars contend that great leaders of nations not only view their decisions from the prism of their impact on them but also think more about how such decisions positively affect their citizens. African political leaders who operate from this perspective will not put their own concerns and interests of their cronies above what is required by the citizens (Dibie 2022). Despite the endowed natural resources in SubSaharan Africa, why do many countries in the continent have high rates of poverty and inequality in healthcare? Jallow (2014) and Obuh et al. (2020) contend that African leaders tend not to be incapable of transforming national economic strategies in the direction that they had promised during the struggle for independence after more than six decades of false promises during election campaigns.

Dibie (2018), Gatwiri et al. (2020), and Van de Walle (2003) contend that some of the driving forces of underdevelopment in many African Countries are lack of effective healthcare system, inequality, high employment, and poverty could be linked to unethical leadership, corruption, policy constraints, and environmental factors. The greatest of these constraints is corruption. While the citizens do not have good and affordable healthcare, many leaders of African countries engage themselves in using public funds to satisfy their personal needs as well as fulfilling the wishes of their family members or promoting nepotism against the wishes of all the citizens of their respective countries (Ajei 2018; Dibie 2018). According to Van de Walle (2001), the underdevelopment situation in Africa is because of deliberate action to prevent the continent's governments from undertaking reforms by societal interest and pressure groups, clientelism within the state elite, and ideological factors. The practice of leaders in many African countries is the determination to acquire wealth while in power, and deliberately pay less attention to engage in economic development, creating job opportunities, and human and institutional capacity building (Dibie 2022; Rowitz 2009). This practice of a government sucking the lifeblood from any economy has been described as a Vampire state (Dibie 2018; Frimpong-Ansah 1992; Van de Walle 2003).

Change is always a challenge to African political leaders. This is because post-independence history has shown that political leaders and senior public administrators have not accepted the task confronting them with respect to transparency and accountability to the citizens (Adedeji 1979; Ake 1996). Contrary to the dependency theory, Claude Ake (1996) argued that development initiatives in African countries must involve the process by which people create and recreate themselves and their life circumstances to realize higher levels of civilization in accordance with their own choices and moral values (Dumede 2016). Thus, development is what the African people must do for themselves by engaging in collaborative governance.

According to the African Development Bank Report (2020) and Ajei (2018), the presence of more active civil society organizations, nongovernment organizations, social media, anticorruption groups, vibrant press, and television media has galvanized more transparency and accountability than what it used to be in many African countries. A transparent and collaborative governance health system encourages a shared vision. According to Dibie (2018), a shared vision in the healthcare system of a nation or any other organization in Africa requires healthcare leaders in both the public and private sectors to understand that the framework for future change in the entire country and citizens being served is paramount to achieving a better result for sustainable development.

The poor in many African countries suffer the worst health challenges and die younger. They have higher than average child and maternal mortality, higher levels of disease, more limited access to healthcare and social protection, and gender inequality disadvantages. Further, the health status of women and girls in rural regions in Africa is terrible (Dibie 2018). For poor people especially, health is also a crucially important economic asset. Their livelihoods depend on it. When a poor or socially vulnerable person becomes ill or injured, the entire household can become trapped in a downward spiral of lost income and high healthcare costs (Gaspar et al. 2019; Patient Beyond Boarders 2024; Wilensky & Teitelbaum 2020). Why do African leaders hide their illness so that they can stay in office for as long as they want?

Furthermore, the perception of African leaders about the quality of their nation's healthcare is mind-boggling. Some African countries such as Nigeria, Ghana, Cameroon, Zimbabwe, Zambia, Kenya, and others have the highest number of foreign doctors in the United Kingdom and the United States. However, most of the political leaders from these African countries often travel to foreign countries for their healthcare from foreign doctors who may not be as qualified as the African physicians but migrated from Africa to practice in Europe and North America (Adeoye 2023; Dibie 2022). Unfortunately, there is no evidence of how African elites have made a major attempt to replicate the positive healthcare system knowledge that they received in foreign countries in their home country in the African continent (Tseane-Gumbi & Ojakorotu 2022).

Conclusion

This chapter has examined why African leaders and elites prefer to seek their healthcare in England, France, Spain, Portugal, Canada, the United States, India, Singapore, and so on. The chapter provides detailed explanations of why factors such as poor funding and infrastructure, adequate regulation and poor standards, lack of highly qualified medical staff, as well as negative perception could be major reasons for a mass exodus of African elite seeking healthcare in countries outside their continent. The chapter also argues that although there are a couple of well-established private hospitals, health centers, and clinics in some African countries; there is still a convoluted perception of poor healthcare services, as well as the fact that patients admitted to such hospitals may not get the value for their money. In addition, it proposed that African leaders must pay attention to their nation's health system rather than snubbing their country's healthcare delivery system to seek health treatment in foreign countries.

Some scholars have described the actions of some African leaders who travel to foreign countries to seek medical treatment as suffering from madness, shameless, preposterous, and overwhelming (Anna 2020; Dibie 2022; Pollard et al. 2023). This is because if the billion dollars that they spend each on medical tourism were invested within the African continent on health infrastructural development, and compelled to receive healthcare in their home country, the general image of some African countries' health system could have been much better than what it is now (Adeoye 2023; Adephagane 2022; Gatwiri et al. 2020; Olanrewaju 2017).

Moving forward, the African nation's political leaders and elites should consider collaborating. to establish public–private partnerships among existing domestic and foreign healthcare providers to build new health facilities. This partnership could help to foster the repositioning of the health systems in some African countries. Thus, the reinvigoration of healthcare could help to build trust and positive perception, as well as motivate more foreign tourists to visit Africa for their healthcare in the future. Thus, building new state-of-the-art medical facilities and modem equipment as well as attracting specialist physicians could be a new mechanism for generating revenue for many African countries in the near future (Dibie 2022; World Bank 2022).

Other solutions to reduce medical tourism challenges in some African countries include a better governance system of healthcare by the Ministry of Health and Agencies, appropriate financing of the healthcare delivery system, and more incentives to attract and retain health workforce personnel. Appropriate health policy should also be enacted, that could encourage multinational corporations to engage in the public–private partnership in the health industry in the provision of modern infrastructure and the promotion of corporate social responsibility. There is also the need for African countries to reverse their rigid health policies and regulations to enhance more investment in the healthcare sector. In addition, trade restrictions need to be revised to enable the promotion of a consistent framework for health professionals with foreign qualifications as well as the encouragement of more foreign healthcare facilities in their respective African countries. The development of vibrant telemedicine and tele-education could also help to mitigate some of the current health challenges in African countries.

According to the scripture God is everywhere around the World. God also created the world, as well as the two first human beings Adam and Eve. However, most African religious people think that without going to Israel, and Mecca respectively, they will not be blessed. Further, the rich industrialized countries around the world, do not pay for their Christian and Muslim citizens to go on religious pilgrimage to Israel, and Mecca. Unfortunately, the poor and developing countries' government in many African countries spend billions of United States dollars each year to sponsor their citizens to pilgrimage. Just like the predicament of medical tourism, the money spent by African governments on these pilgrimages could have been used to build hospitals and other health facilities for their citizens. Dibie (2022) contends that the amount spent for pilgrimage by some African countries is enough to provide free healthcare services to the citizens. These mind-boggling and despicable government appropriation of funding activity in African countries need to stop. People do not have to go on pilgrimage before God can bless them. Whoever wish to go on pilgrimage could save money, and feel free to travel.

Finally, one of the best ways for African nations' governments to dampen corruption and rebellion is to put in place more stringent anticorruption laws that are brutally enforced (United States Department of State 2021; United Nations Development Programme Report 2020; Transparency International 2016). In addition, there is also an urgent need to promote accountability and transparency. Establishing traceability initiatives in all ramifications of the public and private sectors, as well as whistle-blowers' laws could enhance efforts to crack down on culprits of corruption. Foreign firms can also play a key role in this because our research found that mining multinational corporations that practice the ethical principles of corporate social responsibility are less likely to escalate violence (Bryan et al. 2010; Dibie 2018).

References

Abdebayo B. (2020). Africa's leaders forced to confront healthcare systems they neglected for years. https://www.cnn.com/2020/04/10/africa/african-leaders-healthcare-coronavirus-intl/index.html. September 24, 2024.

Adedeji J. A. (1979). Social and Cultural Conflict in Sport and Games in Developing Countries. *International Review of Sport Sociology*, 14(1): 81–88.

Adeoye A. O. (2023). Assessing the associated medical, legal, and social issues in medical tourism and its implications for Nigeria. *Pan African Medical Journal*. Jul 31:45:145. doi: 10.11604/pamj.2023.45.145.41104.

Adephagane L. (2022). Africa: How medical tourism is affecting Africa's healthcare economy. https://allafrica.com/stories/202109060238.html. Accessed January 18, 2024.

African Development Bank (2012). African development report: Towards green growth in Africa. https://www.afdb.org/fileadmin/uploads/afdb/Documents/Publications/African_Development_Report_2012.pdf. Accessed February 23, 2024.

African Development Bank Report (2020). Annual Report 2020. https://www.afdb.org/sites/default/files/documents/publications/afdb_annual_report_2020_main_en_.pdf. Accessed November 14, 2024.

African Development Bank (2022). African economic outlook. https://www.afdb.org/en/documents-publications-african-economic-outlook-2023-previous-african-economic-outlook/african-economic-outlook-2022. Accessed February 23, 2024.

Africanglobe (2012). African leaders agree to more infrastructure spending. https://www.icafrica.org/fr/news-events/infrastructure-news/article/african-leaders-agree-to-more-infrastructure-spending-2694/. Accessed March 15, 2024.

Ajei M. O. (2018). Educating Africans: Perspectives of Ghanaian philosophers. *Phronimon*, 19: 15 pages. https://doi.org/10.25159/2413-3086/5277. Accessed September 28, 2024.

Ake C. (1996). *Democracy and Development in Africa*. Washington DC: The Brookings Institutions.

Anna C. (2020). African elite who once sought treatment abroad are grounded. https://abcnews.go.com/Health/wireStory/african-elite-sought-treatment-abroad. Accessed March 3, 2024.

Anna C., Mednick S., Muhumuza R. (2020). African elite who once sought treatment abroad are grounded. https://apnews.com/article/3fd908519a2a746f965150d8bf1f83ae Accessed September 24, 2024.

Ayittey G. B. N. (2005) *Africa Unchained*. New York: Palgrave Macmillan.

Bachrach C. A., Daley D. M. (2017). Three challenges for population health science. *American Journal of Public Health*, 107(2): 251–252.

Balaban V. & Marano C. (2010). Medical tourism research: A systematic review. *International Journal of Infectious Diseases*, 14: e135–e135.

Beland D., Zarzeczny A. (2018). Medical tourism and national health care systems: An institutionalist research agenda. *Global Health*, 14(68):4–15.

Biz Community (2019). World Tourism Organization Biz Community. https://www. bizcommunity.com/Tag/World+Tourism+Organization. Accessed November 14, 2024.

Bryan L., Conway M., Keesmaat T., McKenna S., Richardson B. (2010). Strengthening sub-Saharan Africa·s health systems: A practical approach. https://www.mckinsey.com/ industries/healthcare/our-insights/strengthening-sub-saharan-africas-health-systems-a-practical-approach. Accessed March 15, 2024.

Buchanan E. (2016). Photos of Tanzania's President Magufuli visiting wife in public hospital go viral. https://www.ibtimes.co.uk/tanzanias-president-magufuli-visits-wife-public-hospital-photos-go-viral-social-media-1591060. Accessed September 24, 2024.

Chiwanza T. H. (2018). The top ten African countries with largest Chinese debt. The African Exponent.

Dalen J. E., Alpert J. S. (2018). Medical tourist; Incoming and outgoing. *The American Journal of Medicine*, 132(1): 9–10.

Deb T. (2024). Medical Tourism Statistics 2024 By Landscape, Healthcare, Treatments https:// media.market.us/medical-tourism-statistics/. Accessed September 24, 2024.

Dibie R. (2022). Healthcare policy and administration in Nigeria. *The Journal of African Policy Studies*, 28(1): 101–139.

Dibie R. (2018). *Business and Government Relations in Africa*. New York: Routledge Press.

Dixit S., Emery N., Kumar C. (2019). Is trade with India changing Africa's healthcare landscape? https://www.brookings.edu/allicles/is-1rade-with-india-cha1lgi1lg-afrkas-hcalthcare-landscape/#. Accessed March 15, 2024.

Ejifoma R. (2021). West Africa: UBTH Set to Curb Medical Tourism in West Africa. This Day Newspaper, Nigeria. https://allafrica.com/stories/202104050095.html. Accessed February 25, 2024.

Ferrell, O. C., & Fraedrich, J. (2019). *Business Ethics: Ethical Decision Making and Cases*. Boston, MA: Cengage Learning.

Ferrell O. C., Fraedrich J., Ferrell L. (2013). *Business: Ethical Decision Making and Cases*. Mason. OH: South-Western/ Cengage Learning.

Frimpong-Ansah J. H. (1992). *Saving for economic recovery in Africa. African Centre for Economic Policy Research*. Ed. by J. H. Frimpong-Ansah. London, United Kingdom: Currey Press.

Froeb L. M., Mccann B. T., Shor M., and Ward M. R. (2018). *Managerial Economics: A Problem Salving Approach*. Boston, MA: Cengage Learning.

Galal S. (2024). Share of travel and tourism in Africa's GDP 2019–2023. https://www.statista. com/statistics/1320400/share-of-travcl-and-tourism-in-africas-grossdomestic-product/. Accessed January 29, 2024.

Gaspar V., Mauro P., and Medas P. (2019). Tackling corruption in government. international monetary fund. https://blogs.imf.org/2019/04/04/tackling-com1ption-in-e:ovcmment/. Accessed September 24, 2024.

Gatwiri K., Amboko J., Okolla D. (2020). The implications of Neoliberalism on African economies, health outcomes and wellbeing: A conceptual argument. *Social Theory Health*. 18(1):86–101,

Glinos I. A., Baeten R., Helble M., Hans Maarse H. (2010). A typology of cross-border patient mobility. *Health & Place*, 16(6): 1145–1155.

Health Tourism (2024). What Drives the Medical Tourism Market in 2024? [[Page1]]Medical tourism and facts. https://www.myshortlister.com/insights/medical-tourism-market#:~:text=The%20 medical%20tourism%20market%20has%20grown%20significantly%20over%20the%20 past,(CAGR)%20of%2023.03%25. Accessed August 29, 2024.

Holsinger J. (2017). *Leadership for Public Health: Theory and Practice*. Chicago, IL: Health Administration Press.

Hotelier (2020). Dubai crowned best medical tourism destination in the region. https://www. hoteliermiddleeast.com/news/dubai-crowned-best-medical-tourism-destination-in-the-region. Accessed August 29, 2024

International Trade Organization (2023). Nigeria country guide: Healthcare. https://www. trade.gov/healthcare-resource-guide-nigeria. Accessed September 24, 2024

Jallow, B.G. (2014). Leadership in colonial Africa: disruption of traditional frameworks and patterns. https://www.semanticscholar.org/paper/Leadership-in-colonial-Africa-%3A-disruption-of-and-Jallow/903e0f9776f6dc605d783b910e141d4a9fb296e3. Accessed November 14, 2024.

Johnson J. A., Stoskopf C. H. (2010) *Comparative Health System: Global Perspectives*. Boston, MA: Jones and Bartlett Publishers.

Keck C. S, Scutchfield F, Holsinger J. (2012). *Future of Public Health*. Ed. Holsinger J. Lexington, KY: University of Kentucky Press, 251 p.

Kim H. L., Hyun S. S. (2022). The future of medical tourism for individual health and well-being: A case study of the relationship between the UAE (United Arab Emirates) and South Korea. *International Journal of Environment Resources Public Health*, 19(9): 5735. DOI: 10.3390/ijerph19095735.

Kraft M. E., Furlong S. R. (2021). *Public Policy: Politics Analysis, and Alternatives*. Thousand Oak, CA: Sage Press.

Kraft M. E., Furlong S. R. (2021). *Public Policy: Politics Analysis, and Alternatives*. Thousand Oak, CA: Sage Press.

Liedong T. A. (2017). African politicians seeking medical help abroad is shameful, and harms health care. https://theconversation.com/african-politicians-seeking-medical-help-abroad-is-shameful-and-harms-health-care-82771. Accessed September 24, 2024.

Longest B. (2016). *Health Policymaking in the United States*. Sixth Edition. Chicago, IL: Health Administration Press.

Martin, K. 2011. TMI (Too Much Information)—The role of friction and familiarity in disclosing information. *Business and Professional Ethics Journal*, 30(1/2): 1–32.

Martin L. M. (2017). The African politicians seeking medical help abroad is shameful, and harms healthcare. https://theconversation.com/african-politicians-seeking-medical-help-abroad-isshameful-and-harms health-care-82771. Accessed March 11, 2024.

Mmotia T. (2019). African leaders prefer overseas to local health care. https://mg.co.za/article/2019-10-07-00-african-leaders-prefer-overseas-to-local-health-care/. Accessed March 6, 2024.

Mogaka J. J. O., Mupara L., Tsoka-Gwegweni J. M., (2017). Ethical issues associated with medical tourism in Africa. *Journal of Market Access & Health Policy*. 5;5(1): 1309770. DOI: 10.1080/20016689.2017.1309770.

Murphy T. (2023). Medical tourism: Traveling outside US for care is common. https://apnews. com/article/mexico-medical-tourism-us-overseas-2abf4d198a3bbad9260bfd9d52067ba2. Accessed August 5, 2024.

Obuh J., Onobun M., Eluwa O., Azama A. A., Aguele O. O. (2020). Medical tourism-issues in Nigeria. *Developing Country Studies*. 10(8): 1–8.

OECD (2007). *Annual Report on Sustainable Development Work in the OECD*. Paris: OECD Publication.

OECD (2009). Trade in health services (medical tourism), in *Health at a Glance 2009: OECD Indicators*. Paris: OECD Publishing.

Olanrewaju A, Woon T. C. (2017). An exploration of determinants of affordable housing choice, *International Journal of Housing Markets and Analysis*, 10(5), 703–723.

Olanrewaju L. (2022). Understanding risk communication effectiveness from public interest, mobility, and COVID-19 cases: A case study of COVID-19 in Nigeria. *Frontiers in Communication*, 7(1). DOI: 10.3389/fcomm.2022.921648.

Oleribe O. O., Momoh J., Uzochukwu B. S., Mbofana F., Adebiyi A., Barbera T., Williams R., TaylorRobinson S. D. (2019). Identifying key challenges facing healthcare systems in Africa and potential solutions. *International Journal General Medicine*. 6(12): 395–403.

Olinos I. A., Baeten R., Helble M. & Maarse H. (2010). A typology of cross-border patient mobility. *Health & Place*, 16, 1145–1155.

Oluwasanmi B. (2020). Thinking with you... Where will president Buhari receive next medical check. https://saharareporters.com/2020/03/24/thinking-you-where-will-president-buhari-receive-next-medical-check-bayo-oluwasanmi#google_vignette. Accessed September 24, 2024.

Patient Beyond Boarders (2024). Medical tourism statistics and facts. https://www.patientsbeyondborders.com/media. Accessed September. 16, 2024.

Piper A. (2023). Medical tourism: Easy steps to penetrate Nigeria patient markets. https://www.magazine.medicaltourism.com/article/medical-tourism-easy-steps-to-penetrate-nigeria-patient-markets. Accessed September 20, 2024.

Pollard K., Jenkins J., Ian Youngman I. (2023). Counting the cost of medical tourism from Nigeria. https://www.laingbuissonnews.com/imtj/news-imtj/counting-the-cost-of-medical-tourism-from-nigeria/. Accessed September 18, 2024.

Rowitz L (2009). *Public Health Leadership: Putting Principles into Practice*. Boston, MA: Jones and Bartlett Publishers.

Stolley K., Watson S. (2012). *Medical tourism. A Reference Handbook*, ABC-CLIO. LLC. ProQuest EBook Central. Santa Barbara, CA: ABC-CLIO Publisher.

Suess C., Baloglu S., Busser J. A. (2018). Perceived impacts of medical tourism development on community wellbeing. *Tourism Management*, 69(I):232–245.

Transparency International (2016). How to stop corruption: Five key ingredients. https://www.transparency.org/en/news/how-to-stop-corruption-5-key-ingredients#. Accessed March 5, 2024.

Tseane-Gumbi L. A., Ojakorotu V. (2022). Medical tourism and African healthcare system: behavioral analysis of the role of African leaders. *Gender and Behavior*, 1(3): 1–9.

United Nations Development Programme Report (2020). World biggest challenges. https://annualreport.undp.org/2020/. Accessed February 23, 2024.

United States Department of State (2021). Combating corruption and promoting good governance. http://www.state.gov/combating-corruption-and-promoting-good-governance. Accessed March 3, 2024.

United States International Trade Commission (2021). Trends in United States travel services trade. https://www.usitc.gov/publications/industry_econ_analysis_332/2021/recent_trends_us services_trade_2021_annual_report.htm. Accessed January 16, 2024.

Van de Walle, N. (2001). *African Economies and the Politics of Permanent Crisis, 1979–1999*. Cambridge United Kingdom: Cambridge University Press.

Van de Walle N. (2003). Presidentialism and clientelism in Africa's emerging party systems. *The Journal of Modern African Studies*, 41, 297–321.

Wilensky S. E., Teitelbaum J. B. (2020). *Essentials of Health Policy and Law: Essential Public Health*. 4th Edition. Boston, MA: Jones and Bartlett Publishers.

World Bank (2023). Combating corruption. https://www.worldbank.org/en/topic/governance/brief/combating-corruption. Accessed September 24, 2024

World Bank (2022). World Development Report 2022: Finance for an equitable recovery. https://www.worldbank.org/en/publication/wdr2022. Accessed September 28, 2024.

World Bank (2015a). Summary on the Ebola Recovery Plan: Guinea [Press release]. https://reliefweb.int/report/guinea/summary-ebola-recovery-plan-guinea. Accessed September 24, 2024.

World Bank (2015b). Summary on the Ebola Recovery Plan: Liberia-Economic stabilization and recovery Plan (ESRP). https://reliefweb.int/report/liberia/summary-ebola-recovery-plan-liberia-economic-stabilization-and-recovery-plan-esrp. Accessed September 24, 2024.

World Economic Forum Report (2014). The Global Competitiveness Report 2014–2015. https://www3.weforum.org/docs/WEF_GlobalCompetitivenessReport_2014-15.pdf. Accessed November 14, 2024.

World Health Organization (2020). A Joint Statement on Tourism and COVID-19 - UNWTO and WHO Call for Responsibility and Coordination. https://www.who.int/ news/item/27-02-2020-a-joint-statement-on-tourism-and-covid-19---unwto-and-who-call-for-responsibility-and-coordination. Accessed November 14, 2024.

World Health Organization report (2022). Putting health at the heart of tourism development in small countries of the WHO European region. https://iris.who.int/bitstream/handle/10665/363672/WHO-EURO-2022-6156-45921-66177-eng.pdf?sequence=2. Accessed November 14, 2024.

World Economic Forum (2024). Davos Forum 2024: Cooperation in a fragmented world. https://www.iberdrola.com/about-us/iberdrola-world-economic-forum-davos. Accessed November 15, 2024.

Zana D. (2017). *Why do Buhari, Dos Santos and Mugabe go to hospital abroad?* BBC News. https://www.bbc.com/news/world-africa-40685040. Accessed March 30, 2021.

INDEX

coronary disease 50, 51, 66, 90, 95, 96, 112, 113, 131, 132, 149, 166, 167, 205, 267, 299, 300, 333

corruption xlii, 3, 5, 19, 44, 64, 65, 78, 79, 81, 110, 111, 123, 129, 130, 133, 140–42, 147, 148, 150, 151, 163, 164, 173, 176, 183–85, 187, 220, 222, 223, 226, 227, 239, 243, 244, 256, 266, 267, 270, 278, 307, 330, 331, 341, 342, 364–66, 368, 371

cost of healthcare 31, 44, 49, 50, 61, 63, 64, 74–76, 78, 79, 94, 110, 111, 129, 130, 143, 144, 147, 148, 164, 178, 199, 243, 244, 260, 262, 263, 328, 330, 331, 334, 339, 344, 349, 360, 369

COVID-19 pandemic 2, 6, 11, 14, 15, 36, 45, 48, 52, 59, 60, 92, 96, 97, 106, 113, 114, 124, 141, 204, 220, 237, 247, 269, 324, 350, 368

crack down 371

D

data analysis 15, 16, 41, 48–52, 63–66, 77–81, 95–97, 110–14, 146–50, 163–67, 185, 203, 220–26, 242–46, 248, 261–69, 283–86, 299–301, 314–16, 330–34, 349–52

degenerative illnesses 363

demography 46, 180, 220, 224

dentist 174

dependency theory 31–33, 368

desertification 58

developing countries 12, 31, 37, 59, 75, 217, 301, 360, 363, 370

diabetes 46, 50, 51, 90, 95–97, 114, 131, 132, 149, 176, 267, 268, 275

diamond 5, 42, 43, 52, 122, 256, 366

diamond mining 44, 52

diarrheal disease 51, 66, 80, 112, 113, 131, 132, 149, 166, 167, 267, 299, 300, 333

dictatorship 73, 157, 187

digital health technology 75

digital healthcare 9, 75, 76, 82

dilapidated 10, 65, 175, 177, 187, 222, 310, 344, 362, 364

disabled person 126

disciplinary board 49, 50, 53, 64, 78, 79, 110, 111, 129, 130, 147, 148, 164, 243, 244, 264, 265, 330, 331

disparities 11–13, 16–18, 28, 45, 53, 57, 59, 60, 65, 71, 73, 82, 90, 91, 114, 115, 121, 124, 125, 139, 142, 150, 158, 168, 176, 177, 198, 201, 218, 242, 253, 256, 259, 269, 270, 277, 278, 301, 305, 308, 309, 312, 316, 323, 326, 334, 335, 344, 346, 364

dispensaries 12, 58, 74, 143, 203, 216, 294, 298

doctors xix, 4, 8–10, 14, 19, 28, 30, 31, 33, 37, 45, 48–53, 59, 63–67, 74, 75, 77–81, 91, 92, 94, 96, 98, 109, 111–14, 125, 127, 129–32, 142, 145, 147–51, 160, 161, 163–66, 174–77, 180–86, 197–99, 202, 204–7, 209, 216, 222, 223, 236–38, 243–47, 254, 256, 260, 262–68, 270, 278, 279, 284, 285, 300, 308, 310, 314, 315, 326, 328, 330–32, 335, 342–44, 346, 349, 350, 352, 353, 360, 363, 365, 369

E

economic consequences 74, 75

economic diversification 6, 324, 360

economic growth xli, 6, 7, 81, 82, 141, 247, 307

electronic health record 9

emergency 9, 16, 63, 91, 97, 110, 127, 133, 145, 162, 168, 181, 182, 200, 204, 206, 219, 220, 222–25, 236–39, 242, 262, 263, 285, 296, 308–10, 321, 324, 345, 348

emergency medical treatment 345

emergency preparedness 324

empowerment of women 218

entrepreneurs xli, 178, 359

environment xix, 1, 3, 6, 8, 15, 16, 27, 29, 31–34, 37, 41, 44, 47, 58, 60, 67, 93, 99, 104, 107, 124, 126, 141, 161, 175, 177, 186, 236, 238, 246, 247, 295, 296, 302, 311, 327, 328, 347, 351, 362, 367, 368

epidemiological sector 46

ethical leadership 53, 133, 368

ethics 53

evidence based healthcare 53, 75, 133

evidence-based performance 45

exemplary stewardship 52